PUBLIC HEALTH PRACTICE
& THE SCHOOL-AGE
POPULATION

PUBLIC HEALTH PRACTICE & THE SCHOOL-AGE POPULATION

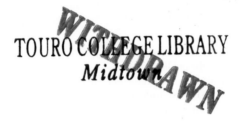

Edited by

Diane DeBell BA (Hons), MA, PhD, FRSA, Director of the Centre for Research in Health and Social Care at Anglia Ruskin University, Chelmsford and Cambridge, UK

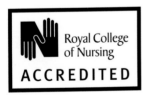

Royal College of Nursing

ACCREDITED

Hodder Arnold

A MEMBER OF THE HODDER HEADLINE GROUP

First published in Great Britain in 2007 by
Hodder Arnold, an imprint of Hodder Education and a member of the Hodder Headline Group,
an Hachette Livre UK Company
338 Euston Road, London NW1 3BH

http://www.hoddereducation.com

British Library Cataloguing in Publication Data
A catalogue record for this book is available from the British Library

Library of Congress Cataloging-in-Publication Data
A catalog record for this book is available from the Library of Congress

ISBN   978 0 340 907207

1 2 3 4 5 6 7 8 9 10

Commissioning Editor: Clare Christian/Jo Koster
Development Editor: Naomi Wilkinson
Project Editor: Clare Patterson
Production Controller: Lindsay Smith
Cover Design: Nichola Smith
Index: Liz Granger

Typeset in 10/12 Agaramond by Charon Tec Ltd (A Macmillan Company) Chennai, India
www.charontec.com
Printed and bound in Malta.

What do you think about this book? Or any other Hodder Arnold title?
Please visit our website: www.hoddereducation.com

This book is dedicated to Alice

CONTENTS

LIST OF CONTRIBUTORS

Jane V Appleton RGN, RHV, PGCEA, BA(Hons), MSc, PhD
Reader in Primary and Community Care, School of Health and Social Care, Oxford
Brookes University, Oxford, UK and Post-doctoral Research Fellow, Centre for Research in
Primary and Community Care, University of Hertfordshire, UK

Simon Bradford MPhil, PhD
Senior Lecturer, Centre for Youth Work Studies, Brunel University, Middlesex, UK

Margaret Buttigieg RGN, RHV, FPCert, PGCEA, DipN(London), BA(Open University), Counselling
Accreditation, NLP Master Practitioner
Independent Consultant, MAB Consulting, UK

Emma Croghan RGN, RSCN, SCPHN, BSc(Hons), PGDip, MPH, PhD
Director of Research and Training, ELC Consultancy Ltd, Staffordshire, UK

Diane DeBell BA(Hons), MA, PhD, FRSA
Professor of Policy in Health and Social Care and Director of the Centre for Research in
Health and Social Care, Anglia Ruskin University, Cambridge and Chelmsford, UK

Maggie Fisher RGN NDN, RHV, BA(Hons)Ed, PGDip
Area Co-ordinator for the Family Links Nurturing Programme, Hampshire Primary Care
NHS Trust, Hampshire, UK and Professional Officer to the CPHVA, UK

Simon Forrest BA(Hons), PGCE, MA(Ed), MA
Faculty of Social Sciences, The Open University and Honorary Senior Lecturer in
Adolescent Sexual Health, Faculty of Health and Social Care Sciences, University of
Kingston and St George's Medical School, London, and Visiting Fellow to the Social
Science Research Unit, Institute of Education, University of London, UK

Leslie Gelling RN, BSc(Hons), MA, PhD
Senior Research Fellow, Faculty of Health and Social Care, Anglia Ruskin University,
Cambridge, UK

Susan Kirk RN, RHV, RM, DNCert, BNurs, MSc, PhD
Senior Lecturer, School of Nursing, Midwifery and Social Work,
University of Manchester, UK

Kathryn Lowe RGN, RNT, FPCert, BSc(Hons), PGDE
Senior Lecturer, Faculty of Health, Edge Hill University, Lancashire, UK

Yvonne McNamara PGCE, DipCounselling, MPhil
Lecturer, Centre for Youth Work Studies, Brunel University, Middlesex, UK

Dinah Morley MSc, BA(Hons)
Former Deputy Director, YoungMinds, London, UK

Tina Moules SRN, RSCN, CertEd, MSc, PhD
Head of Department of Advanced Practice and Research, Faculty of Health and Social Care, Anglia Ruskin University, Cambridge and Chelmsford, UK

Theresa Nash RN, SNCert, FPCert, BSc(Hons), Higher DipHV, PGCert
Principal Lecturer, Primary Care Enterprise Lead, Kingston University and St George's University Medical School, London, UK

Niamh O'Brien BA(Hons), MSc
Research Officer, Faculty of Health and Social Care, Anglia Ruskin University, Chelmsford, UK

Dawn Rees BA(Hons), CQSW, MA, DipM
Acting National CAMHS Implementation Lead, National CAMHS Support Service (part of the Care Services Improvement Partnership), UK

Sarah Sherwin RGN, CPT, BSc(Hons), HEDip, MA, RNT
Senior Lecturer and Pathway Leader, School Nursing, University of Wolverhampton, UK

In early 2007, when UNICEF published its first 'report card' of child well-being in rich countries, there was something of a sharp intake of breath across the four countries of the UK. Using a multi-dimensional overview of the state of childhood, UNICEF was indicating UK child health and well-being as the poorest amongst 21 industrialized nations when measured on overall health factors.

How could this have happened? From 1997, the New Labour government had argued for a series of policy intentions designed to support population health improvement: a public health orientation to services; a recognition of the social and economic dimensions of health determinants; a re-orientation of service delivery designed to eradicate antiquated departmental and professional boundaries. Indeed the Chancellor's comprehensive spending review in January 2007 reported improvement in reducing child poverty.

It would be fair to say that the shift in 1997 to a public health orientation in health and social care delivery systems set the stage for the possibility of a social model of medicine in the UK. Yet, there has been slow progress toward achievement. That slow progress has had much to do with ingrained habits of working; repetitive service re-organizations; government anxiety about the costs of redistributive approaches to the underlying causes of poverty; and an uncertainty about what is meant by a public health orientation to population health when we think about the work of clinicians and practitioners.

This profile applies to whole populations within the four countries. When we focus on child health, we find that the picture is even more alarming. In effect, we are a nation that is storing up health problems that will affect our next generation of adults. Mitch Blair and his colleagues in 2003 set an important lead by specifying a focus on child public health, a focus that had slipped off the public health agenda.

In this book, we examine the health and well-being of children of school age but we do so by re-visiting the full range of public health practice from analysis to action, in other words, from the work of epidemiology to the community interventions that seek to improve health. We do this by locating the child in the family, the school, and the community. These are the three locations that school-age children inhabit as they grow and develop from school entry to emergence into adulthood.

Within this profile of thinking, we also encounter questions about resource distribution and commissioning. Where should we invest in services to improve child health? How should we design programmes that use inter-professional skills? What is the evidence base that we need in order to make such decisions? And what are the factors that most impact on child health?

Yet services are only part of the full picture. Child health is affected by language, culture, gender, ability/disability, immigration status, housing, adult carer health, consumer behaviour, nutrition, sanitation, clean water, transport systems, and the ecology of the immediate environment. And child health issues do not emerge in single focus. It is the constellation of factors in the material and the psychosocial environments that interact to affect a child's ability to grow and develop well or poorly.

This is the first book to open discussion of the public health practitioner's approach to child health during the school-age years. Each chapter is the beginning of an important debate and should be read in those terms. If this book triggers widespread argument and further research, it will have achieved its purpose.

Diane DeBell
Norwich and Cambridge 2007

ACKNOWLEDGEMENTS

This book was partly prompted by Mitch Blair and his colleagues, when they published *Child Public Health* in 2003. It also benefited from an early conversation with Pat Jackson and an American 'road conversation' in Portland, Oregon, with Dawn Rees, particularly over a plate of oysters. A very warm thank you to Naomi Wilkinson, Clare Patterson and Penny Howes of Hodder for their expertise and calm efficiency. And thank you to the contributors to this book. It has been a genuinely collaborative venture.

I owe more than thanks to Alice, Chris, Jenny, Schnig, Jeff and Sara. Very special thanks to Alice Tomkins, who understands children and likes them, who finds them interesting, witty, and 'usually a lot smarter' than adults. And special thanks to Jenny DeBell, who understands both motherhood and also what it means to foster a child. For Jeff and Sara, we are all whispering a fair wind.

Diane DeBell
Norwich and Cambridge

Section 1

THE CHILD IN 21ST CENTURY BRITAIN

1 BACKGROUND AND CONTEXT

Diane DeBell

INTRODUCTION

> *Amy, age 14, and her brother Nathan, age 16, are adoptive children although Nathan is, in fact, his father's birth child from a former relationship. This is a family-held secret. Nathan is currently serving a custodial sentence and Amy has been able to maintain some contact with her brother via letters delivered by her adoptive father. This young sister and brother have always been close. Since Nathan's arrest, Amy has been distressed and angry at home and at school. Her relationships with teachers at school are poor and she frequently truants. She is currently under threat of expulsion and she has few friends. Her relationship with her mother is poor.*
>
> ***(DeBell, 2003, p.10)***

This young girl is failing at school but no one knows why. She is the child of a complicated family profile and a judicial system that neither recognizes nor takes responsibility for its effect on the emotional lives of prisoners' children or siblings. Amy's teachers are not aware that she has a close family member in prison nor do they have experience of the damaging effects the stigma of imprisonment can have on a child. Amy's attempts to keep her brother's imprisonment a secret mean that not even the school nurse knows the nature or cause of her distress. Amy is perceived to be a problem at school and at home.

Does this compilation of circumstances describe a child health problem? And, if it does, how do we understand it in terms of child public health, in terms of preventable illness, in terms of health promotion, and in terms of public health practice?

The answers lie within our definitions of child health and well-being. For example, in contemporary Britain we now collectively agree that child emotional and mental distress is, in fact, a health problem. Indeed, child and adolescent mental health is probably the most pervasive health problem in 21st century Britain. Meltzer *et al.*, for the Office of National Statistics, estimated in 2005 that one child in ten experiences a mental health problem at some point during their school years. The charity YoungMinds has placed that figure at double the estimate of Meltzer *et al.* (see Chapter 8, p.179).

Yet we often have difficulty thinking about 'health' in terms other than physical and endogenous descriptions. To take this one step further, social definitions of health continue to sit uneasily with medical definitions.

> *Health matters have for too long been viewed as somehow separate from the societies in which they are in fact embedded.*
>
> ***(Coburn, 2003, p.338)***

Child public health practice, in keeping with Coburn's observation, starts from the position that each individual child's physical and mental health is a consequence of multiple factors within the settings in which the child lives – the home; the school; the local community and neighbourhood. Furthermore, the child's health is affected by a range of government policies arising from disparate government departments. In Amy's case, Home Office policies on family visiting and contact affect her ability to remain in contact with her brother. Teachers and school nurses play an important part in public health practice for school-age children, but the complexities of a child's family life as an influence on health require considerable cross-boundary thinking.

> *The social environment is a public health issue because it has such a big impact on health and because public health workers can do so much to improve it. Unlike most health professionals, who are restricted to helping individuals on a case-by-case basis, public health workers can change institutions and laws that organize the social environment at a population level.*
>
> ***(Donald, 2006, p.242)***

The questions that follow are twofold:

- Is child health enabled or is it compromised by the economic, social, material and political environment of Britain today?
- Whose responsibility is child health protection and improvement?

And thus the over-riding child public health question:

- Is Britain a toxic environment for children growing up in the 21st century?

When we think about child public health, our starting point is generally the measurable and observable morbidities. This is the traditional work of epidemiology. This necessary stage of measurement means that interventions are, in turn, more likely to be focused on those facets of preventable child ill-health about which we can hope to make a positive difference at the population level (from dental caries to sun protection; from nutrition and exercise to road safety and cycle helmets; from accidental injury to child protection).

But for public health practitioners, it is also the social and political context, not only the clinical profile, that matters when we think about how to prevent ill-health in children and young people of school age. In other words, it is the population-level information that helps practitioners in their work with individual children and families.

A NEW CHILD PUBLIC HEALTH: WHO IS THIS BOOK FOR?

Child public health is emerging – or perhaps re-emerging – as a special-ity of both public health and paediatrics, and as a broadly based inter-disciplinary movement.

(Blair et al., 2003, p.3)

In their comprehensive work of 2003, Blair *et al.* provide us with the ground-ing we need to understand causality and risk, concepts that are fundamental to the work of public health practitioners, who, in turn, seek to develop strategies and interventions to improve and protect child health. But Blair and his col-leagues do not seek to conceptualize childhood nor to differentiate children by age. In this book, we focus our attention on the school-age child (from school entry at age 4 or 5 years to transition into adulthood at age 16 or 18 years). There is a range of reasons for this attention.

The developmental period from neonatal to school age has long been a focus of investment and research; the school-age years less so. Yet the school years are a long period of growth and development during which children, young people and their families often experience changing social circumstances and diverse family formations, and they experience school-led transition points as the child moves toward eventual entry into adulthood and independence.

Many diverse health and social care professionals are involved with child health during the school years. But so too are education professionals, housing and local authority officers, youth and community workers, the criminal just-ice system, voluntary and charitable bodies, and local community groups. This book is for these readers. It also provides a rich resource for service managers and for service commissioning bodies. Furthermore, the contributions in this book indicate many areas of need for targeted research into the issues that affect school-age child health.

This is the first book to focus attention exclusively on public health practice with the school-age population. It thereby provides a basis for debate, research and, particularly, for frontline practice. The book is organized in sections that foreground the three settings in which children grow and develop – the family; the school; and the local community/neighbourhood. But it also opens in Section 1 with analysis of the legal issues affecting child health and the implications of difference and diversity for child health in the UK. The final section of the book specifically addresses four core health issues – child and adolescent mental health; long-term conditions; lifestyle behaviour approaches to health improvement; and the challenges linked to involving children and young people in decision making about their own health needs.

This book is designed to stimulate discussion and debate; to provide a practical agenda for thinking and for argument amongst its readers; and to foreground the health improvement and protection needs of school-age children and young people.

THINKING ABOUT THE SCHOOL-AGE YEARS

This book starts from the premise that our collective understanding of school-age childhood health has been largely under-represented in those critical debates that inform public health thinking at all levels – from epidemiological description to theories of cause for ill-health (health determinants); from intervention designs to measures of their effectiveness; and ultimately, the public health policy direction of current government thinking. We are not arguing a 'failure' of focus, but rather the need to look closely and specifically at the school-age years in public health terms.

To do that we need to think about what we mean by childhood during these years. In developmental terms, this age span (from school entry age to 16/18 years) is the period of transition from full dependence on family and carers to a presumption about transition into adult rights and responsibilities. These school-age years (about 20 per cent of the UK population, or 11.2 million, fall into this group[1]) are a time of dramatic physical and emotional development. And for too many children, these years are not a happy and healthy period of life.

The illnesses, disease, long-term conditions, and thus the morbidities of the school-age years, are largely preventable, yet they are frequently below the radar of mainstream public health planning. Furthermore, when ill-health is not preventable, many of its adverse *consequences* for individual children *are* preventable. The full picture concerns more than healthcare services alone, and child health improvement is dependent on multisectoral analyses and interprofessional service development.

For example, the recently identified child 'obesity epidemic' in both Britain and the US is an example of the way child health tends to be observed in single-issue focus rather than in terms of a complex set of socio-economic and environmental factors that can affect the health of all children and young people of school age. We are only at the starting gate in our understanding of the obesogenic environment.

In other words, the factors behind a rise in childhood obesity are preventable, but only by first identifying the multiple causes, including consumer behaviour; the food industry's role in food production, distribution and advertising; the public sector's investment decisions about food for children at school, in hospital and in care; and the nature of legislation needed to govern the food industry. And even these initially indicative issues do not include those factors

---

[1]Because data are not maintained specifically for school-age children and young people, we have extrapolated this estimate (for age 5 to 18 years) from diverse sources for the year 2006.

that govern child physical activity – access to pleasurable exercise, safe play areas and the school environment. Nor do they reflect the historic shift in the relationship between body weight/stature, the measure of calorie expenditure in contemporary labour, and the cost, supply and availability of food within any particular developed country.

THINKING ABOUT CHILDHOOD

The very concept of childhood is a culturally bound phenomenon. When we speak of contemporary childhood in the developed countries, we tend to oscillate between overly sentimental terms that deny agency, and thus deny voice to this sector of the population on the one hand, while on the other hand, we can quickly find ourselves resorting to blame or ridicule (of the family, of the child) – most notably from the pre-adolescent period. Defining a balance between protecting children and allowing them agency is fraught with cultural as well as political confusion. For example, children are not citizens because they are disenfranchised, yet they are frequently and incorrectly referred to as 'citizens with rights'. In the UK, the concept of children's rights is highly circumscribed, despite Britain's ratification of the UN Convention on the Rights of the Child (1989).

The language of social policy and of healthcare is a language imbued with presumptions about progress. For example, when we speak of the present in developed countries, we tend to comfort ourselves that, in general, the conditions of our lives and the directions of government health and social care policy are improving, are 'for the good'. However:

> . . . it could be argued that if one applies a holistic definition of health, young people now are no healthier than they were a century ago.
>
> **(Hall, 2006, p.i)**

In this book, we take a hard look at two related issues: (1) what is the state of child health in Britain today; and (2) what is the function of child public health practice in improving and protecting the health of school-age children?

No one would seriously argue that a desire to maximize child health is not an *a priori* good. Yet, a close look at the history of child health in the UK, as elsewhere, reveals a strangely haphazard approach to children's health once past the neonatal and early years period. Five milestones thus far in the 21st century indicate a promising shift in this relative neglect of a more holistic and more comprehensive focus on children's health and well-being:

- *Child Public Health* (Blair *et al.*, 2003)
- *Health for all Children* (Hall and Elliman, 2003)
- *The National Service Framework for Children, Young People and Maternity Services* (Department of Health and Department for Education and Skills (DfES), 2004)
- The *Every Child Matters: change for children* framework (HM Government, 2004)
- The Children Act 2004.

We argue in this book that the health of school-age children and young people has not been systematically studied from the perspective of a population cohort. Instead, we have multiple studies of single health issues or of child health and social care delivery systems for specific child health matters. This work is essential but it needs theorizing in terms of public health practice, and it needs intensification of attention on the school-age years.

Yet, we may be at a point of change in that profile. The moment is opportune for development of an integrated approach to child public health. Blair *et al.* (2003), Hall and Elliman (2003) and Cowley (2002, 2007) have set the stage for just such a programme of work. And this book takes those arguments and insights as a starting point for investigating and then setting an agenda for public health practice with the school-age population.

In addition, from a policy perspective, the four countries of the UK have each begun to focus attention on the health implications of the settings in which children live. Specifically, policy in each country has begun to focus on the child from the perspective of service delivery systems and of child health issues (e.g. the recent emergence of public health concerns about childhood obesity, sexual health, risk behaviours linked to alcohol and illicit drug use, child and adolescent mental health and child vulnerability). Furthermore, we see an emerging recognition of the impact that social and environmental factors have on the child's experience of growing up in Britain today.

> *Population health has a troubling blind spot (as does health promotion at times) to work in the political economy area that sheds light on the forces that drive health determinants.*
>
> **(Raphael and Bryant, 2003, p.416)**

School-age children are a population group in need of coherent and systematic attention but, from a public health perspective, the field is still new and fresh.

To address these issues, we consider concepts of childhood alongside the function of public health practice in its efforts to improve and protect the health of school-age children. The studies in this book focus on the four countries of the UK at the outset of the 21st century in its European context. But we also refer to North American models of public health practice, and we do so with reference to international comparators where appropriate or helpful.

CONTEMPORARY CHILDHOOD

We no longer presume that child labour is an acceptable feature of either the formal or informal economies in developed countries. We also argue for a child's human rights alongside adult human rights, and we have statutes to protect children from, at least, physical abuse or harm but also from demands that they 'earn their keep' by labour. To that degree, we formally seek to protect our children. Yet, children of school age in 21st century Britain grow up in an adult culture in which they are largely unprotected from the pressures of consumerism (advertising, publishing, purchasing pressures). Children in Britain share this profile with children in virtually all developed countries.

Furthermore, we infantilize children, while at the same time presuming that their access to adult culture is appropriate. We extend young people's financial dependence on the family into the post-schooling years while at the same time we complain of 'yob cultures' – implying the young person's responsibility to *behave well*, to behave *as an adult*. Our perspectives on child health and our concepts of childhood are contradictory and confusing. We sexualize the child's public and private environment, yet we are squeamish about providing access to effective education about sexual health.

David Hall wrote of school-age children in Britain in March 2006:

> *An alarmingly high proportion of our young people grow up in disrupted and unsupportive families and attend schools where bullying of all kinds is a daily occurrence, gang membership is the key to safety and mediocre education is delivered by an endless succession of supply teachers.*
>
> *They live in an obesogenic environment – the lack of facilities for sport and leisure, the disappearance of family mealtimes and home cooking and the emergence of fast food all contribute. They are exposed to a constant emphasis on the desirability of early sexual activity and subtle advertising encourages the huge increase in alcohol consumption by young people. The end product of this toxic mixture is a mixture of physical and mental ill-health which is outwith the experience of mainstream medical care.*
>
> **(Hall, 2006, p.i)**

THINKING ABOUT PUBLIC HEALTH PRACTICE

> *Preventable diseases can be prevented; curable ailments can certainly be cured; and controllable maladies call out for control. However, investigators tend to shy away from posing the questions in their full generosity. To confront the big picture seems like an overpowering challenge.*
>
> **(Sen, 2005, p.xii)**

The health economist and nobel laureate Amartya Sen has written extensively about the reticulated relationships between social and economic rights and health and well-being. Because Sen is a health economist, he faces no explicit professional demand to look at the humanity of his subject – only to the implications of measurement. Yet his work is deeply humane. He refers to the destructive forces in international health economies as *unfreedoms*.

We have become accustomed to the presence of international child poverty, malnourishment, boy soldiers, child sexual exploitation, poor education systems, child homelessness and family breakdown.

Effective interventions to improve child health are the business of all professionals who work with children, not simply healthcare workers, but we have significant difficulty in establishing what it is that makes an intervention effective – what works to improve and protect child health.

Furthermore, the very concept of public health practice resides in a concept of multiprofessional responsibility (Pencheon *et al.*, 2006). Indeed, in Britain we can track the emergence of child public health as a concept for the organization of health and social care services and of other public services and voluntary agencies from the very end of the 20th century. In only a decade, the terminology of public health has become a core part of UK practice (our downstream activities) in community nursing, in paediatrics, in housing, social care, education, youth and community work, and in a plethora of child therapies, and it is now embedded in a range of government policy documents (upstream activities).

Any 'look' at the wider history of public health leads us to considerations of both a social agenda for health issues and of matters that require political action. As Kate Billingham wrote in 1997, public health is a way of 'seeing' health problems (see Chapter 5).

> *Essentially public health is a distinctive way of seeing health problems: public health nurses and doctors ask different questions about their practice, requiring them to look beyond individuals to populations, such as:*
>
> • *Why is this happening?*
> • *How often?*
> • *What is the social context?*
> • *Who else should be involved?*
> • *What works and what doesn't?*
>
> *They also make different connections: between one individual and another, between individuals and communities, between individuals and social structures, between the stories that people tell them and the epidemiological evidence, between health services and other agencies, between medical and social models of health and between health and social policies . . . [they] tend to have a commitment to a set of values based on equity, justice and work for social change at local and national levels.*
>
> **(Billingham, 1997, p.271)**

THEORIES UNDERPINNING CONTEMPORARY PUBLIC HEALTH

Public health practitioners work from a social perspective on population-level approaches to health and well-being. And in order to make a difference, such perspectives are inevitably driven by political argument. For many public health practitioners, the political push behind their work may be sufficiently muted as to be unconscious. Indeed, public health practitioners tend to work within 'the present', with little knowledge of the history or politics that inform their daily work. One purpose of this book is to provide context of this kind to support the multiprofessional and multidisciplinary work of public health practitioners.

Public health practice has a political dimension, whether that is implicit or explicit within individual workforce planning. It is also based within concepts of social justice. Unlike basic scientific medical research, public health practice is embedded in social interpretations of medical data. This means, for example, that arguments premised on social justice have to be proved. It is insufficient to cite social justice as uncontested territory. It is necessary to make the case and to expose the contradictions we find both in human behaviour and in social and economic policies deriving from national governments.

A number of theorists in Britain (e.g. Wilkinson, 1996; Bartley, 2004; Marmot, 2004) are now articulating arguments about the causes of ill-health (socio-economic, psychosocial, life-course and political economic explanations). Most of these, with the exception of life-course theories, do not yet specify child health separately from analyses of national and local population health comparators.

However, with the contemporary shift in public health focus from conventional analyses of disease and disorder incidence to a strengthened focus on the social determinants of health, not only have analysts highlighted the vast inequalities in health, but recent work has particularly focused on the damaging political and economic systems that govern people's lives and their health.

Poor health tends to cluster in poor communities.

(Coburn, 2003, p.338)

For example, when epidemiologists measure health at the neighbourhood level within a national population, they find that countries with highly competitive economic structures (e.g. relatively unrestrained market economies) have far greater divergence in health outcomes than do societies based on a social imperative to equalize income (Kawachi *et al.*, 1997; Levins, 2003). These analyses coincide with, but also go beyond the theories of Marmot (2004) and Wilkinson (1996), the predominating theorists behind British health policy at the outset of the 21st century. The implications of such arguments press us to think about the determinants of public health from perspectives that question political economies and national government policy direction (Hofrichter, 2003).

In other words, we are beginning to see debates about health inequalities and about social cohesion that challenge more deeply our recent presumptions that income differentials alone are the key determinants of poor health. These debates will matter for child public health practitioners as we move further into the 21st century.

UNDERSTANDING THE SUBJECT

This book is written in a context of debate about (1) the definition of health; (2) the determinants of poor health; and (3) the priorities for child health in the UK and across national borders.

As with any centennial moment in history, the 21st century has about it a tone of 'new' perspectives and 'new' insights into what constitutes health and well-being, and how health might be improved. When we think of children, for example, it is helpful to move to the most current health debates. Contemporary debates tend to articulate health determinants in terms of the relative importance of three factors: genetic inheritance, personal lifestyle behaviours and structural factors, including family income differentials. These are the three key determinants of health that are used to justify and to explain the vertical relationship between local and national service delivery and policy-planning decisions as they affect population health.

It is worth our while to think about each of these in turn. For example, the genetic profile is only a single component in any explanation of health status and it matters, not in terms of itself alone, but in terms of the larger social environment. Skin pigmentation is a useful illustration. This entirely trivial genetic marker matters primarily because of social responses to skin colour within cultures. And a genetic susceptibility to cancer, in turn, is only important if the environmental factors are in place to trigger it (Levins, 2003, p.379). In other words, our predilection for seeking 'cause' often leads us to over-simplification of concepts of cause.

Health-related behaviours, in contrast, are the primary areas in which public health practitioners seek to intervene, but individual human choices are always made from alternatives and within contexts of opportunities. 'Choice' is heavily inscribed by information, knowledge and opportunity.

England, for example, largely (though not wholly) positions its health policy in terms of a focus on individual lifestyle and health-related behaviours (Department of Health, 2004) and also on measures of cost-effectiveness (Wanless, 2001). And the current direction of debate about the 'obesity epidemic' amongst children is a salutary example of what is often referred to as the dangers inherent in context stripping. In other words, weighing and measuring children at school is a valuable tool for epidemiological data gathering. But we need to ask a question about resource distribution, given the multiple factors that need to be addressed by public health practitioners if we are to reverse the current trend in childhood obesity.

In *Child Public Health*, Blair and colleagues signal the shortcomings of context-free public health initiatives by constructing a scenario for public health practice in its efforts to address childhood obesity (Blair *et al.*, 2003, pp.237–42).

MAKING A DIFFERENCE

In other words, most contemporary debates are about what causes ill-health. It is the field of health determinants that draws greatest attention from critical analysts. How to improve poor health is, however, an altogether more difficult matter.

In addition, we are only at the starting gate when we ask ourselves what we mean by 'health and well-being'. The definitional problems behind these concepts are culturally as well as historically shaped. *Every Child Matters: change for children* (HM Government, 2004) provides us with the closest definitional response we have yet achieved, but it is the implementation of appropriate interventions that causes us significant challenges.

This book is a close examination of the *practice* of public health, and it orientates the concept of 'practice' as one step beyond epidemiology. In other words, we examine the work of practitioners who are seeking to discover which/what kind of interventions will improve and protect the health of school-age children. We take as a given the remarkable achievements of more than a century of epidemiology in its ability to identify the locations and the causes of ill-health.

We are fortunate in being able to take such achievements for granted in the developed countries. It is not the case that epidemiology plays such a sophisticated role as a support for health system design in transition economies (e.g. many of the countries emerging from the post-Soviet period) or in the developing countries.

This book is about public health practice that relies on the findings of epidemiology as its starting point. By 'public health', the contributors mean to include (a) the principles that underlie the discipline of public health; (b) the theories that seek to explain the causes (determinants) of ill-health within populations; (c) the practices that seek to develop effective interventions for the improvement and protection of health; and (d) the policies that steer public health practice at any particular historical point and in any particular geographic area.

The conundrum that arises from that perspective, however, is the question of how we link epidemiology, which is a classic system of measurement of disease and disorders, to children's health needs, which often do not necessarily start from 'ill-health'. How do we position children's health needs in terms of exogenous rather than endogenous descriptors?

The great public health pioneers of Europe and North America, for example, have always been concerned with finding the causes of ill-health – what we now refer to as the determinants of health. In so doing, they have also been concerned with how to bring about social and environmental change that can remove those causes.

John Snow was a London general practitioner (GP), whose practice was at the centre of a cholera epidemic in 1854. More than 500 people died in 10 days within a 250 yard radius of Broad Street. By plotting the geographic area, John Snow deduced that the Broad Street pump was the transmission point for infection, and he removed the pump handle (Blair *et al.*, 2003, p.8).

In John Snow's case, his deductive reasoning led him to an experimental action that stopped the spread of infection. In contemporary terms, it is in the understanding of what makes a public health intervention effective that we discover the most difficult challenges for contemporary public health practitioners. And we find that the contemporary field of public health practice abounds with such examples of health and social care workers experimenting with interventions at just such a local level. Yet we have too little knowledge of the effectiveness of these experiments. We know too little about 'what works'.

The difficulty, however, is in proving the effectiveness of any particular intervention. We need to know if X intervention actually caused Y to change. A further difficulty lies in transferring practice from one location to another and in ascribing outcomes to specific actions (the external validity question). Indeed, there is a kind of swashbuckling heroism in the work of these early public health practitioners.

LOOKING TO HISTORY

In Europe, public health pioneers emerged in response to urban industrialization in the 18th and 19th centuries and were, from the outset, concerned with finding the causes of ill-health. Their desire, individually and collectively, was always and continues to be a determination to bring about change that can remove the causes of ill-health – social, material, environmental, even political causes of preventable illness, disease or early death. The great public health pioneers have always been change agents. And change agents of this kind are inevitably at the forefront of controversy, and particularly so when change requires large-scale investment or population interventions that run counter to dominant social patterns of behaviour.

For example, the 19th century sanitation movement was not achieved without struggle. The cost of engineering drains for entire national populations has always been and continues to be high – *vide* the contemporary developing world. Conquering the spread of preventable infectious disease by means of universal vaccination was no less radical a step in the work of public health specialists. Indeed, Edward Jenner (1749–1823) enabled the revolutionary development of an effective smallpox vaccination by using entirely unethical means – if assessed by contemporary guidelines. And, arguably, the eventual success of vaccination to protect against infectious diseases relied on the mid-20th century rise of welfare state economies in developed countries. Indeed, we still measure general child health within a national context in terms of a nation's ability to ensure vaccination rates.

Now, at the beginning of the 21st century, we talk mainly about health inequalities, and the field of debate for the past decade has been focused on understanding the determinants of health and of ill-health as they appear to be a consequence of social and material inequalities within and across national borders. That material deprivation is damaging to health is not in itself a matter of dispute, nor are socio-economic inequalities new. However, why such health inequalities appear to have become increasingly intractable and what needs to be done are matters of considerable debate. For example, the 'war on poverty' and on child poverty is by now familiar. However, national governments do not generally address the issue in terms of income redistribution. Such thinking is mainly absent from 21st century geopolitical thinking. The main exceptions are Cuba, some parts of South America and, to a degree, the Nordic European countries.

But in the 21st century, can we realistically identify the mechanisms that produce compromised health as an outcome of material inequality? Do we understand why material deprivation is so intransigent, not only in the developed countries but particularly in developing and transitional economies, which are, in fact, the homes for roughly 85 per cent of the world's child population? Furthermore, what are the practical interventions that public health practitioners identify that they believe will make a beneficial difference to child health? And how are such interventions designed, how are they practised and what evidence do we have that particular interventions are effective? In Chapters 3, 4, 5 and 11 these questions are approached with a view to indicating for us some of the challenges that contemporary public health practitioners are encountering, particularly in the four countries of the UK.

FEATURES OF PUBLIC HEALTH THINKING

Epidemiological measurement, a discipline now more than a century old, is fully capable of identifying the locations and profiles of mortality and morbidity. What such measurement cannot do is tell us how to reverse the profiles of damage, which can be traced to the complex interaction between location, social relationships, material wealth or want and individual decision making about health-related behaviours. Indeed, national political policy direction combined with the operation of macro-economies by nation states can itself be a cause of ill-health or early death (see Hofrichter, 2003).

In the UK, as is the case internationally, it is material poverty that has become the primary focus of attention in health-improvement debates. Where children are concerned, the current child public health policy position has derived largely from life-course theories of health inequalities, which result in arguments for targeted investment in maternal, neonatal and pre-school investment in child health. The Sure Start programmes in the UK (relatively recent) and Head Start in the USA (dating from 1962) are powerful examples of government policy based on a theory of health inequalities – in these cases, life-course theories.

But the school-age years, as a consequence, have trailed behind in terms of both financial investment and human resource in both the UK and the US.

It is worth thinking about this from a public health measurement perspective. In simple terms, there are two points of measurement that historically have been able to capture a population profile of health status – records of births and deaths (in those countries where these are registered). Thus we derive 'average life expectancy' as an indicator of a whole population's health status.

Of course, no individual is a statistic, nor indeed is a total community's life expectancy inextricably linked to a statistic. These are indicators of underlying health factors and it is the underlying factors that we need to extricate from our explanatory models. What can happen in simple figures of mortality, for example, is the accidental omission of the school-age childhood stage – given our collective assessment of health in terms of neonatal survival (birth to age 5 years) and in terms of adult health as related to mortality and morbidity rates.

Furthermore, the most difficult health field to understand via measurement is the area of long-term conditions and complex illness. These are health problems in which people do not generally feel ill in the sense that acute events are about 'illness'. In the school-age years, however, long-term conditions can be difficult to manage in terms of health care, because of developmental changes in the child's height and weight over more than a decade of growth. Long-term conditions are also complicating factors in the child's emotional and intellectual development and in the child's adaptation to his or her environment (see Chapter 9).

Furthermore, long-term conditions also generate social and environmental challenges in the settings children inhabit – the family; the school; the community neighbourhood. Since the mid-1980s, Britain has moved, more or less efficiently, toward principles of inclusive education, which means that the school setting is theoretically required to accommodate child health needs. This represents a radical conceptual change about child health, ability and disability in educational planning in only two decades. Yet the consequences for the child in the school setting are not yet resolved and these issues are explored in Chapters 5 and 9.

MAKING HEALTHY CHOICES: WHAT DOES THIS MEAN FOR CHILDHOOD?

At the same time, a parallel policy focus on individual 'lifestyle' choices about health behaviours has become a pronounced explanatory system and a particular focus of government policy in Britain in the past decade. What constitutes 'choice' about health-related behaviours is not, however, straightforward.

Indeed, most practical health-promotion initiatives focus precisely on the design of interventions that are believed to have a capacity to change health-related risk behaviours (e.g. seat belt legislation, tobacco control, sexual health education), and to change individual decision making about health-related behaviour choices.

This focus on health-sustaining behaviours has become a focus for contemporary government policies in most developed countries.

It is important to note that transfer of responsibility for health from the state to the person can be argued to be a way of reducing the financial burden of ill-health on government budgets. In other words, the balance between enabling or supporting 'healthy decisions' amongst the populace on the one hand and investing government funds in health-improvement interventions on the other hand is complex. In addition, every intervention to improve population health must itself be tested for effectiveness. This is a research burden representing considerable cost even before the factoring in of both the financial and the political costs of funding population-level interventions.

On the other hand, it is also valid to argue that helping to 'enable' people to make personal choices that sustain their own health is an indication of a mature democracy. But 'choice', as we have already noted, is heavily inflected by material and psychological factors that reside outside notions of individual agency. We might even go further, with some confidence, and suggest that children are much more severely constrained in matters of choice than are adults.

THINKING ABOUT SOCIAL POLICY

One of the tasks of this book is to analyse the mechanisms (their theoretical underpinnings) that drive a contemporary health policy specifically designed to improve the health of school-age children and young people. What presumptions do we make that lie behind our health and social care policies and our public health interventions?

Any 'look' at the history of public health leads us to considerations of both a social agenda for health issues and of matters that require political action, a way of 'seeing' that encourages us to act.

The book is divided into five sections, three of which locate the child in the main settings in which children grow up and develop – the family (Chapter 4); the school (Chapter 5); the local community and neighbourhood (Chapters 6 and 7). Section 1 analyses the legal issues that concern childhood health (Chapter 2); and examines some of the questions of difference and diversity that children and young people negotiate in their growing-up years (Chapter 3). Section 5 investigates key health-related issues – child and adolescent mental health (Chapter 8); long-term conditions (Chapter 9); lifestyle approaches to health improvement (Chapter 10); and some of the challenges we encounter in seeking to involve children and young people in decision making about their own health-related needs (Chapter 11).

CONCLUSION

This book explores public health practice with children and young people of school age. It brings together insights and debates from across diverse disciplines in order to ask questions about the health of our children and young people and about our strategies and practices for improving and protecting their health. Blair *et al.* in 2003 commented that 'child health is emerging – or perhaps re-emerging – as a speciality of public health' (p.3). In this book, we have focused the spotlight on child health in the school-age years.

What do we know? What questions do we need to ask? How do we work across professional, departmental and interest-focused boundaries in order to improve child and adolescent health?

In just a decade, the principles of public health have become a core part of practice in community nursing, in paediatrics, in housing, social care, education, youth and community work, the youth justice system, and in the work of voluntary and charitable bodies (our downstream activities). And public health is at the heart of government policy across a range of departments (our upstream activities).

Public health practice is interprofessional work at its most demanding, and it involves all these actors working together – not an easy agenda. Pencheon *et al.* (2006) refer to the 'eternal verities of public health, in disease prevention, communicable disease control, health protection, and health promotion' (p.xxxi). This book explores these concepts but it does so by placing the school-age child and young person in a social, economic and political context.

Many practitioners tell us that they are still unclear about what a public health approach actually means. Billingham in 1997 referred to it as a way of 'seeing'. And by this she was referring to the connections that public health practitioners make between the individual and the population.

It is, if anything, a reflection of the challenges we confront that interprofessional working can, at times, be so very difficult. How to improve and protect the health of school-age children and young people is a challenge that this book addresses, and to achieve that means highlighting, indeed repeating, the inter-professional agenda.

KEY POINTS

- This book is about public health practice and the school-age population.
- Public health practice arises from a way of 'seeing' the child or young person within a context and an environment, as part of a population profile.
- During the school-age years, the child experiences a long period of growth and development in which we need to make connections between the child's experiences at home, at school and in the local community or neighbourhood.
- Public health practice involves finding strategies to protect and improve health, and for children and young people of school age that involves inter-professional development and cross-agency working at its most demanding.
- Public health practitioners ask themselves difficult questions about their practice. How can I design effective interventions? Who do I need to include in my work? How do I know what works? And, is what I am doing making a difference?

REFERENCES

Bartley M (2004) *Health Inequality: an introduction to theories, concepts and methods.* Cambridge and Oxford: Polity Press.

Billingham K (1997) Public health nursing in primary care. *British Journal of Community Health Nursing* 2:270–4.

Blair M, Stewart-Brown S, Waterston T, Crowther R (2003) *Child Public Health.* Oxford: Oxford University Press.

Coburn D (2003) Income inequality, social cohesion, and the health status of populations: the role of neo-liberalism. In: Hofrichter R (ed.) *Health and Social Justice: politics, ideology, and inequity in the distribution of disease. A public health reader.* San Francisco CA: Jossey-Bass, pp.335–55.

Cowley S (ed.) (2002) *Public Health in Policy and Practice: a sourcebook for health visitors and community nurses.* London: Ballière Tindall.

Cowley S (ed.) (2007) *Public Health in Policy and Practice: a sourcebook* (2e). Edinburgh: Elsevier.

DeBell D (2003) *Starting Where They Are Project: supporting young people with a prisoner in the family.* London: Action for Prisoners' Families.

DeBell D, Tomkins A (2006) *Discovering the Future of School Nursing: the evidence base.* London: McMillan-Scott.

Donald A (2006) Facilitating community action. In: Pencheon D, Guest C, Melzer D, Muir Gray JA (eds) *Oxford Handbook of Public Health Practice* (2e). Oxford: Oxford University Press, pp.240–6.

Department of Health (2004) *Choosing Health. Making healthier choices easier.* London: Department of Health.

Department of Health and Department for Education and Skills (2004) *The National Service Framework for Children, Young People and Maternity Services.* London: Department of Health. www.dh.gov.uk/PolicyAndGuidance/ HealthAndSocialCareTopics/ChildrenServices/ChildrenServicesInformation/ ChildrenServicesInformationArticle/fs/en?CONTENT_ID=4089111& chk=U8Ecln (accessed 17 January 2007).

Hall DMB (2006) Foreword. In: DeBell D, Tomkins A *Discovering the Future of School Nursing: an evidence base for practice.* London: McMillan-Scott, p.i.

Hall DMB, Elliman D (2003) *Health for All Children* (4e). Oxford: Oxford University Press.

HM Government (2004) *Every Child Matters: change for children.* Nottingham: DfES Publications. www.everychildmatters.gov.uk/_content/documents/ Every%20Child%20Matinserts.pdf (accessed 5 February 2007).

Hofrichter R (2003) The politics of health inequities: contested terrain. In: Hofrichter R (ed.) *Health and Social Justice: politics, ideology, and inequities in the distribution of disease. A public health reader.* San Francisco CA: Jossey-Bass, pp.1–56.

Kawachi I, Kennedy BP, Lochner K, Prothrow-Stith D (1997) Social capital, income inequality, and mortality. *American Journal of Public Health* 87:1491–8.

Levins R (2003) Is capitalism a disease? The crisis in US public health. In: Hofrichter R (ed.) *Health and Social Justice: politics, ideology, and inequities in the distribution of disease. A public health reader.* San Francisco CA: Jossey-Bass, pp.365–84.

Marmot M (2004) *Status Syndrome: how your social standing directly affects your health and life expectancy.* London: Bloomsbury.

Meltzer H, Green H, McGinnity A, Ford T, Goodman R (2005) *The Mental Health of Children and Young People in Great Britain 2004.* London: Office for National Statistics.

Pencheon D, Guest C, Melzer D, Muir Gray JA (2006) *Oxford Handbook of Public Health Practice* (2e). Oxford: Oxford University Press.

Raphael D, Bryant T (2003) The limitations of population health as a model for a new public health. In: Hofrichter R (ed.) *Health and Social Justice: politics, ideology, and inequities in the distribution of disease. A public health reader.* San Francisco CA: Jossey-Bass, pp.410–27.

Sen A (2005) Foreword. In: Farmer P *Pathologies of Power: health, human rights, and the new war on the poor.* Berkeley and London: University of California Press Ltd, pp.xi–xvii.

Wanless D (2001) *Securing our Future Health: taking a long-term view. An interim report.* London: HM Treasury.

Wilkinson RG (1996) *Unhealthy Societies: the afflictions of inequality.* London: Routledge.

Website

YoungMinds www.youngminds.org.uk (accessed 5 February 2007).

Act of Parliament

This Act is published by HMSO in London, and can be accessed from the UK Parliament website (www.publications.parliament.uk).

Children Act 2004

2

LEGAL ISSUES AND YOUNG PEOPLE'S HEALTH

Leslie Gelling

INTRODUCTION

Even the briefest consideration of children's and young people's health would be incomplete without an analysis of the many complex legal and ethical issues. The provision of health and social care and the requirements of the law have become inextricably linked to the extent that legal issues are central to the work of all health and social care practitioners. Most importantly, arguments about who should be involved in decision making and who can give informed consent, or refuse consent, have been central to the legal and ethical debate and, therefore, the practice of health and social care practitioners.

The law, especially family law, does not exist in a static state. Rather, it reflects changes in social and cultural attitudes (Bainham, 2005). In addition, it is important to consider the many rapidly changing demographic factors. For example, during the past half-century there has been a gradual erosion of family networks and the very nature of what constitutes a family. This has been influenced by a significant growth in the rate of divorce, more frequent remarriage and increased cohabitation outside marriage. Such events, together with greater appreciation of the fundamental human rights of young people, have changed the whole of the climate in which young people live in developed countries. This change has impacted upon the children, their families and those caring for them.

There can be no doubt that the relationship between the legal capacity of young people and the obligations placed upon those with parental responsibility have been fashioned within the context of medical decision making:

> *This is not really surprising since the health of children is self-evidently the most basic and essential consideration in protecting their welfare.*
> **(Bainham, 2005, p.309)**

This chapter will consider the legal issues and how they relate to young people's health in general, but this will inevitably result in a detailed consideration of how young people are involved in decision making and the role they might play in giving or withholding informed consent. It is important to note that this chapter will not examine the requirement for informed consent to participation in research, which raises many additional complex theoretical, legal and practical dilemmas that are outside the remit of this chapter.

BACKGROUND

First it is important to review the background to the current legal situation in the UK by considering the historical perspective. In doing so the reader will develop a better understanding of how we have got to where we are today. Although health and social care practitioners grapple with this complex and challenging legal framework every day, this is undoubtedly preferable to where we were at the start of the 20th century or earlier.

The rights of children and young people[1] have moved a long way since they were considered the property of adults and were treated and used as the adults saw fit. This frequently meant that young people were uneducated, had to work to bring much-needed income into the household, experienced poor levels of health and were not involved in any decisions about any aspect of their lives. In recent years young people's rights have developed alongside those of consumers of health and social care services, but young people have frequently been left off the agenda (Freeman, 1993). For example, there was no reference to young people in *The Patient's Charter*[2] and although The Health of the Nation[3] stressed the importance of infant and child health, it did so with the aim of achieving success in attaining targets rather than assuring individual rights for young people (Moules, 2006).

If we consider the background to the current legal situation, it is evident that there are still wide-ranging opinions that range from a liberationist view, which proposes that young people should have equal rights with adults and have greater decision-making capacity than is widely believed in today's society. And, in contrast, a paternalistic view argues that young people are incompetent to make decisions for themselves and require adults to protect them and, hence, make decisions for them. In reality and within legal restraints, most young people are treated as being at some point between these extremes. This chapter will provide the briefest introduction to the key legal requirements that are relevant to young people's health and their rights.

---

[1] To avoid unnecessary repetition, the term 'young people' will be used to mean 'children and young people' for the remainder of this chapter.

[2] Launched by the NHS in 1991 and updated in 1995, *The Patient's Charter* was an attempt to set standards for patient care. The Charter was all about the quality of services offered in NHS hospitals and community health organizations. *Patient's Charter: services for children and young people* was not published until 1996.

[3] Between 1992 and 1997 The Health of the Nation strategy was the central plank of health policy in England and formed the context for planning of services delivered by the NHS.

Involving young people in decisions about their lives is now accepted as an integral component in the delivery of health and social care. This approach is believed to promote self-esteem, increase compliance and, therefore, promote improved health. The notion of rights for young people is, however, a relatively new concept that has its roots in the 1924 Declaration of Geneva[4] in which it is stated that 'mankind owes to the child the best it has to give'. The Declaration was based on six core principles with an emphasis on protection of the young person with little regard for their right to participate in decision making (Moules, 2006). This demonstrated a paternalistic attitude, common at the time, in which adults were believed to be the defenders of young people who were incompetent to make decisions for themselves (Freeman, 1983). The Declaration reflected the social circumstances at the time, with an emphasis on ensuring that young people were fed and not allowed to go hungry. Clear in the Declaration was the requirement that all decisions about a young person's health care should be controlled by adults and seldom, if ever, involve a young person in the decision-making process.

The Children and Young Person Act 1933[5] took this one step further in the UK and made it a criminal offence not to take the necessary action to protect young people from harm, or to take any action that might cause harm to a young person. The Act imposed a minimum standard of medical care on those with parental responsibility. Again, the emphasis was on what was required of parents rather than on the rights of young people.

In the 1950s, the United Nation's Declaration on the Rights of the Child[6] further widened the debate on the rights of young people. Despite this, the Declaration still failed to acknowledge that young people had the right to act in an autonomous manner, and the focus was again on the adult's responsibility to ensure welfare and protection (Freeman, 1983; Moules, 2006). This Declaration did, however, take the discussion about the rights of young people further forward by placing the debate firmly in an international context and placing obligations on members of the United Nations.

In the 1960s there was greater recognition that protecting society from juvenile delinquency and the aim of helping young people were essentially complementary. It was also increasingly uncommon to classify young people into one of two groups, the deprived and the depraved (Bainham, 2005). The Children and Young Persons Act 1969 was heavily influenced by these changing views and moved the focus slightly, from only protecting young people to assisting them to become members of society.

The Family Law Act 1969 set a presumptive standard that young people aged 16 and 17 years in the UK are presumed to be competent unless it can be demonstrated otherwise. This is based on the assumption that 16- and 17-year-olds were competent if they could understand and retain information and were able to weigh up that information and the likely consequences of any decision

---

[4] The Declaration of Geneva, also adopted by the League of Nations in 1924, resulted largely from the efforts of the British child's rights pioneer Eglantyne Jebb.
[5] See www.swarb.co.uk/acts/1933CaYPAct.shtml
[6] See www.unhchr.ch/html/menu3/b/25.htm

they might make. Considering age in this way demonstrated a growing appreciation of the need to treat young people as having different levels of competence. It was no longer acceptable to treat all young people, from newborn to 17 years, in the same way.

In a landmark decision, in 1980, the Department of Health and Social Security for the UK issued a notice making it lawful for doctors to give contraception and advice to girls under the age of 16 years. Most importantly, this was allowed without involving the parents and without obtaining their prior consent. This decision was justified on the grounds that the doctors would be acting in the young person's best interests by protecting them from the harmful effects of sexual intercourse. Victoria Gillick, the mother of five girls under the age of 16 years, sought assurances, from her area health authority, that her daughters would not receive such treatment without her permission. This resulted in considerable legal argument during which Victoria Gillick initially lost her case, then had the decision overturned in the Court of Appeal and ultimately lost again in the House of Lords[7].

The House of Lords held that young people, under the age of 16 years, could give consent to contraceptive advice without their parent's knowledge or consent, providing they could demonstrate sufficient maturity and intelligence to understand the proposed treatment. Although the focus of this legal case was on contraceptive advice and treatment, the resulting legal ruling applied to all medical treatment and was a landmark decision acknowledging the right of young people to take some control of their own health care, and introduced the concept of 'Gillick competence', assessed using the following Fraser Guidelines[8]:

- that the young person understands the health professional's advice
- that the professional cannot persuade the young person to inform his or her parent or allow the doctor to inform the parents that he or she is seeking contraceptive advice
- that the young person is very likely to begin or continue having intercourse with or without contraceptive treatment
- that without receiving contraceptive advice or treatment, the young person's physical or mental health or both are likely to suffer
- that the young person's best interests require the health professional to give contraceptive advice, treatment or both without parental consent.

The test of Gillick competence became widely used but there was, and remains, considerable debate about what the concept actually means and what level of competence is required to make important decisions about one's own health. The debate was inevitable because competence varies enormously and is dependent on multiple complex factors, including the nature of the proposed treatment, peer pressure and the family environment (Hendrick, 2006). It is clear, however,

---

[7] *Victoria Gillick* v *West Norfolk and Wisbech Health Authority and Department of Health and Social Security.*

[8] Lord Fraser overturned the Gillick ruling in the House of Lords in 1985 and suggested criteria for best practice for health and social care practitioners.

that the rights of young people received a major boost in the UK as a result of the decision made by the House of Lords. The test of Gillick competence had enabled a large number of young people to participate in decision making about their own health care.

The United Nation's Convention on the Rights of the Child (1989)[9], ratified in the UK in 1991, has been described as the most authoritative and comprehensive landmark statement of the fundamental rights of young people until that point in time (Bainham, 2005). Unlike so many other Conventions and legal provisions, this Convention was universally welcomed and it was signed up to more rapidly and by more countries than any other international instrument (Hendrick, 2006). The Convention was the world's first international legal instrument to focus on young people's rights and was based on the following three core principles:

• young people have special needs which set them apart from adults
• the best environment for a child's development is within a protective and nurturing family
• governments and the adult world in general should be committed to acting in the best interests of the child.

As these principles suggest, the aims and general obligations of the Convention were prevention, protection, provision and participation. In line with the fourth 'p', Article 12 of the Convention set out to assure respect for a young person's views:

> . . . the child who is capable of forming his own views [has] the right to express those views freely in all matters affecting the child, the views of the child being given due weight in accordance with the age and maturity off the child.
>
> **(Convention on the Rights of the Child 1989, Article 12)**

There is, however, a clear and obvious conflict between Article 12, which stresses that young people should be heard, and Article 3, which stresses protection and care with an emphasis on the rights of parents and guardians. Requiring that young people should be heard need not necessarily influence the final decision. Indeed, it could be argued that nothing the young person might say will influence the final decision if the adult does not believe it to be in the young person's best interests. Unlike the later European Convention on Human Rights, this Convention did not result in significant changes to English law but it did establish the important principle that the young person's voice should be heard.

When the Children Act 1989[10] was passed, coming into force in October 1991, it was hailed as a 'children's charter' because it appeared to give young people the absolute right to provide informed consent and informed refusal. The Act pulled together much of the complex and technical law that had

---

[9] See www.unicef.org/crc/
[10] See www.opsi.gov.uk/acts/acts1989/Ukpga_19890041_en_1.htm

grown up during the preceding decades (Bainham, 2005). This new legislation replaced existing law governing the custody and the upbringing of young people and the public law applying to social services. In addition, the Children and Young Persons Act 1969 and the Magistrates' Court Act 1978 were significantly amended in the UK. More than any preceding legislation, the Act highlighted a young person's right to autonomy and acknowledged their independent status. In doing so, the Act legitimized young people as individuals rather than as objects of concern (Hendrick, 2006). Importantly, young people were now allowed to challenge, through the courts, decisions made about their care. For the first time it seemed that young people would truly have a say in decisions about their own care. In reality, however, this has been extremely rare because courts are able to filter out cases in which they believe the young person lacks the necessary understanding of the situation. This filtering process was contrary to the objectives of the Act and again placed the onus of responsibility for decision making with those possessing parental responsibility.

The Act attempted to strike a balance between the role of the state, the rights of young people and the responsibilities of parents. To do this, the Act was founded on three fundamental principles. The first, the welfare principle, emphasized the need to ensure that the interests of young people should be the paramount consideration. The second principle, the primacy of the family, was based on the belief that the best place for young people to grow up is within their family and that the state should only intervene when it is absolutely necessary. The third and final principle, the young person's voice, set out to enhance the young person's legal status and their capacity for independent action. This was to be achieved by giving young people greater rights to have their views taken into account when making decisions about their health care. This final principle potentially marked a further move away from the prevailing notion of paternalism, a notion that had been enshrined in much of the preceding legislation. As with the United Nation's Convention on the Rights of the Child, however, this right to express their views and to have them taken into account only stretched as far as it was deemed not to be interfering with the young person's best interests by those with parental responsibility.

The welfare principle was the main consideration in the Act and was described as the only consideration in any court decision. The Act broke new ground in that it incorporated a statutory checklist of factors that a court should consider when applying the welfare principle. It was not long, however, before the courts demonstrated a willingness to place greater emphasis on the notion of protection and less on hearing the views of young people. In doing so the courts undermined the clear intentions of the Act (Hendrick, 2006). Most clearly, the young person's right to refuse treatment was not upheld by the courts. The Act has also been criticized for not achieving all that it might have done, for privatizing the family, for not obliging parents to involve young people in decision making and for not providing sufficient protection for young people (Fortin, 2003; Hendrick, 2006; Moules, 2006). Such criticisms might help to explain why the child protection framework has required so much amendment in the Children Act 2004[11].

The European Convention for the Protection of Human Rights and Fundamental Freedoms[12] was ratified as the Human Rights Act 1998[13], implemented in October 2000. The Act resulted in major change in the way cases would be argued in court (Bainham, 2005). Although the provisions of the Act altered very few decisions, there had to be greater consideration of the young person's human rights, including the right to be involved in decisions affecting the young person's life.

The Green Paper *Every Child Matters*[14] outlined proposals for information-sharing systems in the UK, holding basic information on all young people with practitioners able to indicate that they were providing a service to a young person and, where appropriate, that they had a concern about a young person. The Children Act 2004 provided the legal framework to enable practitioners to share early information to ensure that young people and families are getting benefit from services such as education and basic health care and to enable them to get the support they need at the right time. In particular, the Act contained provision for the creation and operation of a secure professionally maintained information child index that might be set up at local, regional or national level or a combination thereof. In doing so, the Act provided a legislative foundation for whole-system reform to support this long-term and ambitious programme. One of the key provisions of the Act included the appointment of Children's Commissioners[15] in each of the four countries of the UK and the establishment of structures to promote interagency co-operation and greater protection for young people. Central to the new Commissioner role was the aim of ensuring that the voice of young people is heard. How successful each Commissioner has been in doing this has yet to be determined. It is clear that, although protection remained the primary concern, the right to have one's voice heard was also growing in significance.

Considering the complex legal and ethical background is important for health and social care practitioners because it affects every aspect of their everyday practice and every young person's health care. It also demonstrates that current legal provision has shifted the balance from paternalism to inclusion of young people in the decision-making process, while retaining the paramount requirement to protect the young person.

YOUNG PEOPLE'S RIGHTS

The whole issue of young people's rights has always been extremely complex. As demonstrated above, much legislation has set out to clarify the rights of

[11] See www.opsi.gov.uk/acts/acts2004/20040031.htm
[12] See www.conventions.coe.int/Treaty/en/Treaties/Html/005.htm
[13] See www.opsi.gov.uk/ACTS/acts1998/19980042.htm
[14] See www.everychildmatters.gov.uk/_files/EBE7EEAC90382663E0D5BBF24C99A7AC.pdf
[15] Peter Clarke was appointed the UK's first Children's Commissioner in Wales in 2001. Further appointments were made in Northern Ireland (Nigel Williams) in 2003, in Scotland (Kathleen Marshall) in 2004 and in England (Al Aynsley-Green) in 2005. Independent of government, the Commissioner's remit is to promote awareness of views and interests of children.

young people but this has not always been the outcome. Rather, legislation has highlighted a clear conflict between a young person's rights and the obligations placed on others to provide protection.

Possessing a right requires action or restraint from others and justification for rights are based on either legal or moral principles (Gillon, 1985). Legal rights are created by national governments and are based on what is considered right and wrong according to the law. Moral rights are based on moral principles that are intrinsically specified as 'good' by a particular civil society. Universal moral rights are those that apply to all humans and stem from the one fundamental right of all 'men' to be free (Hart, 1970). This places an obligation on all people to respect others' autonomy. Special moral rights are those possessed by some but not by others, and usually result from prior actions such as promises or contracts. The essential difference between legal and moral rights is that legal rights can be abolished and are subject to change, according to the will of the government of the day. It has been argued that these are the only true rights that exist (Bentham, 1970). It is these legal rights that can be enforced. In contrast, moral rights are intrinsically agreed as a collective 'good' and are not, therefore, subject to change. The preceding section demonstrated changes to the legal status of young people's rights, marking a theoretical bridging of the gap between legal rights and moral rights.

The rights of young people have only been high on the agenda within the UK in recent years, given a particular boost by the Gillick case and the Children Act 1989. English law has been paternalistic or protectionist in orientation and it has been argued that this has resulted in a focus on safeguarding the welfare of young people above any consideration of their rights. The concept of young people's rights is extremely complex and cannot be looked at in a one-dimensional way (Bainham, 2005). Any consideration of young people's rights should include elements of both protection and self-determination:

> *It can be cogently argued that the welfare of children dictates that they are allowed a degree of self-determination or qualified autonomy.*
> **(Bainham, 2005, p.100)**

These concepts should not be considered as existing at the two extremes of a continuum. The concepts do, however, result in potential conflict between a young person's right to self-determination and their right to be protected.

The nature of young people's rights has been a matter of considerable controversy and theoretical debate. Bainham (2005) highlights three influential British theories on rights for young people that merit brief consideration here. Neil MacCormick explored 'Will theory' and 'Interest theory' (MacCormick, 1984). 'Will theory' was based on the notion that to possess a right one has to be able to exercise individual choice over enforcement by others. The essence of this theory is the pre-eminence of the right-holder's will over the will of others. The 'Interest theory' focuses on the protection of an individual's interests by imposing duties on others. The critical difference between the two theories is that the 'Will theory' involves the capacity for individual autonomy, whereas in the 'Interest theory' it is sufficient for the existence of a right that there is an identifiable interest and a corresponding duty (MacCormick, 1984). This suggests that the

'Interest theory' is more relevant to a consideration of young people's rights than the 'Will theory' because law dictates that, although young people's opinions should be taken into account, it is the will of others, those with parental responsibility, that will ultimately make or legitimize the decision.

In the second theory, John Eekelaar, like MacCormick, focused on the interest theory of rights but places particular emphasis on the need to ensure that an individual's interests are capable of being isolated from the interests of others (Eekelaar, 1986). When considering the rights of young people this is extremely complicated because a parent has the legal power to make decisions for a young person and this power is exercised in the young person's best interests or based on the welfare principle. This is problematic because the young person's interests will not always be identical to the parent's interests. Eekelaar argues that, because no young person can claim parental independence, a young person's principal right should be to have the best medical decisions made for them by someone with parental responsibility. This paternalistic approach is also extended to young people who are perceived to be competent because Eekelaar suggests two limitations that restrict a young person's right to make decisions and have them respected. First, the decision should be compatible with the general law and the interests of others. Second, the young person should not make a decision that is contrary to his or her physical or mental well-being. This again suggests that a competent young person is only allowed to make a decision if those with parental responsibility concur with that decision.

In the third theory, Michael Freeman adopted a more practical approach and focused on the need to ensure that young people have participatory rights (Freeman, 1983). It was emphasized that the implementation of legal rights could become an abstract consideration of theoretical principles if the will of others is lacking to put the principles into practice. Freeman produced the following four classifications of young people's rights:

- rights to welfare
- rights to protection
- rights to be treated like adults
- rights against adults.

Consideration of these individual rights results in multiple conflicts about who should be making decisions and about who has the right to overturn a decision made by a young person. This again marks a leap between the preferred situation and the real-world situation faced by families and health and social care practitioners every day.

There is some common ground amongst these three theoretical perspectives. First, young people possess a fundamental human right to be involved in decision making. Second, this right is restricted by the requirement to adhere always to the welfare principle and the need to protect the best interests of the young person. Third, this right places an obligation or duty on someone with parental responsibility to ensure that decisions are always made in the young person's best interests. These three points emphasize the need to embrace both 'qualified self-determination' and 'limited paternalism' (Bainham, 2005). These theories, and others, offer some clarity about young people's rights, but there remains much controversy about the basis upon which paternal or court intervention can be justified.

There is greater theoretical merit underpinning the principle that those with parental responsibility should consider what the young person would ideally want for themselves if they were sufficiently mature or competent to make the decision for themselves. In theory, this principle may require someone to balance what they believe the young person might wish in, what they perceive as, their own best interests and what the individual with parental responsibility might believe is actually in the young person's best interests, again demonstrating the potential conflict highlighted previously. In reality it is more likely that decision making will reflect the values and beliefs of the legal decision maker and will be based upon what they perceive to be in the young person's best interests.

The notion of possessing rights implies the existence of legal and moral duties in someone and immediately focuses on rights that exist in the adult world. These rights will often clash with the rights that might be given to young people (Bainham, 2005). One of the main problems when considering young people's rights is that they do not exist in a vacuum. They have to be considered alongside the rights and interests of others and in the light of many other potential complex factors.

AUTONOMY

Obtaining informed consent to treatment requires the application of both legal and ethical principles that are founded on the central principle of respect for autonomy. Respecting a young person's autonomy or right to self-determination risks causing tension between the young person and those with parental responsibility. As already demonstrated, it can sometimes be difficult to decide when a parent's legal right to make a decision should yield to the young person's right to make their own decisions (Henricson and Bainham, 2005). This is further complicated because the extent to which a young person's rights are upheld may depend on the views of the adults around them. There is a danger that an existing power relationship between an adult and a young person could result in even a well-reasoned argument being dismissed by the adult. This clearly presents a dilemma for health and social care practitioners who are obliged to encourage the young people's views to be heard, but ultimately have to concede that parents probably know the young person best and are better placed to judge their competence to make important decisions. Parents may also feel uncomfortable about the notion of involving young people as active participants in decision making (Diduck and Kaganas, 2006).

Thus far in this chapter it has been demonstrated that there are three basic possibilities for making decisions, within an appropriate legal framework, about a young person's health:

• decisions made by parents
• decisions made by the young person

- decisions made by outside agencies, including courts, usually to resolve disagreement between or within the above parties or when health and social care practitioners might disagree with the above decisions.

These points demonstrate that, irrespective of who might be involved in the decision-making process, someone must have the final say. If at all possible, the young person's right to make autonomous decisions should be respected, or they should at least have their opinions taken into account.

There are, however, a number of reasons why young people may not have their opinions taken into account (Hendrick, 2006). The greatest obstacle arises from unfounded prejudices about young people's abilities and the belief that it is unwise, unkind or a waste of time to listen to young people, especially when considering complex medical or health issues. This belief has been demonstrated to be false and evidence has been provided to indicate that young people are able to make complex decisions and plan for the future (Fortin, 2003). Other reasons limiting the involvement of young people in decision making might include:

- lack of time and resources to facilitate decision making
- lack of confidence, on the part of health and social care practitioners, in communicating with young people
- lack of skill in communicating with young people
- language barriers between the young people and adults
- failure to recognize non-verbal communications
- tension between adults and young people
- a need for adults to feel in control.

Respecting autonomy and gaining freely given informed consent from young people is theoretically important but can also be beneficial to all involved for three main reasons (Hendrick, 2006). First, health and social care practitioners will be protected from legal action. Second, it will have beneficial therapeutic effects because it helps to secure the individual's co-operation and trust. Finally, individuals are responsible for their own decisions, which promote self-esteem. Practitioners are required to be familiar with legal requirements to ensure lawful practice but they also need to be aware of the multiple benefits of promoting autonomous decision making. Balancing these can be problematic and requires careful consideration of each situation.

AGE OF CONSENT

Defining what constitutes a 'young person' or a 'child' is a legal concept that requires detailed consideration of multiple social factors. Furthermore, as demonstrated elsewhere in this chapter, such definitions can be changed. In the Children and Young Persons Act 1969, the status of childhood was redefined with the age of majority being reduced from 21 to 18 years. This is fraught with complication because young people vary considerably in their legal capacity to make certain decisions and to take certain actions, with the result that a young person's competence is determined by the context in which it is being considered.

It is important that young people are not forced to make decisions against their will because respect for autonomy is not an absolute principle but is a matter of degree (Hendrick, 2006). If the treatment is complex and carries serious risks, respect for autonomy might be about letting them express their opinion, but the final decision will be made by the individual with parental responsibility. If the treatment is relatively minor, the young person's wishes can determine the final decision in many instances. In determining a young person's competence to participate in decision making, their age will undoubtedly be taken into account.

Like the Children and Young Persons Act 1967, the Children Act 1989 defined children as those under the age of 18 years. These young people can be further divided into three broad age-based groups: those aged 16 and 17 years; those under 16 years of age and considered Gillick competent; and those under 16 years of age and not considered Gillick competent. It is generally agreed, and in accordance with the Family Law Act 1969, that 16- and 17-year-olds are competent to make decisions about their health and to give informed consent to treatment. Despite this, courts retain the right to their protective role and can veto this consent if it is deemed contrary to the young person's best interests. Parents do not have the same right to veto but they can act as a proxy consenter if the young person is deemed incompetent to do so.

The right to give informed consent should also carry the right to refuse to consent to an investigation or treatment, but this is not straightforward in this age group. Although a young person might be considered competent, their right to informed refusal can be overruled by the courts, by their parents or by someone with parental responsibility. In such circumstances, health and social care practitioners can obtain proxy consent that over-rides the young person's refusal to consent. Again it must be demonstrated that such decisions are made in the young person's best interests. Overturning a young person's decision in this way might be lawful, but it fails to demonstrate respect for the young person's right to self-determination.

The right of a young person under the age of 16 years to consent was established in the Gillick case (discussed earlier in this chapter). Young people demonstrated to be Gillick competent and to meet the Fraser guidelines are assumed to be able to consent for themselves but, as with older children, they are unable to refuse consent to treatment if the decision is perceived to be against their best interests. The result is that they can be treated against their wishes. In such circumstances the courts have stressed the need to ensure that the young person's wishes are considered, but the degree to which the young person's wishes influence the final decision is unclear.

Proxy informed consent is required for young people under the age of 16 years and deemed not to be Gillick competent. Again the core principle is that all decisions are made in the young person's best interests. In most cases this will be unproblematic, but if health and social care practitioners believe that a parent's decision, or the decision of the person with parental responsibility, is not in the young person's best interests, they can apply to a court to have the decision overturned. Making such a decision risks causing considerable distress to all involved, including the young person, and risks damaging the relationship between the family and the health and social care practitioners.

In all circumstances it is necessary to assess a young person's level of competence, which requires consideration of their ability to understand their choices and their willingness to make a choice based on that information. It should not be assumed that all young people wish to make choices about their health care, and it is important that they are not pressurized into making decisions. To do so risks causing greater distress than results from removing the young person from the decision-making process. For example, a young person may be torn between what they might wish to do and a desire to please their parents. Such situations require careful management by practitioners, who need to balance legal requirements and the need to ensure that the young person receives the best possible care.

PARENTAL RESPONSIBILITY

Parental responsibility is central to the Children Act 1989 in which it is described as the legal authority parents have over young people and the phrase 'parental rights' is replaced with 'parental responsibility'. Parental responsibility is defined as:

> *All rights, duties, powers, responsibility and authority which by law a parent of a child has in relation to the child and his property.*
>
> **(Children Act 1989, Section 3(1))**

The concept of parental responsibility emphasizes the duties of parents rather than their rights. This duty is to take all possible actions to protect the young person from possible harm.

The Act has been criticized because it does not go into detail about what parents can or cannot do. Instead, it has been argued that the Act exhibits 'misplaced complacency over the existing state of family values' and emphasizes the privacy of the family (Fortin, 2003). It is further argued that detailed legislation would have been more useful to parents and health and social care practitioners, and failing to provide such detail has resulted in continuing uncertainty about what constitutes parental responsibility.

Despite this, it is generally agreed that those with parental responsibility can make decisions about many aspects of a young person's life, including giving informed consent to medical treatment or a healthcare intervention. Although the scope of parental responsibility is broad, it is not absolute and is subject to two main restrictions (Hendrick, 2006). First, the welfare principle requires that those with parental responsibility act always in accordance with the young person's best interests. Second, parental responsibility diminishes as the young person matures and becomes more capable of making independent decisions. Even this, however, is not straightforward because detail is lacking about how competence might be judged, especially in complex situations where competence might be temporarily or intermittently reduced.

Situations may also arise where those with parental responsibility disagree on the decision to be made. As in all other situations, it is the welfare of the young person that should be of paramount importance. Even the application of this principle, however, is not always sufficient to resolve a dispute. For the sake of all concerned, especially the young person, it is essential to make every effort to try and resolve any dispute that might arise. When resolution is not possible, it may be necessary to resort to arbitration through the courts but this should always be a last resort.

CONFIDENTIALITY

The principle of confidentiality is one of the oldest in medical and healthcare ethics and has become one of the central principles in professional codes of practice. The strict requirement to ensure confidentiality is justified on two main grounds, the utilitarian and deontological arguments (Hendrick, 2006). The utilitarian argument focuses on the need to ensure that patients feel they can trust health and social care practitioners with information they may reveal. If they feel they cannot trust practitioners, they may not be willing to reveal sensitive information or may be deterred from seeking assistance at all. If either situation should occur, the young person's health may be adversely affected. Deontologists believe that confidentiality should be respected because it is inherently right to do so irrespective of welfare considerations. This latter argument fails to recognize the need to balance the young person's right to have their voice heard and their right to be protected from danger.

Confidentiality is a universally accepted principle and, although there is no specific statute in English law to define or enforce it, Article 8 of the Human Rights Act 1998 protects respect for private life. Despite this, it is generally accepted that a formal level of confidentiality exists between a patient and health or social care practitioner. This right to confidentiality is owed as much to a young person as it is to any other person, if they are sufficiently mature to form a relationship of confidence with another person. It is important to distinguish between a young person's competence to give informed consent to treatment and their right to confidence.

There are circumstances when the duty of confidentiality is not absolute (Bainham, 2005). The right to have one's confidence respected can be breached for two main reasons, to protect a patient's best interests and in the public interest (Hendrick, 2006). In all circumstances a decision to breach a confidence must be justified. The disclosure of confidential information in the patient's best interest is paternalistic and limits the young person's autonomy, in an attempt to protect a young person's health, their safety and their welfare. For example, if it is suspected that a young person is being abused then breaching confidentiality is a legitimate action because it is acting in the young person's best interests. This situation is more complicated if the young person is Gillick competent and does not wish an aspect of their health to be discussed with a parent.

Disclosure of confidential information in the public interest is more complicated because its scope is much less certain. It can be invoked to justify any breach of confidence if it is thought to be in the public's best interest. In case law, it is required to demonstrate a 'real' and 'genuine' risk of danger to the public to justify a breach of confidence.

In English law there has been no authoritative ruling on when a young person is entitled to have information kept confidential from parents. In general, however, there is agreement that competent young people have the same right to confidentiality as adults (Bainham, 2005). The situation is much more complicated when considering the rights of incompetent young people, if young people are to be able to retain some control over their person health information (Hendrick, 2006). If young people do not possess control of their health information, they also are unable to make truly informed decisions about their own health care.

CONCLUSION

The law has become so important in the provision of health and social care for young people that it is now central to the practice of all health and social care practitioners. In every aspect of their working lives, practitioners have to grapple with the application of legal requirements while always trying to ensure that the young person receives the best possible care. This chapter has explored just some of the legal complexities.

KEY POINTS

- Any consideration of young people's health would be incomplete without an analysis of the complex legal and ethical issues, especially concerning decision making, informed consent and informed refusal.
- Legal and ethical issues are central to the everyday practice of health and social care practitioners.
- Young people should, as far as possible and within current legal frameworks, be involved in decision making and providing informed consent to health and social care investigations and interventions.
- If a young person is unable to be involved in decision making, through lack of competence, proxy decisions can be made on their behalf.
- The welfare of the young person must always be the principle that guides decision making.

REFERENCES

Bainham A (2005) *Children: the modern law* (3e). Bristol: Family Law.

Bentham J (1970) Anarchical fallacies. In: Melden AI (ed.) *Human Rights*. Belmont: Wadsworth, pp.28–39.

Diduck A, Kaganas F (2006) *Family Law, Gender and the State* (2e). Oxford: Hart Publishing.

Eekelaar J (1986) The emergence of children's rights. *Oxford Journal of Legal Studies* 6:161–82.

Fortin J (2003) *Children's Rights and the Developing Law* (2e). London: Lexis Nexis Butterworths.

Freeman M (1983) *The Rights and Wrongs of Children*. London: Frances Pinter.

Freeman M (1993) Laws, conventions and rights. *Children and Society* 7:37–48.

Gillon R (1985) *Philosophical Medical Ethics*. Chichester: Wiley.

Hart H (1970) Are there any natural rights? In: Melden AI (ed.) *Human Rights*. Belmont: Wadsworth, pp.61–78.

Hendrick J (2006) Legal and ethical issues. In: Moules T, Ramsey J (eds) *The Textbook of Children's Nursing* (2e). Cheltenham: Nelson Thornes.

Henricson C, Bainham A (2005) *The Child and Family Policy Divide: tensions, convergence and rights*. York: Joseph Rowntree Foundation.

MacCormick N (1984) *Legal Right and Social Democracy: essays in legal and political philosophy*. Oxford: Oxford University Press.

Moules T (2006) Children's rights. In: Moules T, Ramsey J (eds) *The Textbook of Children's Nursing* (2e). Cheltenham: Nelson Thornes.

Acts of Parliament

All these Acts are published by HMSO in London, and all can be accessed from the UK Parliament website (www.publications.parliament.uk).

Children and Young Person Act 1933
Children and Young Persons Act 1967
Children and Young Persons Act 1969
Family Law Act 1969
Magistrates Court Act 1978
Human Rights Act 1998
Children Act 1989
Children Act 2004

3

DIFFERENCE AND DIVERSITY AS DETERMINANTS OF HEALTH: ETHNICITY, GENDER AND DISABILITY

Simon Forrest and Theresa Nash

INTRODUCTION

Although attention to difference and diversity as determinants of child public health has sharpened in recent years, the issues are not new. Awareness that there are population sector differences in the ability to gain access to health services and to positive health outcomes is not a preserve of contemporary political and academic life. In fact, more than a century has passed since the vulnerability of some minorities to poorer health and higher mortality was first observed. And, in striking resonance with contemporary analysis, the connection between health inequalities and the social, economic and environmental deprivations experienced by these minority groups was initially elaborated in the 19th and early 20th centuries (Trask, 1916; Engels, 1987; Acheson, 1998).

Yet, despite this impressive heritage, there is no doubt that public health interest in difference and diversity has increased greatly in recent years as society itself has been perceived to become more diverse. By talking about perceptions of increasing diversity it is not our intention to suggest that this is some ways artifactual, but to signal from the outset that we understand that difference and diversity are historically and socially specific constructs. This means that what constitutes difference, how and which groups of people are categorized as different and how these differences are responded to is context bound.

Clearly, societies are not stable and unchanging entities in which a limited variety of diverse groups are simply waiting to be discovered by increasingly subtle investigative technologies. The very investigative technologies with which we explore society are, at least to some extent, the means by which we construct groups, and even where differences within society are apparently self-evident, like the differences between men and women, how we define those categories, how we impose them and how we regard people within them reflect ideological, political and cultural investments and assumptions about what constitutes norms and hence what (or whom) is different from the norm. For example, as Liz Stanley's elegant analysis of studies of sexual attitudes and behaviours within Britain across the last 80 years demonstrates, there is a complex and dynamic relationship between the acts of scientific categorization, social norms and ideology and, moreover, these acts of constructing difference and diversity feed back into public consciousness of norms. They become benchmarks by which people define their own and others' values, identities and behaviour in terms of difference from one another (Stanley, 1995).

In this chapter, we explore the implications of taking the view that difference and diversity are experienced by children and young people as dynamic dimensions of their sense of identity. For public health practice, particularly service development and delivery, how children and young people understand and experience their place in a social world is what matters. This is not to assert that children and young people do not belong to groups or that they cannot be categorized as different from one another in terms of dimensions like ethnicity, gender and (dis)ability, but that the homogenizing of individuals through grouping can unhelpfully smooth over the realities of lived experience in which children and young people develop a sense of identity that is similar to or different from others, more or less strongly according to the particularities of specific social interactions, circumstances and contexts.

In terms of public health practice, this means that their encounters with health and other professionals and their understanding of public health messages are all contexts in which their sense of difference and diversity may be more or less accentuated according to a whole range of factors. Thus, targeting children and young people solely by some putative group identity may mean that they do not recognize that services or messages are relevant for them.

THE EMERGENCE OF DIFFERENCE AND 'DISCOVERY' OF DIVERSITY

Approaching a consideration of child public health from this perspective involves us in exploring some of the influences that have contributed to the emergence of increased awareness of difference and diversity within the field, and which represent social sites where children and young people may experience a sense of their difference and diversity from others.

As we have already suggested, advances in behavioural and disease epidemiology have a constructive role to play in the development of increasingly sophisticated ideas about difference and diversity. The capacity to access more data about the health of the nation, and our ability to subject it to more subtle and complex interrogation, has enabled public health analysts to identify ways of characterizing vulnerability to disease or ill-health by factors that are associated with the increasing fragmentation of society into groups. It is possible to talk about differences and diversity in health not only by gender and age, but also by locality, ethnicity and (dis)ability. Moreover, increasing subcategories of the population can be created by exploring the interactions between these dimensions of difference.

These changes have been linked to changes in the nature of public health as a practice *per se*. In the UK and other rich developed countries, this has been particularly marked in relation to children and young people where public health has widened its scope in terms of both the topics with which it is concerned and the variety of agencies engaged in this work (Blair *et al.*, 2003). The effects of broadening both the 'what' public health is and the 'who' is involved in securing and promoting it have inevitably increased the potential for identifying different and more diverse target groups and settings.

Changes in public health have, of course, not taken place in isolation. The trend towards a 'rights-based' inflection in the development of public policy has also sharpened attention to difference and diversity. In the last decade, the UK has enshrined in its own statutory law a commitment to global and regional declarations on human and children's rights (Council of Europe, 1950, 1961; United Nations, 1989; Human Rights Act 1998). The effect of spelling out the rights of the individual and pledging to ensure that these are equitably available naturally causes a spotlight to fall on those groups and individuals who are denied the entitlements associated with these rights. This 'rights-based' agenda within public policy both sets the tenor for public health practice and has a very direct influence on it by committing the UK Government to take steps to ensure that the health of all children and young people is protected and promoted.

The rise of 'rights-based' inflections within public policy can also be connected with the increased emergence of social movements that aim to achieve recognition and equality for a wide variety of groups. Putting human rights on a legal footing gives extra political leverage to individuals and groups who feel militated against or denied entitlements that they perceive to be their due. Some of these have had a very direct bearing on public health practice. To take one example, the political movements among gay men in the wake of the emergence of the HIV/AIDS epidemic, for equal recognition of their identity and acknowledgement of their particular vulnerability to HIV, illustrate a sense of the way group identity can be galvanized through threats to individual health and well-being. One potential effect of the mobilization of minority groups is the destabilization of norms in the wider population and the creation of yet more diversity and difference. The emergence and success of the gay rights movement has contributed to the liberalization of thinking about sexual identity as a whole as well as the fragmentation and multiplication of sexual identities since the 1980s (Forrest and Ellis, 2006).

Awareness of the political dimension to the emergence of difference and diversity alerts us to the wider historical processes of struggle against stigmatization and oppression that often form their backdrop. This is particularly important because there is a tendency to lose sight of that fact, that the history of many forms of difference and diversity reveals that they have associations with negative experiences for minorities so defined. For example, when we talk about ethnicity as a dimension of difference in public health, we tend to regard it as fairly neutral. We see it as a term that emphasizes socially constructed differences between people associated with their group and individual origins, shared social background, cultures, traditions and sense of identity (Senior and Bhopal, 1994). However, ethnicity has only relatively recently replaced 'race' as the preferred lexical construct for dealing with these forms of difference between people. Despite its redundancy in public health terminology, what the term 'race' reminds us is that, when we talk about ethnic minorities in the UK and across Western Europe as whole, we are generally talking about people whose experiences of their ethnic difference has largely been associated with a history of colonialism, nationalism, racism, the exploitation of the labour of poorer nations by richer nations and, more particularly in recent times, the flight of people from persecution, poverty, unrest and war.

Understanding this history enables us to track its effects on contemporary debates about health issues. For example, the migration of people to Western European countries from the poorer East and South often stimulates debate about the relationship between nationality and entitlement to health services and the extent to which immigrant people are identified as a potential source of disease. Attempts to explore and address the links between the spread of HIV and the mobility of infected people to Western European countries from Eastern Europe and Sub-Saharan Africa, which takes place at both national and pan-European levels, illustrate the way that pejorative and generalizing views of immigrants as posing a risk to indigenous populations and placing a burden on health services can enter the public realm and thereby configure debate in ways that straggle effective political and strategic action on health (see, for example, Nicole and de Groot, 2003).

Finally, changes in the nature of social institutions and cultural practices also influence our understanding of social diversity and difference. Among the most significant of these changes are those that have taken place in the nature of the family and childhood. While we can still talk about 'the family' in public health analysis and practice, the term now refers to a wide range of social, economic and relational arrangements between people. Families not only comprise men and women and their biological offspring, but they also comprise same-sex couples, single parents, non-biological parents and a variety of reformed families who parent both their own biological and other children.

The nature of childhood has altered too. Whereas it once referred to a relatively short period of life ending around the early teenage years, it has now expanded and diversified such that it extends into the teenage years and beyond, thus resulting in the creation of whole new social groups of young people (the 'tweenies' and the 'teenagers'), for example, who may as a group display as much diversity within the group of 'children' as difference from other groups (Hendrick, 1997).

DIMENSIONS OF DIFFERENCE AND DIVERSITY

This overview aims to provide a broad context for thinking about difference and diversity in the context of a public health focus that targets children and young people. We have attempted to elaborate an argument that, while diversity is a 'real' social fact, it is also a dynamic construct influenced by social, cultural, ideological and economic processes. We have also sought to emphasize that dimensions of difference and diversity have a historical basis that is characterized by the marginalization of individuals and groups who depart from some social norm and who struggle for recognition and equality. We have sought to destabilize any notion that difference and diversity are fixed, static concepts that enable the neat categorization of people into a variety of historical pigeon-holes.

We recognize that trying to apply this conceptualization of difference and diversity in the context of public health is no easy task. Public health traditionally relies on the generation of categories of people in order to target policy, planning and service delivery, and we are not arguing for the abandonment of that approach but rather its refinement. Prior to coming to back to this issue, we present some information below about five of the major dimensions of difference and diversity that concern public health policy makers and practitioners, and preface this with commentary on the public policy context.

THE POLICY CONTEXT

Our objective here is to outline the UK public policy context around difference and diversity, with a focus on public health. We are aiming to be neither exhaustive nor to limit ourselves to policy that explicitly and solely relates to health, since difference and diversity and health are a cross-cutting theme in contemporary public policy development. Recent moves to enable parents to achieve a better balance between working and home life, in order to enable children to access the social, educational, welfare and *health* benefits that can accrue from parental involvement demonstrates this (Work and Families Act 2006).

Social inclusion

The cross-departmental approach to tackling social issues and taking into account difference and diversity in public policy development is a particularly marked characteristic of British legislative activity under the successive New Labour governments, which have been in power since 1997. This approach flows from a series of broad ideological commitments to reducing social exclusion and inequalities that are claimed to orient and underpin public policy. According to its definition of social exclusion as 'when people or places suffer from a series of problems such as unemployment, discrimination, poor skills, low incomes, poor housing, high crime, ill-health and family breakdown', the New Labour government has placed difference and diversity in terms of inequalities and disadvantages associated with specific demographic characteristics and localities firmly at the heart of its conceptualization of policy development (Social Exclusion Unit, 2006).

Equality, difference and diversity

Social inclusion foregrounds achieving equality as a cross-cutting driver of policy. This has a direct influence on public health activity. Alongside developing a broad-based statutory framework of human rights, the government has placed statutory responsibilities on national and local government and statutory sector bodies including the health service to take into account inequalities (both of outcome and access to services). It has also put in place responses that take into account diversity and difference, because these are so frequently associated with disadvantage and social exclusion.

Within the health services, the goal of health equality, and the extent to which a failure to acknowledge and respond to diversity and difference, presents a barrier to achieving it, are recognized in a variety of policy directives and guidance documents. The *National Service Framework for Children, Young People and Maternity Services* (NSF) (Department of Health and Department for Education and Skills, 2004) and the Children Act 2004 make explicit the aims of providing a universal service that is needs led and tackles health inequalities, thus implying responsiveness to diversity of need among children and young people (Children Act 2004).

A further significant lever on achieving equality has come into place with the ratification of the single Equality Act in 2006, which will lead to the formation of a Commission on Equality and Human Rights (CEHR). From 2007, this Commission will subsume the responsibilities of the Equality Opportunities Commission, the Disability Rights Commission and the Commission for Racial Equality. The CEHR is being set up with the general duties of encouraging respect for difference and diversity, challenging prejudice and discrimination and ensuring mutual respect between groups 'based on understanding and valuing of diversity and on shared respect for equality and human rights'. The CEHR will take on the powers of the existing Commissions as well as new powers to enforce legislation more effectively and promote equality for all (Equality Act 2006, Part 1 Section 3). The CEHR will provide the centralizing authority responsible for monitoring and helping to enforce various laws on discrimination including the Race Equality Duty of 2001, the Disability Equality Duty, which came into force in 2006, and a Gender Duty which will come into force in 2007. The health and social care services are bound by these duties and therefore become liable to scrutiny by the CEHR.

Children, difference, diversity and health

The influence of these policies is very clear in areas like the NSF and in guidance on specific health topics relating to children and young people. To take two examples, the NSF has an overall aim of improving equality of access to health services and health outcomes, and identifies respecting difference and diversity and making appropriate responses to it as an important objective on the road to its fulfilment. In the foreground of the framework stand commitments to make services needs led, to increase the level of children's and parents' participation in decision making, and to tackle inequalities. Within these over-arching aims and objectives, several sections of the NSF deal explicitly with aspects of difference and diversity – age; children from groups that are at risk of harm; disabled children; and those with complex needs.

With regard to age, the NSF recognizes that children and young people are receptive to health-promotion messages about different topics at different ages, and that at some point in late childhood a smoother transition to adult services needs to be accomplished. The framework also takes a fairly holistic view of children's and young people's needs, demanding better linking of health and education, welfare and employment-related services. In the context of age-related difference and diversity, the framework also draws attention to the special and potentially acute needs of specific groups including disabled children and young people, those living in rural areas and those who are looked after by local authorities and/or are leaving care. With regard to children and young people at risk of harm, the NSF sets outs specific steps to be taken in order to ensure they are identified earlier and are provided with more effective and appropriate support. With regard to disabled children and those with complex needs, there are commitments to achieving their integration into mainstream services coupled with requirements to make these more needs led with an increase in the degree of active involvement of children and their families in decisions that affect them. The additional exclusion of disabled children from families of ethnic minorities is also noted.

The NSF illustrates how difference and diversity are conceptualized and reflected at the level of health-specific policy, but it is to guidance on specific health-related topics that we must look to see in detail how difference and diversity are to be addressed. To take one example, ethnic diversity and difference among children and young people is a recurrent theme in health policy, and the strategy and guidance on teenage pregnancy demonstrates how this dimension of difference is conceptualized and how responses to it are envisioned. Within the Teenage Pregnancy Strategy, young people from some ethnic minorities are identified as groups who are particularly vulnerable to early parenthood, which both reflects and can compound their vulnerability to social exclusion (Social Exclusion Unit, 1999). Guidance supporting the implementation of the strategy approaches ethnicity as a component of individual and group identity that influences health-related attitudes, values, beliefs and behaviour. The strategy notes that ethnicity and cultural and religious beliefs are often connected in the context of specific cultural heritages and traditions that carry with them particular configurations of attitudes towards health issues. Guidance in this area has also highlighted the role that discrimination can play in breeding distrust of statutory organizations among young people from ethnic minorities, and the potential ignorance among professionals of ethnic minority community and family values (Teenage Pregnancy Unit, 2000, 2002).

There are many other dimensions of difference and diversity reflected in the public policy context, including gender and sexuality, and an even greater number of specific target groups that are all perceived to have particular needs that diverge from those experienced by other children and young people.

Despite the diversity of difference noted, we can identify some common themes across the field. In short, the public policy context that bears on children and young people and health in the UK is characterized by the following:

- a recognition that access to health services and positive health outcomes is inequitable in the UK and that dimensions of difference and diversity are associated with these inequalities. The major underlying concern is with the stark (and increasing) differences between children and young people from richer and from poorer backgrounds. However, ethnicity, disability, social marginalization and exclusion, gender and sexuality are all recognized to varying degrees as relevant dimensions of difference and diversity in the efficient and effective targeting of public health activities.

In this context, policy aims tend to constellate around the following:

- ensuring that access to health and services is equitable
- recognizing that children and young people from marginalized and minority groups (ethnic minorities, disabled children, those in care and young prisoners, among others) are often disadvantaged in terms of the quality of their health and access to health services
- and, that this disadvantage is rooted in a number of factors, including some that are directly within the influence of public health practice, such as discriminatory practices within health and social care services and by health and social care professionals, and the accessibility and acceptability of health provision to people from minority groups.

CHILDREN, YOUNG PEOPLE, ETHNICITY AND HEALTH

Data derived from the 2001 Census report that around 8 per cent of the population come from 'non-white' ethnic backgrounds, of which the largest proportion, comprising around a half, are described as Asian or Asian British with another quarter described as Black or Black and British. People described as Chinese make up a further 5 per cent of the non-white population.

Demographic data from the same source have identified the younger population as more ethnically diverse than the older population, although age distribution is not similar across all ethnic minorities. Trends reflect waves of immigration such that the population of people categorizing themselves as Irish, for example, have the oldest age structure, followed by people from the Caribbean. People from Africa and the Far East tend to be younger than the population as a whole. The 'Mixed' group have the youngest age structure with half being under the age of 16 years. The Bangladeshi, 'Other Black' and Pakistani groups also have young age structures: 38 per cent of both the Bangladeshi and Other Black groups were aged under 16 years at 2001 and 35 per cent of Pakistanis also fell into this age group. This was almost double the proportion of the White British group where one in five (20 per cent) were under the age of 16 years. Ethnic diversity within the UK also has a strong geographical character with around 45 per cent of all 'non-white' people living in London (Office for National Statistics, 2001).

In recent years, increasingly detailed research on ethnicity has emerged, which has identified and explored the epidemiological, behavioural and social aspects of differences in health status and service use between and within ethnic groups (see for example, Health and Social Care Information Centre, 2005; Neale et al., 2005; Wardle et al., 2006). With regard to children and young people, evidence has emerged of an association between some conditions and diseases and ethnicity. For example, children from Indian, Pakistani, Bangladeshi and Chinese backgrounds have been found to be less likely to report acute sickness than other ethnic groups. Indian and Pakistani boys are more likely to be overweight than boys in the general population. African-Caribbean and Pakistani girls are more likely to be obese than girls in the general population (Office for National Statistics, 2004a).

Explanations for the inequitable distribution of ill-health among children and young people from ethnic minorities are the subject of some dispute, although there seems to be consensus that the effects of ethnicity cannot easily be disaggregated from other social factors, particularly socio-economic disadvantage. It has been suggested that aspects of ethnic heritage, genetic predispositions, behavioural norms within communities, the impact of racism and inequalities in uptake and experiences of health care and socio-economic status may all be influential factors. Furthermore, problems with disaggregating ethnicity as a single influencing factor reflect limitations in both the data available for analysis and the theorizations of socio-economic status and ethnicity that are being used (Smith et al., 2000).

Research on service uptake among ethnic minority groups also suggests links with socio-economic status, although ethnicity does seem to emerge as a factor in its own right in some studies. Evidence suggests that Indian and Pakistani children are more likely to have visited their general practitioner in the preceding fortnight than children in other ethnic groups, and that they and Bangladeshi and Chinese children are less likely to have attended an outpatient clinic in the preceding quarter. Such results would be more meaningful if other factors such as perceptions of health status were also taken into account (Cooper et al., 1998, 1999; Saxena et al., 2002).

What evidence there is on this score suggests that health status varies by ethnic group, and that, while children from Asian ethnic groups report better health, African-Caribbean children report worse health than the population in general (Saxena et al., 2002). However, both health needs and perceived susceptibility may vary by gender at least as much as by ethnicity, and gender may be more influential than ethnicity in determining the views of young people with regard to some health issues, particularly sexual health (Connell et al., 2004). Parents' and carers' roles in assessing the health status of children and young people, and in facilitating their access to health services, are poorly understood. Yet some research suggests that they play a major role in deciding when young people access health services, which services they then access, and in organizing appointments and accompanying young people to the majority of consultations. How this affects consultations, confidentiality and young people's preparedness to disclose their concerns remains to be subjected to any robust investigation (Jacobson et al., 1994).

Qualitative studies on attitudes to health and service uptake among young people provide some illumination on the range of factors that may inform differences in health and social care service use, although they rarely adopt any specific focus on ethnicity. A body of work on the accessibility and acceptability of health services with a focus on general practice suggests that, although satisfaction with services is high, health professionals are generally perceived as providers of advice on biomedical problems rather than on disease prevention. In addition, significant minorities of young people experience problems in consultations, ranging from ambivalence about whether they are given enough time, to difficulties with expressing personal concerns. There are also problems associated with believing that they are being taken seriously, and young people express serious reservations about achieving privacy in the reception areas of surgeries and about the maintenance of patient confidentiality (Atkinson *et al.*, 2003; Churchill *et al.*, 2000; Jacobson *et al.*, 1994; Malik *et al.*, 2002).

REFUGEE AND ASYLUM-SEEKING CHILDREN

Because the majority of refugees and asylum-seeking children and young people originate from ethnic minority groups, there is a tendency to conflate their needs with those of resident ethnic minorities despite significant differences. There are a considerable number of unaccompanied children and young people among refugees and asylum seekers (around 3000 annually) and antipathy within sections of the indigenous population compounds their already considerable vulnerability to ill-health (Refugee Council and the British Council for Adoption and Fostering, 2001).

Many child and young refugees are at risk of having been exposed to infectious disease and either have not been vaccinated or have uncertain medical histories. They may be or may have been malnourished and may have witnessed or been subject to violence and torture. Girls and young women may have been subject to female genital mutilation and/or domestic violence (Burnett and Peel, 2001). Research has shown that a disproportionately high number of child refugees display signs and symptoms of severe trauma and experience mental and emotional ill-health. This not only includes various forms of depression, anxiety and agoraphobia but is also manifest in problems impacting on their ability to integrate with other young people and society more widely, including problems with peers, hyperactivity and conduct disorders (Fazel and Stein, 2002).

It can be difficult to respond to these complex and sometimes acute needs because of language barriers and cultural issues that can hamper intercultural communication. Refugee children and young people may not be clear about their entitlements or what services are available to them or how to access services. The importance of interpreters and the advocacy and social and emotional support provided by appropriate cultural organizations based in the community has been highlighted, and web-based resources are playing an increasingly significant role in supporting refugees and asylum seekers, as are professionals working with them in health and welfare services (for example, HARP: Health for Asylum-seekers and Refugees Portal, www.harpweb.org.uk).

CHILDREN, YOUNG PEOPLE, GENDER AND HEALTH

Areas of major gender difference include susceptibility to accidents and resultant disabilities. Research suggests that over three times as many road traffic fatalities involve boys as girls between the ages of 15 and 19 years. A gender differential, albeit smaller, is also reflected in other accidents among 2- to 15-year-olds, which may reflect the greater involvement of boys in sports and outdoor activities.

Cancer is relatively rare among children, although cancers account for 23 per cent of all deaths among girls between the ages of 5 and 15 years. Cancer affects a similar proportion of boys, but is overtaken as the main source of mortality by accidents. There are some gender differences in the kinds of cancer that affect children and young people, with leukaemia and bone and brain tumours twice as likely to affect boys as girls (Office for National Statistics, 2002).

Obesity also has a strong gender dimension among 2- to 10-year-olds, with a trend since 1995 for a greater increase in the proportion of boys who are obese from 10 per cent to 16 per cent, while the proportion of girls has remained stable at 12 per cent. Looking at a wider age range, the differentials close slightly, but there is still evidence that the rate of increase in obesity is greater among boys than girls, particularly in the early teenage years (Information Centre for Health and Social Care, 2006). Problems with weight and obesity are clearly linked to exercise and diet but also to self-image, which is highly gendered. Young men tend to see themselves as fitter than women see themselves and boys are less likely to see their diet as important to their well-being.

The influence of self-image is also discernible in the prevalence of eating disorders, notably those associated with attempts to lose weight, which are much more prevalent among girls and young women. Nevertheless, there may be signs of rise in eating disorders among boys and young men (Gregory et al., 2000). Work on the link between diet, weight, eating disorders and attitudes toward food suggest that there are distinct gender differences in views about and motivations for eating behaviours, with girls most likely to cite emotional reasons for over- or undereating and boys more likely to cite social reasons. Young people seem well aware of the social expectations that feminine physical beauty is associated with being thinner and masculine attractiveness with being heavier, more muscular and taller (MacKinnon et al., 2002).

Smoking, drinking and drug use are all patterned by gender. Although there has been a steady rise in drinking alcohol by quantity by age, such that nearly half of 15-year-olds self-report having been drunk at least once and around a quarter in the last week, the proportion of boys between the ages of 11 and 15 years drinking ten units a week has remained fairly stable. In contrast, the proportion of girls drinking more is rising quickly towards parity. There has been a particularly steep rise in the reported number of 14-year-old girls drinking alcohol. Girls remain much more likely to be tobacco smokers than boys, although boys are much more likely to have used drugs, with the greatest differential in the teenage years where 31 per cent of boys compared with 24 per cent of girls reported using drugs in the last year (Office for National Statistics, 2004b).

Boys are more likely than girls to suffer from a recognizable mental disorder. Among 5- to 10-year-olds, 10 per cent of boys and 5 per cent of girls have a mental disorder. Among 11- to 16-year-olds, the reported proportions are 13 per cent for boys and 10 per cent for girls. Overall hyperkinetic and conduct disorders are much more common among boys than girls between the ages of 5 and 16 years and girls are much more likely to report emotional problems between the ages of 11 and 16 years (Office for National Statistics, 2004c).

We also know that sexual health issues have a strong gender dimension, with boys and young men much less likely to know about sexually transmitted infections and to know that they are infected, than girls and young women. They are also less likely to know about and to seek treatment (Lloyd et al., 2001).

Despite these significant differences in health outcomes and behaviours by gender, robust analysis of the reasons behind them is remarkably rare. An exception would seem to be recent work on boys and young men (a potential gender bias in itself), which has found that beliefs about and the acceptability of risk-taking among boys and young men plays a part in some aspects of their susceptibility to accidents. Their tendency towards 'physicality' might also account for their disproportionate representation in conditions like hyperkinetic disorders. This work also points to the need for a subtle and sophisticated model of gender that can take into account both individual factors and social norms when service provision issues are being considered. For example, services may be practically and qualitatively more acceptable and accessible to girls and young women, while boys and young men may perceive expression of concern about health issues and the use of services as signalling weakness and a failure to cope that conflicts with their understanding of masculinity (Lloyd et al., 2001).

CHILDREN, YOUNG PEOPLE, SEXUALITY AND HEALTH

In addition to gender, sexuality is an important dimension of diversity among young people, with particular significance for public health practice. For some time there has been a focus on the promotion of sexual health among young gay men because of their vulnerability to sexually transmitted infections, including HIV. This focus is associated with efforts to develop specialist services, targeted health awareness and informational/education materials. At a more general level, attempts to reach young gay men with better prevention earlier have been given some support by more liberal guidelines on sex and relationships education in schools (Department for Education and Employment, 2000).

However, a proper consideration of sexuality from a public health perspective implies much more than thinking about appropriately targeted measures for older, sexually at-risk young gay men. Sexual identity is more diverse and includes young lesbian women and bisexual young people. For many young people, long in advance of their sexual debut, uncertainty about sexual identity can make them vulnerable to mental health problems associated with defining their sexuality and coping with other people's reactions to them (Forrest et al., 1997). Well- and widely reported problems with homophobic bullying (for both gay and non-gay children and young people) are known to have a significant impact on young people's mental well-being. There is an inverse relationship between their willingness to discuss their concerns about sexual identity and ill-health (Ellis and High, 2004). Despite making some inroads through activities like the Healthy Schools initiatives, it is evident that there is scope for public health practice to adopt a wider and more active approach to challenging heterosexism and homophobia within and outside health and social care services.

CHILDREN, YOUNG PEOPLE, DISABILITY AND HEALTH

Estimates of the number of children and young people with disabilities vary considerably, according to which definitions are being used. Under the fairly narrow definition used in the Disability Discrimination Act 2005, it is estimated that there are at least 320 000 children and young people under the age of 16 years living with a disability in the UK. Assessments that use a wider definition of disability capable of articulating discriminatory treatment and stigmatization of a person based on their physical, mental and/or emotional capacities cause the estimates to rise to nearly double this number (Office of the Deputy Prime Minister *et al.*, 2005).

Disability among children and young people tends to have a different profile from disability in the older population. Children and young people are more likely to have a recognized learning difficulty than is the case with older people (Social Exclusion Unit, 2004). There has also been a marked increase in recent years in the numbers of children and young people diagnosed with an autistic spectrum disorder (ASD), or with other behavioural difficulties, and those experiencing clinically defined mental health problems. Similarly, the number of children and young people with a statement of special educational need (SEN) has risen. Notably, of those children between the ages of 4 and 15 years with a statement of SEN, more than two-thirds are boys and an increasing proportion of all children with disabilities come from an ethnic minority group. We also know that disability issues cluster in families and that over 17 500 families include more than one disabled child (Office of the Deputy Prime Minister *et al.*, 2005; Smyth and Robus, 1989; Walker *et al.*, 2002).

Among disabled children and young people with either physical needs that require a medical response or support (and hence bring them into frequent contact with health services) or with needs that do not require a medical response, research consistently demonstrates that it is failure to take account of their social needs that most affects their views on services. This, ultimately, has an impact on their access to good health and better life opportunities. For example, disabled people recall their experiences of growing up quite differently, depending on two main factors: first, how they saw themselves and were seen and treated by others; and second, the extent to which they experienced practical and emotional difficulties resulting from being a disabled child. Those people who reported that they were seen and treated differently from their friends and family during childhood tended to see themselves as disabled, and this feeling was compounded if they received ongoing medical treatment or personal care (Grewal *et al.*, 2002).

In addition, many disabled children and young people experience particular difficulties with accessing appropriate health support during the transition from childhood to the greater independence associated with adolescence and early adulthood. They already face difficulties with achieving independence because of the intrinsic discrimination within the labour market and the emphasis on educational attainment. Research has concluded that the extent to which young people feel that they are supported in trying to achieve their aims and fulfil their desires (economic, personal, social, sexual and relational aspirations) has a direct impact on their expectations and whether they enter adulthood from solid or shaky ground (Grewal *et al.*, 2004; Heslop *et al.*, 2001; Molloy *et al.*, 2003). Evidence suggests that steps to improve disabled children's and young people's experiences of health and social care services involves achieving consistency of contact between professionals and families, such as improved consultation skills (e.g. directly addressing the child); using appropriate language; and taking a positive view of the individual as a person rather than an impairment (Connors and Stalker, 2002).

A FOCUS ON FIELD RESEARCH

Through the course of this chapter we have spelled out some of the broad conceptual considerations that public health practitioners and policy makers need to take into account when developing an understanding of the significance of difference and diversity as determinants of health. We have also outlined some of the epidemiological and analytical data that relate to five major dimensions of diversity in the young population. Although we have been neither comprehensive nor exhaustive in our selection, we have attempted to provide some indication of areas of need for particular public health attention. Moreover, to support the framing of an argument with which we opened this chapter, we have provided a view of difference and diversity that takes into account the fact that these are 'real' social facts but that they are experienced as dynamic constructs influenced by social, cultural, ideological and economic processes. We asserted that, from this point of view, placing too much attention on categorical forms of difference runs the risk of smoothing over the social realities that children and young people experience in feeling similar to or different from others, more or less strongly, according to the particularities of specific social interactions, circumstances and contexts.

In order to illustrate this point in a very concrete way, we want to preface some concluding statements about difference and diversity and child public health with one example derived from some small-scale, qualitative research on health service access issues that we have undertaken with young people from ethnic minorities.

This involved a questionnaire survey of all the young people registered with three general practices in a locality in South West London, followed by face-to-face interviews with a subsample. The second element of the study set out to enable us to explore the specific questions of 'if and how' ethnicity related to attitudes to and use of services (Forrest *et al.*, 2005; Nash and Smith, 2003).

In the interviews, we found that young people in general had concerns about several areas of health service provision, including the confidentiality of access and consultations, the qualitative aspects of interaction with health professionals and the practical accessibility of services (appointments, opening time, location and so on). Ethnicity as a dimension of diversity did seem to be associated with views and experiences of these issues in some obvious ways, especially around language barriers and the (very few) experiences of racism. However, it was evident as we worked on the data that the nature of the interaction between ethnicity and health concern and service access issues was not always consistent outside these specific areas. It became clear, when we began to look at situations where ethnicity was most powerfully experienced as a dimension of difference relating to health, that there were several other factors in play, including the topic of health concern and gender and age issues.

It was clear that in cases where young women from ethnic minorities accessed health services for sexual health advice and care and entered into consultations with health professionals from the same ethnic and cultural backgrounds as themselves, ethnicity was strongly experienced as an aspect of identity and a potential determinant of health. In these situations, young women felt most conscious of attitudes towards femininity and female sexuality embodied in their cultural traditions and experienced the tension between wanting to take control of and care for their sexual health at the same time as not overtly challenging these norms. We concluded that the study demonstrated that, although there are situations and circumstances under which dimensions of difference and diversity have a very obvious and concrete implication for public health activity, such as barriers to communication when a child and health professional do not share a common language, there are other circumstances in which difference is experienced in a much less categorical way. In other words, an effective use of services is highly dependent on the context of the engagement between the child or young person and health service professionals.

CONCLUSION

The implication of this research and the findings in this chapter for public health practice is that it is necessary to interleave categorical views of difference and diversity with a more subtle view of these concepts as a dynamic aspect of identity when targeting children and young people with public health activities. This is important not only in relation to developing and providing frontline health services. It is also an important insight for public health activity through other vectors such as schools and the mass media. Children and young people's recognition of the relevance to them specifically of information or interventions will depend on a range of contextual factors that bring to the fore different aspects of their sense of belonging to one, another or several social groups.

KEY POINTS

- Public health practice needs to take difference and diversity among children and young people into account in order to understand and respond to inequities in access to health services and positive health outcomes.
- The public policy context in the UK provides a broad platform for this in terms of drawing increasing attention to human rights and respect for different needs and reducing social exclusion.
- Health-specific policy places specific demands on service planners and providers to respond positively to difference and diversity.
- Although this chapter has explored five major dimensions of difference and diversity among children and young people – ethnicity, refugee status, gender, sexuality and disability – it is important to recognize that diversity is not experienced only in these categorical terms but as dynamic aspects of personal and group identity in the context of specific social interactions and settings.

REFERENCES

Acheson D (1998) *Great Britain Independent Inquiry into Inequalities in Health*. London: The Stationery Office.

Atkinson K, Schattner P, Margolis S (2003) Rural secondary school students living in a small community: their attitudes, beliefs and perception towards general practice, *Australian Journal of Rural Health* 11:73–80.

Blair M, Stewart-Brown S, Waterson T, Crowther R (2003) *Child Public Health*. Oxford: Oxford University Press.

Burnett A, Peel M (2001) Asylum seekers and refugees in Britain: health needs of asylum seekers and refugees. *British Medical Journal* 322:544–7.

Churchill R, Allen J, Denman S *et al.* (2000) Do attitudes and beliefs of young teenagers towards general practice influence actual consultation behaviour? *British Journal of General Practice* 50:953–7.

Connell P, McKevitt C, Low N (2004) Investigating ethnic differences in sexual health: focus groups with young people. *Sexually Transmitted Infections* 80:300–5.

Connors C, Stalker K (2002) *Children's Experience of Disability a Positive Approach: Interchange 75*. Edinburgh: Scottish Executive Education Department.

Cooper H, Smaje C, Arber S (1998) Use of health services by children and young people according to ethnicity and social class: secondary analysis of national data. *British Medical Journal* 317:1047–51.

Cooper H, Smaje C, Arber S (1999) Equity in health service use by children: examining the ethnic paradox. *Journal of Social Policy* 23:457–78.

Council of Europe (1950) *Convention for the Protection of Human Rights and Fundamental Freedoms.* http://conventions.coe.int/Treaty/en/Treaties/Html/005.htm (accessed 9 January 2007).

Council of Europe (1961) *European Social Charter.* http://conventions.coe.int/Treaty/en/Treaties/Html/035.htm (accessed 9 January 2007).

Department for Education and Employment (2000) *Sex and Relationship Education Guidance: 0116/2000.* London: Department for Education and Employment.

Department of Health and Department for Education and Skills (2004) *National Service Framework for Children, Young People and Maternity Services.* London: Department of Health. www.dh.gov.uk/PolicyAndGuidance/HealthAndSocialCareTopics/ChildrenServices/ChildrenServicesInformation/ChildrenServicesInformationArticle/fs/en?CONTENT_ID=4089111&chk=U8Ecln (accessed 5 February 2007).

Ellis V, High S (2004) Something to tell you: gay, lesbian or bisexual young people's experiences of secondary schooling, *British Educational Research Journal* 30(2):213–25.

Engels F (1987) *The Conditions of the Working Class in England.* Harmondsworth: Penguin.

Fazel M, Stein A (2002) The mental health of refugee children. *Archives of Disease in Children* 87:366–70.

Forrest S, Ellis V (2006) The making of sexualities: sexuality, identity and equality. In: Cole M (ed.) *Education, Equality and Human Rights: issue of gender, 'race' sexuality, disability and social class* (2e). London: Routledge, pp.89–110.

Forrest S, Biddle G, Clift S (1997) *Talking about Homosexuality in the Secondary School.* Horsham: AVERT. www.avert.org/media/pdfs/homosexualityinschool.pdf (accessed 9 January 2007).

Forrest S, Nash T, Greenwood N (2005) *Young Person's Health Service Development Project: Black and Ethnic Minority Groups.* London: Faculty of Health and Social Care Sciences, University of Kingston and St George's Hospital Medical School.

Gregory J, Lowe S, Bates CJ *et al* (2000) *National Diet and Nutrition Survey: young people aged 4 to 18 years.* London: HMSO.

Grewal I, Joy S, Lewis J, Swales K, Woodfield K (2002) *'Disabled for Life?' Attitudes towards, and experiences of disability in Britain: DWP research report 173.* London: Department of Work and Pensions.

Grewal I, McManus S, Arthur S, Reith L (2004) *Making the Transition: addressing barriers in services for disabled people: research report 204.* London: Department of Work and Pensions.

Health and Social Care Information Centre (2005) *Health Survey for England 2004: the health of minority ethnic groups – headline tables.* London: NHS Health and Social Care Information Centre, Public Health Statistics.

Hendrick H (1997) *Children, Childhood and English Society 1880–1990.* Cambridge: Cambridge University Press.

Heslop P, Mallett R, Simons K, Ward L (2001) *Bridging the Divide: the experiences of young people with learning difficulties and their families at transition.* Bristol: Norah Fry Research Centre, University of Bristol.

Information Centre for Health and Social Care (2006) *Health Survey for England 2004. Updating of trend tables to include 2004 data.* www.ic.nhs.uk/pubs/hlthsvyeng2004upd (accessed 9 January 2007).

Jacobson LD, Wilkinson C, Owen PA (1994) Is the potential of teenage consultations being missed?: a study of consultations in primary care. *Family Practice* 11:296–9.

Lloyd T, Forrest S, Davidson N (2001) *Boys and Young Men's Health: literature and practice review interim report.* London: Health Development Agency.

MacKinnon D, Shucksmith J, Spratt J (2002) *Young People and Health in Scotland: what matters to young people about their health and well-being: research in Brief 3.* Edinburgh: Health Board for Scotland.

Malik R, Oandasan I, Yang M (2002) Health promotion, the family physician and youth. Improving the connection. *Family Practice* 19:523–8.

Molloy D, Knight T, Woodfield K (2003) *Diversity in Disability: exploring the interactions between disability, ethnicity, age, gender and sexuality.* London: Department of Work and Pensions.

Nash T, Smith E (2003) *Young People's Health Practice Development Project: Merton, Southwest London: project report.* London: Faculty of Health and Social Care Sciences, University of Kingston and St George's Hospital Medical School.

Neale J, Worrell M, Randhawa G (2005) Reaching out: support for ethnic minorities. *Mental Health Practice* 9:12–16.

Nicole P, de Groot K (eds) (2003) Report: *HIV/AIDS Care for People with a Precarious Residence Status in Europe.* European expert meeting: Amsterdam, 19–21 June 2003. Woerden: European Project AIDS and Mobility, NIGZ. www.strategy.gov.uk/downloads/work_areas/disability/disability_report/pdf/disability.pdf (accessed 22 January 2007).

Office for National Statistics (2001) *Population Size 7.9 per cent from a minority ethnic group.* Census, April 2001. www.statistics.gov.uk/cci/nugget.asp?id=273 (accessed 9 January 2007).

Office for National Statistics (2002) *Social Focus in Brief: children.* www.statistics.gov.uk/downloads/theme_social/social_focus_in_brief/children/Social_Focus_in_Brief_Children_2002.pdf (accessed 9 January 2007). www.strategy.gov.uk/downloads/work_areas/disability/disability_report/pdf/disability.pdf (accessed 9 January 2007).

Office for National Statistics (2004a) *The Health of Children and Young People.* www.statistics.gov.uk/children/ (accessed 9 January 2007).

Office for National Statistics (2004b) *The Health of Children and Young People: Drug use: girls aged 11–15 more likely to smoke.* www.statistics.gov.uk/cci/nugget.asp?id=719 (accessed 22 January 2007).

Office for National Statistics (2004c) *Survey of Smoking, Drinking and Drug Use Among Young People in England,* available at www.statistics.gov.uk/cci/nugget.asp?id=1328 (accessed 9 January 2007).

Office of the Deputy Prime Minister/Department for Work and Pensions/Department of Health/Department for Education and Skills (2005) *Improving the Life Chances of Disabled People: final report.* London: The Stationery Office.

Refugee Council and the British Council for Adoption and Fostering (2001) *Where are the Children? A mapping exercise on numbers of unaccompanied asylum-seeking children in the UK: September 2000–March 2001.* London: Refugee Council and the British Agencies for Adoption and Fostering.

Saxena S, Eliahoo J, Majeed A (2002) Socioeconomic and ethnic group differences in self reported health status and use of health services by children and young people in England: cross sectional study. *British Medical Journal* 325:520–6.

Senior P, Bhopal R (1994) Ethnicity as a variable in epidemiological research. *British Medical Journal* 309:327–30.

Smith GD, Chaturvedi N, Harding S, Nazroo J, Williams R (2000) Ethnic inequalities in health: a review of the UK epidemiological evidence. *Critical Public Health* 10(4):375–408.

Smyth M, Robus R (1989) *The Financial Circumstances of Families with Disabled children living in private households. Report 5. OPCS Social Survey Division.* London: HMSO.

Social Exclusion Unit (1999) *Teenage Pregnancy.* London: HMSO.

Social Exclusion Unit (2004) *Mental Health and Social Exclusion.* London: HMSO: London

Social Exclusion Unit (2006) *What is Social Exclusion?* www.socialexclusion. gov.uk/page.asp?id=213 (accessed 9 January 2007).

Stanley L (1995) *Sex Surveyed 1949–1994: From mass-observation's 'Little Kinsey' to the National Survey and the Hite Reports.* London: Taylor and Francis.

Teenage Pregnancy Unit (2000) *Guidance For Developing Contraception and Sexual Health Advice Services To Reach Black And Minority Ethnic (BME) Young People.* London: Teenage Pregnancy Unit.

Teenage Pregnancy Unit (2002) *Prevention Work with Black and Minority Ethnic Communities, Resources – Prevention and Black and Minority Ethnic Groups.* http://www.dfes.gov.uk/teenagepregnancy/dsp_content.cfm? pageid=148 (accessed 22 January 2007)

Trask JW (1916) The significance of the mortality rates of the coloured population of the United States. *American Journal of Public Health* 6:254–60.

United Nations (1989) *Convention on the Rights of the Child.* www.ohchr.org/english/law/pdf/crc.pdf (accessed 9 January 2007).

Walker A, O'Brien M, Traynor J *et al.* (2002) *Living in Britain: results of the 2001 General Household Survey.* London: National Statistics.

Wardle J, Brodersen NH, Cole T, Jarvis M, Boniface D (2006) Development of adiposity in adolescence: five year longitudinal study of an ethnically and socioeconomically diverse sample of young people in Britain, *British Medical Journal* 332:1130–5.

Acts of Parliament

All these Acts are published by HMSO in London, and all can be accessed from the UK Parliament website (www.publications.parliament.uk).

Human Rights Act 1998
Children Act 2004
Disability Discrimination Act 2005
Equality Act 2006
Work and Families Act 2006

Section 2
THE CHILD IN THE FAMILY

4 APPROACHES TO PARENTING

Maggie Fisher and Diane DeBell

INTRODUCTION

The most important and probably the most influential setting for childhood during the school-age years is the home environment, whether that setting is with the child's natural or adoptive parent(s), reconstituted families, carers, extended family members, foster parents, or within the supervision of the state (children in care). But what do we mean when we refer to the parenting role and why is there such a burgeoning contemporary interest in parenting within government policy, the media and the general public?

Bornstein (2002) defined parenting in the following way:

> *Parents create people. It is the entrusted and abiding task of parents to prepare their offspring for the physical, psychosocial and economic conditions in which they will eventually fare, and it is hoped flourish . . . parents are the 'final common pathway' to children's development and stature, adjustment and success.*
>
> ***(Bornstein, 2002, p.ix)***

> *Parenting is something that parents do, not something they have.*
>
> ***(Quinton, 2004, p.27)***

Parenting involves tasks such as physical care, boundary setting and the teaching of social behaviour. Optimal child and adolescent behaviours such as responsiveness, affection and positive regard are, of course, the ideal outcome of parenting. In theory, those relationship qualities that indicate emotional security and secure attachment are the aspiration *for* parenting.

However, parental ability to achieve this ambitious agenda is influenced by many factors, including genetics; childhood experiences of the parenting role; socio-economic circumstances such as relative poverty; housing; culture; the community/neighbourhood environment; and the health or ill-health of the child or the parent(s). And these factors rarely remain stable throughout the school-age years. The child, furthermore, is a purposive actor in this relationship and we find that individual children respond in different ways to the parenting they experience. Some children are more resilient than others and the parenting role can, intentionally or not, support that resilience or it can introduce risks that the child or adolescent is unable to negotiate. We still know little about the factors that produce resilience in individual children (Ghate and Hazel, 2002; Bartley, 2006).

The Green Paper *Every Child Matters* (Chief Secretary to the Treasury, 2003) specified the importance of the parental relationship in a child's growth and development in the UK:

> *The bond between the child and their parents is the most critical influence on a child's life. Parenting has a strong impact on a child's educational development, behaviour and health.*
>
> **(Chief Secretary to the Treasury, 2003, p.39)**

Government policy in all four countries of the UK during the 21st century has been moving rapidly to a position of concern about the parenting role; about what the state's responsibility for assisting parents to carry out this role should be; and the design of legislation that can support parenting (e.g. the Carers and Disabled Children Act 2000 and the Children Act 2004). It is a policy position we find repeated by the Department of Health, Department for Education and Skills (DfES), the Treasury, the Social Exclusion Unit, the Home Office Family Policy Unit, the Children and Young Persons Unit, the Children and Families Directorate within the DfES and other governmental agencies and departments, including the integrating role now assigned to the four Ministers for Children – one in each of the four countries of the UK.

In January 2007, the Treasury and the DfES published an evidence-based discussion paper, *Policy Review of Children and Young People* (HM Treasury and DfES, 2007) in preparation for the 2007 Comprehensive Spending Review. The intention was to plan family support investment for the years 2008–09, 2009–10 and 2010–11.

This work marks an important recognition of the need for sound evidence about *how best* to assist parents in their work with children and young people. Also see Quinton's valuable overview of research in 2004. Writing in 1999, DeBell found little evidence of agreement about either the value base or the relative effectiveness of work by professional and voluntary or community agencies in delivering parenting support initiatives:

> What is also needed, in addition to shared definitions of what parental support means, is greater clarity about the specific objectives of individual programmes or interventions. The currently poor research knowledge about the relative effectiveness of different approaches is directly linked to poor articulation of the desired outcomes of both individual and joint services.
>
> The evidence also suggests that there is no agreed philosophy or shared vision of parenting. In other words, for partnership working to succeed, a shared understanding of the value base of parenting programmes is needed.
>
> **(DeBell, 1999: 4)**

Much work has been conducted since 1999 in an effort to probe these questions, but, writing specifically about the critical issue of child abuse and neglect in *The Lancet* in 2005, Barlow and Stewart-Brown repeated this discouraging picture:

> Whilst there is some evidence emerging about the potential effectiveness of preventive initiatives, there is considerably less consensus about what works when abuse has already occurred.
>
> **(Barlow and Stewart-Brown, 2005, p.1750)**

This chapter explores the child and young person in the context of 'the family'; the many influences that impact on the family; how 'parenting' affects the child's health and well-being; and the role of the public health practitioner in the broad field known as parenting support.

THEORIES OF PARENTING AND OF CHILDHOOD

Parenting is a complex matter that generates extensive debate. It is an activity in which parents engage almost unconsciously. Historically and, indeed in contemporary Britain, parenting skills and knowledge are passed on through families from generation to generation.

It was with the emergence of psychology and psychoanalysis in the latter part of the 19th century that parenting practices began to be studied as a factor that affects a child's health and development. The very concept of childhood itself did not emerge as a focus for philosophical debate in western nation-states until the 18th century with writers such as Adam Smith, Rousseau, Blake, Boswell and Hume. These earlier philosophical enquiries were largely concerned with the relationship between child development and educational philosophy but, together, they early theorized childhood as a separate sphere from the adult world and one that is shaped by adult actions.

Blake's *Songs of Innocence and Experience* (1788 and 1794) broke important ground when he posed the sentimental view of childhood unworldliness against the reality of what he saw of childhood in the streets of London.

> I wander thro' each charter'd street,
> Near where the charter'd Thames does flow
> And mark in every face I meet
> Marks of weakness, marks of woe.

In every cry of every Man,
In every Infant's cry of fear,
In every voice; in every ban,
The mind-forg'd manacles I hear . . .

(Blake, 1794, Songs of Innocence and Experience)

To put it very simply, the child in Blake is conceived and made manifest as a consequence of how the adult organizes the world.

It was not until the 1970s that a new sociology of childhood emerged, which broke free of the concept of the child as a consequence, primarily, of adult imagination and control – in other words, the child as actor in his or her own life placed the child's voice and the child's active volition at the centre of attention (MacKay, 1973; Speier, 1976; Qvotrup *et al.*, 1994; James and Prout, 1997; Christiansen and James, 2000; Alderson, 2001; Mayall, 2002). This is to oversimplify complex arguments but it is an important concept when we talk about parenting. The child's physical, emotional and psychological vulnerability is set within a context of both the parental function and the child's own strategies for negotiation of, and response to, parental actions. In other words, parenting is a dynamic between the child and the adult.

Following three centuries of theorization in western cultures about the child in relation to the parental figure, we have recently become accustomed in Britain to thinking about the child–parent relationship from a mainly behaviourist approach in classical learning theory. In other words, the thinking here is that parents who behave toward their children in unhelpful ways, either through ignorance or intention, are generally believed to produce behaviours in their children that are counterproductive to the child's health and wellbeing. It is fair to say that this is the starting point for contemporary government policy in Britain and for public health interventions that seek to 'support parents'. In fact, from the softer world of how to manage emotional and behavioural problems in young children and adolescents to the harsher world of antisocial behaviour orders (ASBOs) as well as the realities of child abuse and neglect, the behaviourist approach is dominant in contemporary thinking about how to support parenting.

In this approach to parental support, reward is encouraged, such that it should bring about desired behaviour and ignore undesirable behaviour. It is based on the principle that what you pay attention to is what you get more of. Supporters of this approach believe that teaching parents behaviour management techniques is the most effective way of changing unhelpful parenting practices. (Utting *et al.*, 1993: Webster-Stratton, 1999). Such thinking goes back to Skinner in the 1950s and 1960s, and it is a powerful voice in contemporary government policy. It is also a fairly rapid approach that can be 'taught' quickly and can be 'taught' to parents as a group. It is thereby a cost-effective approach for statutory services in providing parenting support interventions.

The psychotherapeutic approach, on the other hand, attributes unhelpful parental behaviours to parental distress. Here the argument is that effective parenting is, in contemporary popular language, 'emotionally literate'. Attending to the emotional relationship between the parent and the child is argued to be the key to supporting parents. Holistic qualities such as empathy, respect and genuineness are here emphasized and parents are encouraged to understand the *feelings* that cause their children's behaviour. In this way, parents are encouraged to respond in helpful ways to children (Gordon, 1975; Bavolek, 1990; Gottman and Declaire, 1997). The argument is that adult self-reflection and analysis can enable parents to help their children manage their own feelings in emotionally positive ways and can thus improve children's and young people's relationships with others. Praising desirable behaviour and ignoring unhelpful behaviour, as in the behaviourist approach, is also advocated as a strategy and is designed to help foster positive parent–child relationships that can lead to emotional well-being.

A further school of thought suggests that difficulties begin with the baby and the 'goodness of fit' (Thomas and Chess, 1977) between parent and infant. Temperamental or genetically determined neuropsychological differences can here make parenting more or less challenging and can be the cause of unhelpful parenting practices.

> *Parents' perceptions of their child are known to be important factors in influencing parenting behaviours.*
>
> **(Ghate and Hazel, 2002, p.15)**

All the proponents of the different approaches agree that changing parental behaviour can have a critical impact on children's behaviour, and that low self-esteem, feelings of guilt and inadequacy in parents and in children can be substantial barriers to positive behavioural change in the child. The varying schools of thought, however, begin from different theories of childhood, and thereby describe different approaches to the most expedient way of changing parental behaviour and thus child or adolescent behaviour where that would benefit the child. There are various studies that provide evidence to support each model.

What is common to these different approaches is that parenting can be defined as the feelings, attitudes, behaviours and beliefs that parents have with regard to their children, including rejection of the child. Researchers examining parenting and parenting programmes have identified a number of adult attributes that arguably are necessary for successful parenting and healthy parent–child relationships. But there is also much that is in common between parent–child relationships and social well-being within communities and societies (Wilkinson, 1996) and within schools (Weare, 2000). In other words, articulations of the determinants of healthy adult relationships are identical between those needed for healthy parenting and those needed for effective teaching and for healthy communities. The argument is that the critical skill needed for creating emotional well-being in the home, at school and in the community is reciprocity in human relationships.

APPROACHES TO PARENTING STYLES

Diverse research programmes have theorized parenting styles (e.g. the statistical classification generated by Stevenson *et al.*, 2004). In 1973, Diana Baumrind identified three parenting styles that are frequently used as a point of reference by public health practitioners. She argues that parenting styles derive from parental behaviours along the four dimensions below:

- warmth and responsiveness or nurturance – often reflected in the emotional tone of a family
- parental expectations of a child ('is this a realistic expectation for a child of this age?')
- clarity and consistency of rules
- style and level of communication between parent and child.

Using the above four dimensions, Baumrind described three specific combinations of these features and referred to them as 'parenting styles':

- the permissive style, which is high in nurturance, but low in parental expectation, control and communication
- the authoritarian style characterized as high in control and parental expectation, but low in nurturance and communication
- the authoritative style, which is high in all four dimensions.

In 1983, Maccoby and Martin took Baumrind's (1973) model a step further and identified a fourth category: the neglecting style. This insight has been widely accepted and underpinned by research findings (Dornbusch *et al.*, 1987; Glasgow *et al.*, 1997; Lamborn *et al.*, 1991; Steinberg *et al.*, 1989, 1991, 1992, 1994, 1995). Maccoby and Martin (1983) adjusted Baumrind's dimensions in order to propose a two-dimensional model along a continuum from level of control/demand to acceptance/rejection or responsiveness as depicted in Fig. 4.1. Where these two dimensions intersect they create four distinctive parenting styles, which are similar to Baumrind's (1973) original three styles described above.

It is frequently argued that parenting *styles* can be highly predictive of particular outcomes for children but these assertions, significantly, focus attention on family systems rather than on individual parental behaviours. And, of course, parents do not fall neatly into these categories. Parenting styles vary and change in response to the child's age, behaviours, temperament and health profiles (e.g. child or parental ill-health or disability). Indeed, individual children within the same family act, respond and see their worlds differently from each other. Nevertheless, the following styles provide us with a way of organizing and thus describing diverse parental behaviours in relation to the child.

- *Authoritarian parenting* can be characterized by an insistence on unquestioning obedience, order and respect for authority. Authoritarian parents make high demands on their children and can be emotionally unresponsive. This style of parenting is associated with children who perform less well in school, have less social competence with peers and have lower self-esteem (Maccoby and Martin, 1983; Baumrind, 1991). Children of authoritarian parents may appear subdued or, conversely, may display high aggression or appear to be out of control.

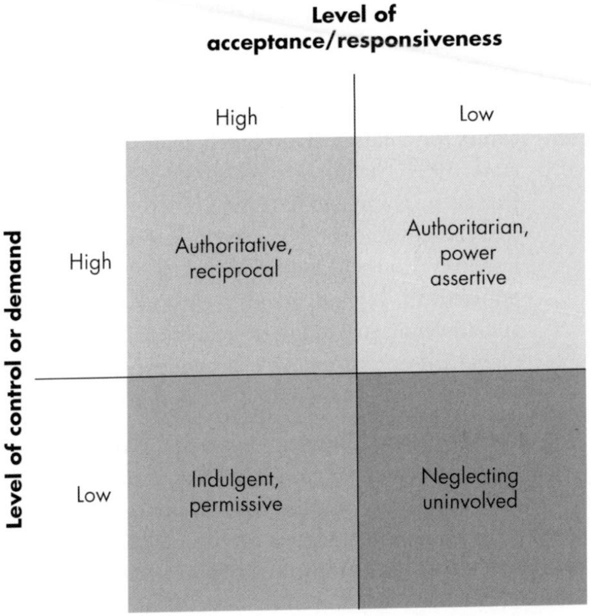

**Level of
acceptance/responsiveness**

Figure 4.1 Parenting styles. (Reproduced with permission from Bee (2000) *The Developing Child* (9e). Boston: Allyn and Bacon, p.385; adapted with permission from Maccoby E, Martin J (1983) Socialization in the context of the family: parent–child interaction. In: Hetherington EM (ed) *Handbook of Child Psychology: socialization, personality and social development Volume 4*. New York: Wiley, p.39.)

- *Permissive parenting* may also be associated with some poor outcomes for children such as underperformance at school during adolescence or tendencies toward aggression if the parents are very lax about aggressive behaviour. Children of permissive parents are more likely to be immature, to evade responsibility and to be dependent on others for help (Maccoby and Martin, 1983).
- *Parents who neglect their children* can trigger disruptive child behaviours and there is a high association between neglect and delinquent behaviours (Patterson, 1992). These children often display disturbance in their relationships with peers and adults. Children of uninvolved, emotionally abusive or neglecting parents can be impulsive and/or antisocial and tend to be less motivated at school (Block, 1971; Pulkkinen, 1982; Lamborn *et al.*, 1991). Parents who neglect their children are often themselves overwhelmed by their own complex problems; may be suffering from mental health problems; may be repeating family patterns of parenting; and can be psychologically or emotionally unavailable to the child. In other words, the parent who neglects a child is likely to have little emotional connection to the child. These children are often described as 'insecurely attached' (Ainsworth *et al.*, 1978). Steele (2002) argued the importance of fathers in the attachment role, while Utting

and Pugh (2003) extended this to include friends and communities. Sanders (2004) also investigated the ways in which sibling relationships can compensate for or can become congruent with parental relationships.

• *Authoritative parenting* is consistently associated with the most positive outcomes for children (Dornbusch *et al.*, 1987; Glasgow *et al.*, 1997; Lamborn *et al.*, 1991; Steinberg *et al.*, 1989, 1991, 1992, 1994, 1995). Authoritative parents are warm and nurturing. They set clear limits and boundaries and positively reinforce desirable behaviour. These parents are characterized as highly responsive to their child's individual needs and are less likely to use physical punishment. High demands are placed on the child to achieve realistic social and academic goals. Children experiencing this type of parenting tend to show higher self-esteem, greater independence and self-confidence and more altruistic behaviour. Academically they perform better (Steinberg *et al.*, 1992).

One disadvantage in using this model is that it cannot capture important patterns of family interaction in diverse cultural or ethnic groups. For example, in some Asian cultures, expectations about strict obedience are often understood by the child to be aspects of parental caring and concern, and may not be perceived to be demonstrating lack of warmth.

NEGATIVE CONSEQUENCES OF PARENTING STYLES

Nevertheless, parenting style is repeatedly associated with outcomes that can affect child health and well-being. Desforges and Aboiuchaar (2003) identified parenting as one of the most important determinants of educational achievement:

> The most important finding . . . is that parental involvement in the form of 'at-home good parenting' has a significant positive effect on children's achievement and adjustment, even after all factors shaping attainment have been taken out of the equation.
>
> **(Desforges and Aboiuchaar, 2003, p.4)**

Parental involvement in a child's schooling between the ages of 7 and 16 years is a more powerful predictor of attainment than family background, family size and level of parental education (Feinstein and Symons, 1999). In particular, a father's interest in a child's schooling is strongly linked to good educational outcomes for the child (Hobcraft, 1998; Flouri and Buchanan, 2001; Goldman, 2005).

Neglectful, permissive and authoritarian parenting are linked with antisocial behaviour (Sanders *et al.*, 1996); low self-esteem (McClun and Merrell, 1998); and drug and alcohol abuse (Cohen *et al.*, 1994). Conversely, authoritative parenting is predictive of good peer relationships and educational achievement (Baumrind, 1978; Steinberg *et al.*, 1992).

Research by Patterson *et al.* (1989) indicates that a combination of coercive parenting, poor supervision and lack of parental warmth or affection could account for 30–40 per cent of antisocial behaviour and criminality, delinquency and violence in adolescence. Child abuse (Egeland, 1997) and family conflict/domestic violence, even if children are not directly involved, have been found to be contributory causes of mental health and social problems in later life (Amato *et al.*, 1995).

Furthermore, studies by Wilkinson (1996) and Brummer (1997) indicate that emotional distress can cause physical illness by affecting the immune response. Smoking, drinking in excess and the consumption of high-fat foods were also found to be valued by young people and adults for their ability to relieve emotional distress (Cameron and Jones, 1985). Stress caused by school examinations has indicated susceptibility to viral infections (Cohen *et al.*, 1994), while Marmot and colleagues (Marmot, 2005; Marmot *et al.*, 1991) early argued that lack of control over life events (also see Rosengren *et al.*, 1933) can create long-term vulnerability to cardiovascular disease. The collective picture indicates a link between emotional distress and physical illness and disease, both in children and long into adulthood.

Research has also repeatedly found greater vulnerability to physical and mental ill-health in boys than in girls. Boys are at greater risk of developing seizure disorders; autism and related problems; dyslexia; hyperactivity; and are more susceptible to maternal mental health problems (Murray and Cooper, 1997). Boys have been found to be more likely to develop conduct disorders, to be involved in criminality and to be more likely to attempt suicide (Lewis and Slogget, 1998).

Hodgson *et al.* (1996) suggest that social and psychological factors are linked in the aetiology of mental health and illness. How individuals respond to stressful events is dependent on their individual strengths or vulnerabilities, which in turn will determine their coping styles and resilience. This is influenced by individual personality profiles that have a genetic component, but is also powerfully shaped by the social and emotional environment in which children grow and develop.

The child is not, however, a passive actor in these profiles. We have called attention to the dynamic that develops between child and adult carer, and we have also referred to the resilience versus risk factors that operate to help or hinder the child in his/her negotiation of the familial, social and psychosocial environment. See Chapter 8 for discussion of these factors in the context of child and adolescent mental health. Figure 4.2 is a visualization of that dynamic in terms of the child's environment and its potential for impact on the child.

THE INTERACTING ECOLOGICAL FRAMEWORK – THE CHILD WITHIN THE FAMILY SYSTEM

Bronfenbrenner's model (1979) of the ecology of human development takes these arguments further by producing a useful framework for considering the child in its real-world setting, because it helps us to understand how interrelated and complex systems outside the family connect in ways that affect the child and the family. Bronfenbrenner argued that the ecology of human

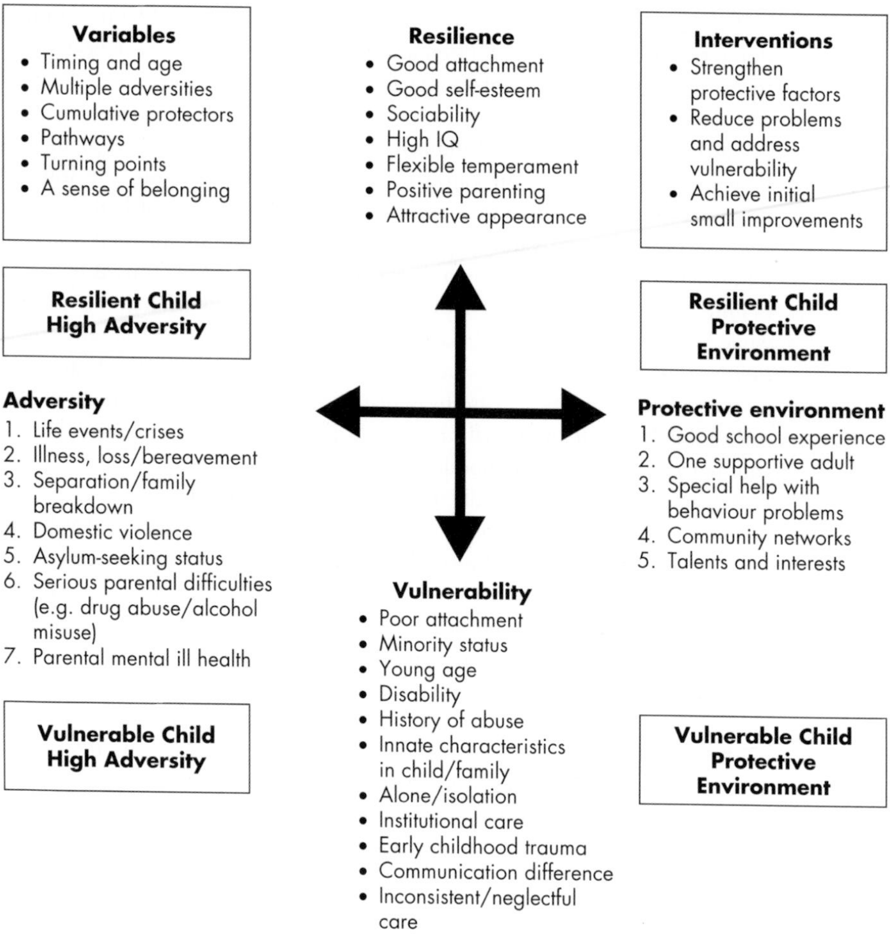

Variables
- Timing and age
- Multiple adversities
- Cumulative protectors
- Pathways
- Turning points
- A sense of belonging

Resilience
- Good attachment
- Good self-esteem
- Sociability
- High IQ
- Flexible temperament
- Positive parenting
- Attractive appearance

Interventions
- Strengthen protective factors
- Reduce problems and address vulnerability
- Achieve initial small improvements

Resilient Child High Adversity

Resilient Child Protective Environment

Adversity
1. Life events/crises
2. Illness, loss/bereavement
3. Separation/family breakdown
4. Domestic violence
5. Asylum-seeking status
6. Serious parental difficulties (e.g. drug abuse/alcohol misuse)
7. Parental mental ill health

Protective environment
1. Good school experience
2. One supportive adult
3. Special help with behaviour problems
4. Community networks
5. Talents and interests

Vulnerability
- Poor attachment
- Minority status
- Young age
- Disability
- History of abuse
- Innate characteristics in child/family
- Alone/isolation
- Institutional care
- Early childhood trauma
- Communication difference
- Inconsistent/neglectful care

Vulnerable Child High Adversity

Vulnerable Child Protective Environment

Figure 4.2 Risk and resilience. From Becker F, Gordon R (2000) adapted from Daniel B et al., (1999). (With permisson from the authors, The University of Sheffield and the NSPCC.)

development consists of four distinct but interrelated systems or types of settings (see Fig. 4.3). The child is at the centre of the model and the child affects and is affected by the settings in which that child spends time. The family is, arguably, the most important setting for the child because this is, quite simply, where the child spends the most time and has strong emotional ties.

- The *microsystem* consists of the child in the family but also includes the immediate settings with which the child has direct personal experience such as the family, the school, after-school activities and the neighbourhood/ community setting. The family, however it is articulated, is the major microsystem for child development in Britain and in many parts of the world.

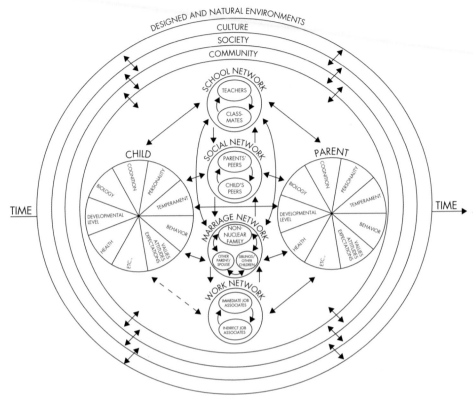

Figure 4.3 Ecology of human development. (Reproduced with permission from Lerner *et al.* (1995) Developmental contextual perspective on parenting. In: Bornstein M (ed.) *Handbook of Parenting* Vol. 2. New Jersey: Lawrence Erlbaum Associates, p.297.)

- The *mesosystem* was described by Bronfenbrenner as:

  > . . . the interrelations among major settings containing the developing person at a particular point in his or her life.
  >
  > **(Bronfenbrenner, 1977, p. 515)**

For example, an interaction between a parent and a child can be influenced by what has happened to the parent at work that day. Or a change in family organization or circumstances, including bereavement or parental divorce can disrupt the child's understanding of his or her world.

- The *exosystem* is an extension of the mesosystem and refers to all the outside influences that the child does not experience directly but which affect one of the microsystems of which the child is part, particularly the family. We can think here of housing, financial resources, adult employment, education and family history.
- The *macrosystem* is the larger cultural setting in which all the other systems are embedded. It includes the neighbourhood in which the family lives; the

family's social circumstances; the family's ethnic identity, cultural values, beliefs, political philosophies; the family's economic circumstances; and the larger cultural/historical events such as war, civil strife, famine, floods or environmental catastrophe that may affect the other ecological systems.

Bronfenbrenner's model allows us to represent the reality that bidirectional socialization (the child and the family) is embedded in a more complex system of social networks, and societal, cultural and historic influences.

THE FAMILY IN THE UK

The family in the UK is understood to be the basic social formation responsible for the growth and development of children and young people. Such is generally the case across all developed countries. The family is a biological reality for most children, and children are generally cared for in a social context, in which their survival depends on a family formation. In fact, children in the care of the state are theoretically placed in a context that is designed to replicate the biological family. However, there are alternatives to the conventional family, which presume a collectivist approach to child rearing such as Kibbutzim, The Nayar of Malabar, collective communities in North America, and the continued existence of large-scale residential care in many of the post-soviet countries of Eastern Europe and in China.

The family takes many forms within the four countries of multicultural Britain, but it is a vital influence on a child's well-being and health. Nevertheless, socio-biologists suggest that the 'mother–child' relationship represents the basic family unit and that it is predetermined by nature. This gender bias is reflected in much government parenting policy. The weight of parental responsibilities, apart from financial responsibility, generally appears to fall upon women. For example, parenting orders have been described as 'mothering orders', simply because they are mainly made against mothers. Some professionals have expressed concern that parenting orders can be seen as discriminatory in practice because they criminalize mothers (Coleman *et al.*, 1999; Ghate and Ramella, 2002). In reality, of course, many of these mothers are the sole carers of these children and the fathers may be non-resident or absent.

Changing social expectations and values, attitudes to gender, marital and relationship breakdown have all had an impact on the family as a unit in Britain and on contemporary government policy. In the UK, roughly 40 per cent of first marriages end in divorce, and the number of lone parents has been on the increase for the last three decades at least. Parents may be divorced, single, same-sex or adoptive. Many children live in reconstituted families with step-parents and step-siblings. Many children live between different homes, with parents who do not live together, and do so without apparent distress. Nevertheless, family breakdown and marital discord have been associated with an increase in disorders such as child depression and anxiety (Wallace *et al.*, 1997; Harold *et al.*, 2001).

The traditional two-parent nuclear family is often argued in developed countries to be the ideal arrangement for raising children. This view is supported by evidence suggesting that there are better outcomes for children raised in these circumstances (Morgan, 1999; Rowthorn, 2001; Wells and Rankin, 1991). Government policy across the UK, however, also acknowledges the private domain of the family by recognizing the rights of individuals to be self-determining within a landscape of changing social mores. This is reflected, for example, in government policy that argues its support for lone parents and for families in relationships other than marriage.

As Bronfenbrenner's model (1979) demonstrates, however, the child is embedded in the family in a context in which there are many interacting pressures, including socio-economic and psychosocial factors that arise from the surrounding culture and the implicit values of the political system of the day – all exerting influences on the family system itself.

> *The whole premise of the 'ecological' framework – in terms of the way people experience everday life – is that children and parents inhabit ecological systems where these levels flow into, and interact with, one another to produce complex nested relationships and layered or overlapping effects.*
> **(Ghate and Hazel, 2002, p.100)**

GOVERNMENT POLICY AND PRACTICE: PARENTAL EMPOWERMENT OR SOCIAL CONTROL?

The Beveridge Report (1942) recommended that the government of the time should find ways of fighting the five 'giant evils' of want, disease, ignorance, squalor and idleness (Timmins, 1996). The outcome was the British welfare state and the establishment of the National Health Service (NHS) in 1948, providing free medical care for all at the point of access. The NHS was part of Beveridge's crusade to tackle disease. Squalor and idleness were tackled by a massive post-war building programme to improve housing, schools, the roads and the nation's infrastructure at a time when the country was near bankruptcy. National Service was also introduced with a view to reducing idleness and unemployment as well as ensuring a standing army. The 1944 Education Act introduced by Rab Butler sought to tackle ignorance and to reduce unemployment. The school-leaving age was raised to 15 in 1944, and universal free schooling was provided in grammar, secondary modern and technical schools. The school-leaving age was raised to 16 in 1972. In 1952 the last workhouse was closed.

Since the Second World War, government interest in parenting has sharply increased. It has been fuelled more recently by concerns about social exclusion, social cohesion, the criminal justice agenda and the potential links between the quality of parenting and the potential for better outcomes for children.

> *Parenting is probably the most important public health issue facing our society. It is the single largest variable implicated in childhood illness and accidents, teenage pregnancy and substance misuse, truancy, school disruption and under achievement, child abuse, unemployability, juvenile crime and mental illness. These are serious in themselves but are even*

> *more important as precursors of problems in adulthood and the next generation.*
>
> **(Hoghughi, 1998, p.1545)**

The concerns reflected here have provided impetus for government policy intervention in the parenting role in the UK and internationally. The New Labour government of 1997 placed an early priority on parenting support (*Supporting Families*; Home Office, 1998), and there has been a steep rise in the range and scale of parenting support interventions since the late 1990s. In 2005, the Treasury with the DfES published *Support for Parents: the best start for children*, and in 2007 a *Policy Review of Children and Young people: a discussion paper* (HM Treasury and DfES, 2005, 2007).

These publications are linked and they contextualize children's and young people's ability or not to thrive within four factors: family prosperity; parenting; the wider community; and services. It is fair to say, however, that greatest attention is focused on parenting rights and responsibilities, with concomitant government investment in parent education, usually time limited.

Some observers have suggested that parent education is a form of social control, and it is important to consider who benefits (Smith, 1997). There are contradictions and tensions in government policy and legislation. Policy makers are faced with the need to juggle contradictory pressures about adult employment (e.g. women's employment and methods to improve men's involvement in the care of their children); a liberal approach to ensuring parental autonomy; and, at the same time, rationales for government interventions in the private sphere of parenting and the family).

The Crime and Disorder Act 1998; the Anti-Social Behaviour Act 2003; the Criminal Justice Act 2003; the Respect Action Plan 2006 (Home Office, 2006); and the Social Exclusion Action Plan 2006 (Cabinet Office, 2006) indicate a move toward direct intervention in parenting work. The National Children's Bureau (2007) argues the need for government investment in evaluations to determine the impact of these measures on children and families.

Furthermore, concerns about child protection have increased since 1989 when the UK Government became a signatory to the UN Convention on the Rights of the Child (UN, 1989). The Laming Report (Department of Health and Home Office, 2003) marked a turning point in recognition that statutory services have a responsibility to protect children from harm by carers (see Chapter 7). Yet the current government has not provided children with the same protection from assault as adults, including assault by a parent.

By failing to give children equal protection under the law, the UK breaches obligations under the UNCRC, the European Social Charter, the International Covenant on Economic, Social and Cultural Rights and other human rights treaties. In 1995, the UN Committee on the Rights of the Child, the Human Rights Treaty Body for the UNCRC, made a formal recommendation to the UK Government to prohibit corporal punishment and raised the following concerns over the use of reasonable chastisement:

> *The committee is worried about the national legal provisions dealing with reasonable chastisement in the family. The imprecise nature of the*

expression of reasonable chastisement as contained in these legal provisions may pave the way for it to be interpreted in a subjective and arbitrary manner. This committee is concerned that the legislative and other measures relating to the physical integrity of children do not appear to be compatible with the provision and principles of the convention, including those of articles 3, 19, and 37.

(Henricson, 2003, p.48)

Other contradictions in government policy can be found in the targeting of parents to provide sex and relationship education in the home, whilst simultaneously bypassing the family when providing confidential sexual health services to children. However, control of children is an issue for which the UK Government has attributed primary responsibility to parents who are then to be supported by schools and the youth justice system.

Families are the core of our society. They should teach right from wrong. They should be the first defence against antisocial behavior.

(Labour Party, 1997, p.19)

The Crime and Disorder Act 1998 introduced parenting orders. Magistrates can direct a parent to attend some form of counselling if their child has committed an offence or has frequently truanted from school. However, the parent cannot be compelled to receive help until help has been offered and rejected by the parent. Many observers have expressed concern about holding parents responsible for their children in this way. Henricson (2003) summarized:

A critical element of parent education programmes is that they should engage parents in the process; this is unlikely to be achieved if parents are having to attend under compulsion and in the context of a humiliating court order.

(Henricson et al., 2000)

There is the possibility that the parenting order could be challenged from a legal and human rights perspective because it attributes blame for the conduct of one person to another, and in effect criminalises a parent without their having committed a crime.

The approach rests on an assumption that the primary responsible relationship in bringing up children rests with parents. This undermines the role of the wider community. It also undermines children's agency.

(Morrow, 1999)

The burden of responsibility in the execution of the legislation tends to fall on the mother with the majority of parenting orders being made against mothers rather than fathers. This has adverse implications for equal opportunities and equality under the law.

(Ghate and Ramella, 2002; Morrow, 1999)

This is another stick with which to beat disadvantaged parents where supportive carrots are to be preferred. It continues a regrettable trend of intervening in the family life of the least well-off in society.

(Henricson, 2003, p.46)

Despite these protestations over compulsion, the evaluations from parenting orders have found that parents who have been required to attend a programme have, nevertheless, reported a benefit from them (Ghate and Ramella, 2002). The Scottish Government has not adopted parenting orders because of its reservations about the efficacy of coercing parents.

Parliament has not tightened definitions of parental responsibility on child safety, such as the age at which a child may be left alone at home. In the absence of government guidelines, the National Society for the Prevention of Cruelty to Children (NSPCC) has produced a code recommending that babies and very young children should not be left unattended, while children under 13 years should not be left at home alone for long periods. The code suggests that children under 16 years should not be left alone overnight or in charge of younger children (Papworth, 2002). Parental rights and responsibilities are, effectively, ill-defined. It has been suggested that Parliament should conduct a policy review to reconcile 'disparate strands of policy', and should produce a parental code to define parental rights and responsibilities, thereby enhancing relations between government and parents (Henricson, 2003)

FAMILY RELATIONSHIPS AND CHANGE DURING CHILDHOOD: THE ROLE OF PARENTING SUPPORT

As children grow and develop from dependent infant to independent adult, the relationship between child and adult inevitably changes. This requires an adjustment in parenting skills for each stage of a child's life. During the cycle of child growth and development, parents themselves also develop and change as they cope with their own life-cycle stages and the changes that occur in their circumstances. This profile can have a significant impact on how parents actually parent their children and how they manage their children's lives and their children's changing relationships to the world in which they are growing up and learning to negotiate.

The concept of parenting support at a whole-population level is relatively new as a feature of government policy. It is also, as we have already noted, a difficult concept to define. What we can do is describe diverse approaches to intervention.

Quinton (2004) argued that parenting support tends to fall into three categories: formal; informal; and semi-formal. In this profile, it is the work of professionals that constitutes formal support (e.g. mainly delivered by health, social care and education practitioners but also by the youth justice system). Informal support is that help and assistance coming from family, friends and neighbours. Semi-formal support is generally provided by voluntary, charitable or faith-based organizations. There is, however, little systematic co-ordination between these sources of assistance for parents. And there is little systematic and co-ordinated training for parenting support, even for professional services. The exceptions tend to be health visiting, and child and adolescent mental health services (CAMHS). And, in some cases, school nurses are trained in parenting support skills. Telephone and internet links are a further form of growing assistance to parents.

There is also repeated evidence that parents who have access to one form of support tend also to use multiple forms of assistance – formal, informal and semi-formal. In other words, 'relationships lie at the heart of support' (Quinton, 2004, p.130), and those parents who are more socially effective are also more likely to receive help. This implies that the most severe parenting problems are often closely linked to isolation of the adult parent(s)/carer(s) from family and/or community networks. (See 'Thinking about risk in approaches to parenting' below.)

In 2004, Whittaker (in Bidmead and Whittaker, 2004) designed a model of both formal and informal approaches to parenting education and support (see Fig. 4.4). 'Informal' here subsumes Quinton's (2004) concepts of 'informal' and 'semi-formal' approaches, by collapsing these into one category. Whittaker's model reflects a birth-to-adolescence perspective and is useful as a starting point for visualizing the structure of parenting support in Britain. What it cannot do is fully reflect the internal system of support that accrues from family members, friends and neighbours, who are integral to any analysis of parenting support. What Fig. 4.4 also disguises is the accidental nature of support systems across the country. In other words, where a family lives will largely determine the scope, scale and accessibility of services, including family and community assistance.

Furthermore, gender bias toward support for mothers has been repeatedly identified in research evidence. On the whole, professionals and community groups tend to focus their work on mothers and do so at the expense of fathers. Williams (1999) identified the process of exclusion of fathers that tended to occur in home visiting. This 'father-blind' approach by public services has been identified by Ferri and Smith (1996); Barclay and Lupton (1997); Burghes *et al.* (1997); Grimshaw and McGuire (1998); Warin *et al.* (1999); Williams and Robertson (1999); Ghate *et al.* (2000).

Professionals who work with families wrestle with many complex issues and need to become adept at managing that complexity (see 'The concept of need in parenting children and young people' below).

Hall and Elliman (2003, p.34) suggest that success in providing parental support is determined not only by what potential helpers do but by the characteristics of the person/people providing the service. The relationships they develop with the parents are critical to the success or failure of the intervention and to the parent's ability to implement effective strategies for parenting. For example, the style of relationship that professionals establish with parents will influence how the professionals are perceived, and will influence parental expectations of their role. This is repeated throughout much of the most recent evidence (e.g. Ghate and Hazel, 2002; Quinton, 2004; Bartley, 2006).

Cunningham and Davis (1985) identified three parent–professional relationships:

- the *expert model* in which the professional feels he/she has all the expertise; takes control of the situation; and makes the decisions. Mutual respect, sharing of information, negotiation and parental views are given low priority. This approach can undermine parental confidence and/or create dependency.

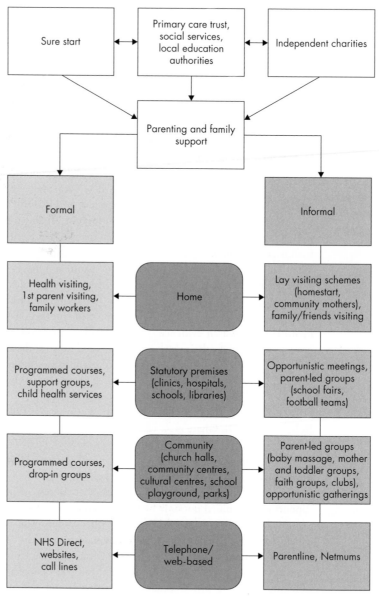

Figure 4.4 Formal and informal facilities for parenting education and support. (Reproduced with permission from Bidmead and Whittaker (2004) *Positive Parenting: a public health priority.* London: CPHVA, p.30.)

It may also lead to important information and problems being missed. It is not a holistic view and pays little attention to the environmental context in which the family lives.

- the *transplant model* sees the parent as having useful skills to augment the professional's skills. Here, the professionals see themselves as 'transplanting' skills to the parent in their absence (e.g. carrying out treatments for technology-dependent children – see Chapter 9). In such cases, professionals understand themselves to be managers of family situations. In this profile, the professional retains overall control and identifies objectives, treatments and teaching methods. The parents may not share these aims and objectives, yet the professional may expect the client to comply with the instructions and to become competent. Furthermore, the family may not have the necessary physical, practical or emotional resources to comply. If excessive demands are made on the family, the outcome can be hostility and a breakdown in the professional–parental relationship.

- the *consumer model*, which evolved to become the *parent advisor model* (Davis *et al.*, 2002), and subsequently developed further to become the *family partnership model*. This approach is based on a shared partnership between professional and parent. Control remains with the parent, and the professional's role is to share information with the parent and to explore options. In this model, the professional acknowledges the parent's expertise, skills and depth knowledge of the family/child situation. The professional acts as a 'skilled helper', with an emphasis on understanding the needs of the family/parent, and negotiates a way forward, a form of counselling. In order to establish this partnership approach, the professional must have appropriate personal qualities such as respect, empathy, personal integrity and excellent communication skills. In such cases, the parent selects the parenting options that most suit the family's needs. The professional's skills lie in establishing the negotiating process and helping to find solutions. In this model, aims and expectations are openly stated and explored, and this forms the basis of a contract. The professional also needs to have an understanding of the helping process, the skills and qualities necessary to enable families to change their practices.

These relationship skills are important for professionals working with parents either on an individual basis or in groups. Parenting UK (formerly the Parent Education Support Forum) advocates specific training for all those who offer parent support and who facilitate parent groups. Parenting UK has developed National Occupational Standards (NOS) for Working with Parents (www.parentinguk.org/2/standards). Training includes provision of adequate supervision for the practitioner and encourages reflective practice and professional development.

Research rarely concentrates on the process of help itself and the parent–helper interaction, elements that can determine success or failure. In such cases, the context of the relationship will determine the outcome. Fonagy *et al.* (2001), for example, argued that positive outcomes in specialist treatments are dependent on the style of treatment rather than the choice of treatment. The core skills he identified were listening to and respecting children and parents and valuing their views and experience. Quinton (2004) also argued that how professionals work with parents is as important as what they do.

Crowley (personal correspondence) suggests that parenting education and support is like performing heart surgery, where professionals are delving into the most intimate relationships between parent and child. Everyone feels vulnerable.

The expectation from the public is that the surgeon will be suitably qualified to perform such operations. So it is with providers of parent education and support. Practitioners need to have the skills and personal attributes appropriate to working with parents. The NOS for Working with Parents supports this contention.

Similarly, Sue Miller in a presentation to the Parent Child Conference (Miller, 2002) reported research carried out in Newcastle and commissioned by the Healthy Action Zone in the North East in 2000. From the findings, she identified three types of approaches to parental perceptions of parent education. This qualitative study interviewed parents from four target groups comprising teenage parents, school children, pre-school children and parents of children with special educational needs. The following models were developed:

- *the dispensing model*: parents ask 'What can I do to change my child?' Parent educators focus on the child as a problem. Surface learning only takes place at this level, and this type of learning is viewed as instruction by an expert.
- *the relating model*: parents ask 'How do I feel about this situation?' Parent educators focus on the parent as a problem. This stimulates a different type of learning.
- *the reflecting model*: parents ask 'Why is this happening?' Parent educators focus on the relationships in the family as a legitimate area for exploration. A deep level of learning can take place. This type of learning is associated with skilled facilitation and an ongoing supportive relationship.

One repeated criticism of research studies (Hall and Elliman, 2003) is that the interventions under study often use highly skilled facilitators, who are well trained, have regular quality supervision and support and are often from a mental health background. When such programmes are replicated, they are often facilitated by less well-qualified staff who have infrequent supervision and operate in less well-organized work environments. As a consequence, the outcomes can be disappointing because replication is not possible. The skill and ability of the facilitator is one of the most critical ingredients in successful outcomes (e.g. the ability to recruit and retain parents from the outset, notably when trying to work with families most in need).

THINKING ABOUT RISK IN APPROACHES TO PARENTING

Despite the generic and the public health definitions of risk, thinking about approaches to parenting actually involves thinking about factors that can cause risk to the parenting function. By this we do not refer to risk in terms of child protection only. Rather, we are concerned with those families who are most in need, whether as a consequence of material or emotional need. What we mean by this is to indicate those factors that complicate the difficult work that parenting involves for all parents.

> *Parenting in a modern industrial society includes a formidable range of tasks and responsibilities. For parents to pull these off requires sufficient resources and social supports, that can be drawn on to help them.*
>
> **(Quinton, 2004, p.180)**

Quinton's work is a useful starting point because it is an overview of 14 studies (in addition to Ghate and Hazel's work, 2002) of diverse challenges that parents encounter. Its purpose is to try to identify the kinds of support that parents themselves want and might use, including how such support is or should be organized. The determination in Quinton's work was to provide an analytical addition to systematic literature reviews, which tend to foreground analyses of interventions themselves (e.g. Barlow and Stewart-Brown, 2001; Patterson *et al.*, 2002; Moran *et al.*, 2004; Sanders and Morawska, 2006). In other words, Quinton and his team were asking broader questions about the parenting experience, and they did this by commissioning individual studies from expert teams (on behalf of the DfES).

> *Research on the effects of supportive interventions – i.e. on 'what works' – needs more specific attempts to understand the direction of effects through well-evaluated trials of different approaches.*
>
> **(Quinton, 2004, p.181)**

Much of the work discussed in Quinton (2004) indicated severe problems with public services. Perhaps one of the most striking studies involved South Asian parents' experiences of living with a child with severe disabilities. The incidence of disabilities amongst South Asian families is three times the national average. This is a public health matter. The findings of Hatton *et al.* (2004) are alarming. They found that these families are not provided with the diagnostic information from healthcare professionals that they need from the outset of diagnosis, nor do they receive information about services that might help them. Many in the study did not speak English and, contrary to popular perceptions, most did not have extended families to assist them. The emotional support that parental partners provided for each other was a key feature of these parents' ability to parent their disabled children in severely adverse circumstances.

Of the commissioned studies, imprisoned fathers were the least likely group to be assisted in their parenting role (Boswell and Wedge, 2004). This confirms work by DeBell (2003) that studied the effect on adolescents of having a close family member in custody. Approximately 125 000 children each year will have a parent in prison (Brown, 2003, p.4). But this figure increases when close family members are included (e.g. siblings, mothers, uncles, grandfathers). The stigma attached to imprisonment means that most children at school who have a close family member in custody do not reveal this fact to the school. Yet, the distress caused by imprisonment of a close family member can lead to poor health, poor educational attainment because of exam disruption, and either social isolation or truancy, anxiety, distress or inability to manage anger. Considerable recent work is focusing on the potential relationship between sibling custody and child and adolescent delinquency (Murray and Farrington, 2006), and between parental imprisonment and children's own eventual criminal behaviour (Murray *et al.*, 2007).

What interventions would be appropriate in each of these cases? Little work has focused on these kinds of difficulty that are encountered by parents attempting to manage their parenting role effectively. The reason is largely linked to the isolation caused by the way these problems are handled by public agencies such as the criminal justice system and the healthcare system. From a public health practice perspective, these examples are neither intractable nor insolvable. But they do tend to be invisible.

Quinton speaks of parental support as a process, and this fits with our earlier argument that the parenting role is itself a process over time, affected by the ecology of the family system itself and the changes experienced by all members of a family as children grow and develop, as family circumstances change and mutate.

Families coping with disabilities (in the child or in the parent/carer) are a stark example of the long-term issues implied by a process approach to parenting development (see Chapter 9). The findings suggest little interagency co-ordination and poor information to assist children and their parents/carers. For example, the tendency to medicalize such experiences fails to take into account the social context in which these families lead their lives.

THE CONCEPT OF NEED IN PARENTING CHILDREN AND YOUNG PEOPLE

The following is a real case study in the UK, but rendered anonymous.

Case Study 4.1

The Jones family is Mum (Marie) age 29 and Dad (Tom) age 31. Marie has two sons (Daniel, age 12 and Mark, age 10) fathered in an earlier relationship that was characterized by domestic violence. The boys no longer have contact with their birth father. Together, Marie and Tom have a daughter (Kylie, age 4). Marie's first child was born when she was 17. Her own mother is remote and Marie was sexually abused by her step-father. Marie and Tom are heavy smokers and Marie suffers from depression. Husband Tom drinks in excess and is an occasional drug user. He has spent time in prison for theft and drug dealing.

The family lives in a three-bedroom house rented from the local authority, located in what is characterized as a deprived estate. They are in rent arrears and are threatened with eviction. Debt is a serious problem. The house is in poor structural condition, is uncared for and is unsafe. The family has a number of pets living in the house with them.

Daniel's behaviour is difficult for his Mum to manage. He has been excluded from school in the past and he often clashes with his brother. Daniel at age 12 is enuretic and has been in trouble with the police for stealing from local shops and fighting with other boys.

Mark has been diagnosed with attention deficit hyperactivity disorder (ADHD) and is currently prescribed with Ritalin. His mother says that she cannot 'handle him', and her husband Tom shows little interest in either of the boys. Mark is a poor sleeper and frequently wanders the house at night.

Kylie is her father's favourite. She is about to start school but is a fussy eater, goes to bed late and wakes frequently in the night.

Marie is six months pregnant and has had a difficult pregnancy. There have been medical concern about the baby's growth and Marie often forgets to attend antenatal appointments.

The complexity of this family's situation and their children's needs will have attracted attention from a range of service providers, including school, health, social care and community services, as well as housing and police officers. The challenge is twofold. On the one hand, the parents and their children can only be assisted in so far as they seek assistance. On the other hand, without assistance, they could potentially be subject to legal interventions – from local authority housing offices, debt agencies and/or the police.

This one family's situation has virtually all the elements that public health practitioners highlight in their work. School nurses, health visitors, CAMHS teams, midwives, children's services, education welfare officers (EWOs) and crisis support teams are all orientated toward assisting with one or more of the presenting problems. The difficulty from a service provision perspective is that the over-riding need is co-ordination and interagency work. A lead professional could be helpful in such a profile of need, but local authority and integrated children's services, across the UK, are new; they are stretched; they are under-funded and under-resourced.

> Time and again, our research revealed that those welfare professionals who listened, who were not judgemental, gave their clients time, who were prepared to advocate for their clients and seek solutions which were appropriate to their needs, were highly valued and made a positive difference to their lives. These were the exception, however, and when interviewed it was often the case that state welfare workers felt that their approach was despite their employing agency, rather than positively endorsed by the agency.
>
> **(Bartley, 2006, p.23)**

The challenge is and, it remains, to determine:

> The extent to which there is overlap between what parents want, what services provide and 'what works'. . . a more thorough understanding of all three should help considerably in our efforts to improve the way in which we deliver services in this field.
>
> **(Ghate and Hazel, 2002, p.10)**

Having said that, we do not know what forms of help and assistance the Jones children have or do not have from relatives, from friends and from schools. Furthermore, the danger is that public policy tends to focus on the parental difficulties, without thinking about each child's individual perspective on the problems he/she is confronting, whether that method of confrontation is successful for the child or not. 'Behavioural problems', for example, are the presenting and public manifestation of the child's experience. And behavioural problems are the generic term with which children like those in our case study will find themselves generally labelled – for the simple reason that it is their behaviour that is public and observable.

Ghate and Hazel (2002) conducted the most extensive new research we currently have about the experiences of families who live and parent their children in poor environments in 21st century Britain. Their findings reveal the stunning capacity that parents actually demonstrate in managing family life in the most adverse circumstances – situations that include seriously poor housing; very low income; parental and child ill-health; an absence of safe play areas outside the home; insufficient resources for food and clothing. These would be risk factors for successful parenting for any parent.

> *The results of the study confirmed that parents living in poor environments are typically exposed to high levels of risk factors at all levels of the ecological model. Whether we explore stressors at the level of the individual, the level of the family and household or at the level of the community and environment, we find clear evidence of elevated levels of adversity for parents and their children relative to the wider population. Based on the data we gathered, there can be little doubt that parenting in a poor environment is a particularly difficult job.*
>
> **(Ghate and Hazel, 2002, p.233)**

There are two obvious approaches that we can take to child poverty: invest in removing material poverty; invest in strengthening resilience and capability in the child and family. This is not an either/or agenda. There is emerging evidence of links between the two in some few deprived areas of the UK where communities, and thus families within them, are being strengthened by developing civil society strategies that start from co-ordinated service delivery (Stewart *et al.,* 1999; Mitchell, 2003; Mitchell and Backett-Millburn, 2006).

In addition, considerable research is being undertaken in an effort to understand the factors that produce 'the enormous capabilities and resilience that people show in their everyday lives and under crisis conditions' (Bartley, 2006, p.3). Thus far, the evidence suggests two common factors that can make resilience in the child or young person more likely.

> *Those mostly have to do with the quality of human relationships, and with the quality of public service responses to people with problems. . . . Good public services enable and encourage people to maintain social relationships, but badly provided ones can create social isolation.*
>
> **(Bartley, 2006, p.3)**

CONCLUSION

We intentionally chose to title this chapter 'Approaches to parenting' and not to use the term 'parenting support'. The latter, as Quinton (2004) argues, is a conceptually problematic term. Furthermore, we have argued that the issue is not merely a matter of parenting skills, important though they are. Children and young people thrive or fail to thrive as a consequence of multiple factors within the ecological framework in which the family finds itself. And child well-being in the family setting is rarely examined from the child's or young person's perspective.

Our purpose in this chapter has been to explore the public health practice issues that arise from the school-age child's home environment, whatever form that might take. In doing this, we sought to explore the factors within family life that can affect the health and well-being of children and young people of school age.

The public health practice perspective on the school-age child requires us to consider the three settings children and young people inhabit during their school-age years: the home; the school; the neighbourhood/community. Within the home setting, the features that matter are the approach to parenting that the child experiences and the social and material circumstances that constitute the family environment, including the services the family can draw upon within the local community. The child and his or her carer(s) live within an ecological framework that interacts with and has consequences for the family unit and thus for children and young people.

We have emphasized the dynamic between the child and the adult carer(s), and we have sought to explore the way in which the child as actor in the family setting has a consequence for the approach to parenting. There is, of course, an imbalance of power within the home, but it remains the case that how a child responds to the carer(s) can affect the approach to parenting, and practitioners need to be sensitive to that dynamic.

It is also widely recognized that individual children and young people have various degrees of resilience when confronting emotional and/or material risk in the family setting. Yet we know little about the delicate balance between risk and resilience. For public health practitioners, the task is to build resilience in whatever way possible. It is this ingredient that public health practitioners need to nurture in children and young people whose home lives are difficult. To do that requires services that are not judgemental, that listen to the child and to the family and that act as advocates for the family. This means reorienting much existing practice.

KEY POINTS

- It is the *quality of human relationships* that determines the health and well-being of the family. All child outcomes eventually flow from the nature of reciprocity that develops within the family, the community within which the family lives, and with the public and voluntary services that seek to support families.
- The quality of public service responses to children, young people and their families, when they encounter problems, is determined by the nature of the relationship that develops between service providers and the individual members of the family. In contemporary Britain, public services are still far from integrated across government departments in most communities.

- Parenting is a process over time and is affected by the ecology of the family system itself, the changes experienced by all members of the family as children grow and develop, as family circumstances change and mutate.
- Children and their parents/carers live family life as a dynamic between the child and the adult. Furthermore, sibling relationships can help or hinder the child's experience of family life. Having said that, children and young people are ultimately vulnerable to adult carer(s)' behaviours.
- We know little about how capability and resilience develop in individual children who are faced with risks from or within family life. Yet it is resilience that helps to protect children and young people in circumstances where the family is potentially damaging.
- Public health practitioners need to start their work with families from the position of relationship building, and they need to help families to create environments that can build resilience in children and young people. This means listening to the child's perspective on family life and creating contexts of assistance that can start from the child's innate strengths (the child's capacity for resilience).
- Service delivery to assist children, young people and their families in the UK is not yet generally integrated or effectively focused.

REFERENCES

Ainsworth M, Blehar M, Waters E, Wall S (1978) *Patterns of Attachment.* Mahwah New Jersey: Lawrence Erlbaum Associates.

Alderson P (2001) Research by children. *International Journal of Social Research Methodology* 4:139–53.

Amato P, Loomis L, Booth A (1995) Parental divorce, marital conflict and offspring wellbeing during early adulthood. *Social Forces* 73:895–915.

Barclay L, Lupton D (1997) *Constructing Fatherhood: discourses and experiences.* London: Sage.

Barlow J, Stewart-Brown S (2001) Understanding parenting programmes: parents' views. *Primary Health Care Research and Development* 2:117–30.

Barlow J, Stewart-Brown S (2005) Child abuse and neglect. *The Lancet* 365:1750–2.

Bartley M (ed.) (2006) *Capability and Resilience: beating the odds.* London: UCL Department of Epidemiology and Public Health on behalf of the ESRC: Priority Network on Capability and Resilience (2003–2007). www.ucl.ac.uk/capabilityandresilience (accessed 19 January 2007).

Baumrind D (1973) The development of instrumental competence through socialization. In: Pick AD (ed.) *Minnesota Symposium on Child Psychology* 7:3–46. Minneapolis: University of Minnesota Press.

Baumrind D (1978) Parental disciplinary patterns and social competence in children. *Youth and Society* 9:239–75.

Baumrind D (1991) The influence of parenting style on adolescent competence and substance use. *Journal of Early Adolescence* 11:56–95.

Bavolek S (1990) Parenting: theory, policy and practice. *Research and Validation Report of the Nurturing Programmes.* Wisconsin: Eau Claire.

Becker F, Gordon R (2000) *The Child's World.* Training pack produced by NSPCC, DOH and The University of Sheffield.

Bee H (2000) *The Developing Child* (9e). Boston: Allyn and Bacon.

Bidmead C, Whittaker K (2004) *Positive Parenting: a public health priority.* London: CPHVA.

Beveridge W (1942) *Social Insurance and Allied Services.* Cmnd 6404. London: HMSO.

Block J (1971) *Lives through Time.* Berkeley: Bancroft.

Bornstein MH (2002) *Handbook of Parenting* (2e). Mahwah: Lawrence Erlbaum Associates.

Boswell G, Wedge P (2004) The parenting role of imprisoned fathers. In: Quinton D. (ed.) *Supporting Parents: messages from research.* London: Jessica Kingsley Publishers, pp.247–51.

Bronfenbrenner U (1977) Toward an experimental ecology of human development. *American Psychologist* 32:513–31.

Bronfenbrenner U (1979) *The Ecology of Human Development.* Cambridge MA: Harvard University.

Brown K (2003) Introduction. In: DeBell D *Starting Where They Are Project: supporting young people with a prisoner in the family.* London: Action for Prisoners' Families, pp.4–5.

Brummer E (1997) Stress and the biology of inequality. *British Medical Journal* 314:1472–5.

Burghes L, Clarke L, Cronin N (1997) *Fathers and Fatherhood in Britain.* London: Family Policy Studies Centre.

Cabinet Office (2006) *Reaching Out: an action plan on social exclusion.* London: The Cabine Office.

Cameron D, Jones ID (1985) An epidemiological and sociological analysis of alcohol, tobacco, and other drugs of solace. *Community Medicine* 7:18–29.

Chief Secretary to the Treasury (2003) *Every Child Matters* (Cm 5860). London: Stationery Office. www.everychildmatters.gov.uk/_content/documents/EveryChildMatters.pdf (accessed 17 January 2007).

Christiansen P, James A (2000) *Research with Children. Perspectives and practices.* London: Falmer Press.

Cohen D, Richardson J, Labree L (1994) Parenting behaviours and the onset of smoking and alcohol use: a longitudinal study. *Paediatrics* 94:368–75.

Coleman J, Henricson C, Roker D (1999) *Parenting in the Youth Justice Context.* London: Youth Justice Board.

Cunningham C, Davis H (1985) *Working with Parents: frameworks for collaboration.* Oxford: Oxford University Press.

Daniel B, Wassell S, Gilligan R (1999) *Child Development for Child Care and Protection Workers.* London: Jessica Kingsley.

Davis H, Day C, Bidmead C (2002) *Working in Partnership with Parents: the parent advisor model.* London: The Psychological Corporation.

DeBell D (1999) *What Do We Know About The Effectiveness of Parenting Support Initiatives: a review of research in the field.* Norwich: Healthy Norfolk 2000.

DeBell D. (2003) *Starting Where They Are Project: supporting young people with a prisoner in the family.* London: Action for Prisoners' Families.

Department of Health and Home Office (2003) *The Victoria Climbié Inquiry. Report of an Inquiry by Lord Laming.* London: HMSO.

Desforges C, Aboiuchaar A (2003) *The Impact of Parental Involvement, Parental Support and Family Education on Pupil Achievement and Adjustment: a literature review.* Report no 433. London: Department for Education and Skills.

Dornbusch S, Ritter P, Liederman P, Roberts D, Fraleigh M (1987) The relation of parenting style to adolescent school performance. *Child Development* 58:1244–57.

Egeland B (1997) Mediation of the effects of child maltreatment on developmental adaptation in adolescence. In: Cicchetti D, Toth SL (eds) *Rochester Symposium on Developmental Psychopathology. Volume VII: the effects of trauma on the developmental process.* Rochester New York: University Press, pp.403–34.

Feinstein L, Symons J (1999) *Attainment in Secondary School.* Discussion Paper 341. London: Centre for Economic Performance, London School of Economics and Political Science.

Ferri E, Smith K (1996) *Parenting in the 1990s.* Family and Parenthood series. London: Family Policy Studies Centre.

Flouri E, Buchanan A (2001) *Father Involvement and Outcomes in Adolescence and Adulthood.* Oxford: Oxford University Press.

Fonagy P, Target M, Cottrell D, Phillips J, Kurtz Z (2001) *A Review of Outcomes of Psychiatric Disorder in Childhood. Final Report to the National Health Service Executive. Project ID MCH 17-33.* London: Department of Health. www.info.doh.gov.uk (accessed 27 January 2007).

Ghate D, Hazel N (2002) *Parenting in Poor Environments: stress, support and coping.* London: Jessica Kingsley Publishers.

Ghate D, Ramella M (2002) *Positive Parenting: the national evaluation of the Youth Justice Board's Parenting Programme.* London: Youth Justice Board for England and Wales.

Ghate D, Shaw C, Hazel N (2000) *Fathers and Family Centres: engaging fathers in preventative services.* York: Joseph Rowntree Foundation.

Glasgow K, Dornbusch S, Troyer L, Steinberg L, Ritter P (1997) Parenting styles, adolescents' attributions and educational outcome in nine heterogeneous high schools. *Child Development* 68:507–29.

Goldman R (2005) *Father's Involvement and Outcomes in Adolescence and Adulthood.* Oxford: Oxford University Press.

Gordon T (1975) *Parent Effectiveness Training.* New York: Peter Wyden.

Gottman J, Declaire J (1997) *The Heart of Parenting: how to Raise an Emotionally Intelligent Child.* London: Bloomsbury.

Grimshaw R, McGuire C (1998) *Evaluating Parenting Programmes.* London: National Children's Bureau.

Hall D, Elliman D (2003) *Health for all Children* (4e). Oxford: Oxford University Press.

Harold G, Pryor J, Reynolds J (2001) *Not in Front of the Children? How conflict between parents affects children.* London: One Plus One.

Hatton C, Akram Y, Shah R, Robertson J, Emerson E (2004) Supporting South Asian families with a child with severe disabilities. In: Quinton D (ed.) *Supporting Parents: messages from research.* London: Jessica Kingsley Publishers, pp.235–40.

Henricson C (2003) *Government and Parenting: is there a case for a policy review and parents' code?* York: Joseph Rowntree Foundation (for the National Family and Parenting Institute).

Henricson C, Coleman J, Roker D (2000) Parenting in the youth justice context. *The Howard Journal* 39:325–8.

HM Treasury and Department for Education and Skills (2005) *Support for Parents: the best start for children.* London: HMSO.

HM Treasury and Department for Education and Skills (2007) *Policy Review of Children and Young People: a discussion paper.* London: HMSO.

Hobcraft J (1998) *Childhood Experience and the Risk of Social Exclusion in Adulthood.* CASE Briefing. Centre for Analysis for Social Exclusion. London: London School of Economics.

Hodgson R, Abbasi T, Clarkson J (1996) Effective mental health promotion: a literature review. *Health Education Journal* 55:55–74.

Hoghughi M (1998) The importance of parenting in public health. *British Medical Journal* 316:1545–50.

Home Office (1998) *Supporting Families: a consultation document.* London: The Stationery Office.

Home Office (2006) Respect Action Plan. The Respect Task Force, 2 Marsham St, London 5W1 4DF. www.respect.gov.uk.

James A, Prout A (eds) (1997) *Constructing and Deconstructing Childhood: contemporary issues in the sociological study of childhood* (2e). London: Falmer Press.

Labour Party (1997) *New Labour Because Britain Deserves Better. Labour Party Manifesto.* www.psr.keele.ac.uk/area/uk/man/lab97.htm (accessed 19 January 2007).

Lamborn S, Mounts N, Steinberg L, Dornbusch S (1991) Patterns of competence and adjustment among adolescents from authoritative, authoritarian, indulgent and neglectful families. *Child Development* 62:1049–65.

Lerner RM, Castellino DR, Patterson AT, Francisco AV, McKinney MH (1995) Developmental contextual perspective on parenting. In: Bornstein M (ed.) *Handbook of Parenting* Vol. 2. New Jersey: Lawrence Erlbaum Associates, pp.287–97.

Lewis G, Sloggett A (1998) Suicide, deprivation and unemployment: Record linkage study. *British Medical Journal* 317:1283–6.

Maccoby E, Martin J (1983) Socialization in the context of the family: parent–child interaction. In: Hetherington EM (ed) *Handbook of Child Psychology: socialization, personality and social development Volume 4.* New York: Wiley, pp.1–102.

MacKay (1973) Conceptions of children and models of socialization. In: Dreitzel HP (ed.) *Childhood and Socialisation.* New York: Macmillan, pp.22–43.

Marmot M (2005) Presentation to the Tackling Health Inequalities Governing for Health Summit. In: The Cabinet Office *Reaching Out: an action plan on social exclusion,* 46. London: The Cabinet Office.

Marmot MG, Davey Smith G *et al.* (1991) Health inequalities amongst British civil servants: The Whitehall study II. *The Lancet* 337:1387–93.

Mayall B (2002) *Towards a Sociology for Childhood. Thinking from children's lives.* Buckingham: Open University Press.

McClun L, Merrell K (1998) Relationship of perceived parenting styles, locus of control orientation and self-concept among junior high age students. *Psychology in the Schools* 35:381–90.

Miller S (2002) *Parental Perceptions of Parenting Education.* Paper presented at the National Family and Parenting Institute, The Parenting Education and Support Forum, One Parent Families, The Open University and the Trust for the Study of Adolescence Parent Child Conference, sponsored by The Children and Young People's Unit, HSBC Bank, The Teenage Pregnancy Unit and the Home Office, 18–19 April 2002, London.

Mitchell R (2003) *Greater Expectations: the parts of Britain where people live longer than they should. RUHBC findings series 4.* Edinburgh: University of Edinburgh.

Mitchell R, Backett-Millburn K (2006) *Health and Resilience: what does a resilience approach offer health research and policy? RUHBC findings series 11.* Edinburgh: University of Edinburgh.

Moran P, Ghae D, Van der Merwe A (2004) *What Works in Parenting Support? A review of the international evidence.* Research report 574. London: Department of Education and Skills.

Morgan P (1999) *Farewell to the Family? Public policy and breakdown in Britain and the USA.* London: London Institute of Economic Affairs.

Morrow V (1999) Conceptualising social capital in relation to the well being of children and young people: a critical review. *The Sociological Review* 47:745–65.

Murray J, Farrington DP (2006) Evidence-based programs for children of prisoners. *Criminology and Public Policy* 5:721–36.

Murray J, Janson C-L, Farrington DP (2007) Crime in adult offspring of prisoners. A cross-national comparison of two longitudinal samples. *Criminal Justice and Behaviour* 34:133–49.

Murray L, Cooper P (1997) Effect of postnatal depression on infant development. *Archives of Disease in Childhood* 77:99–101.

National Children's Bureau (2007) *NCB response to the Comprehensive Spending Review 2007: joint policy review on children and young people.* London: National Children's Bureau.

Papworth J (2002) When you are old enough? *The Guardian* 19 June 2002. www.guardian.co.uk/parents/story/0,,739853,00.html (accessed 19 January 2007).

Patterson G (1992) *Antisocial Boys.* Eugene Oregon: Castalia Press.

Patterson G, DeBaryshe B, Ramsey E (1989) A developmental perspective on antisocial behaviour. *American Journal of Psychology* 44:329–35.

Patterson J, Barlow J, Mockford C *et al.* (2002) Improving mental health through parenting programmes: block randomised controlled trial. *Archives of Disease in Childhood* 87:472–7.

Pulkkinen L (1982) Self-control and continuity from childhood to late adolescence. In: Baltes P, Brim G Jr (eds) *Lifespan Development and Behaviour* Volume 4. New York: Academic Press, pp.64–107.

Quinton D (2004) *Supporting Parents: messages from research.* London: Jessica Kingsley Publishers.

Qvotrup J, Bardy M, Sgritta G, Wintersberger H (eds) (1994) *Childhood Matters. Social theory, practice and politics.* Aldershot: Avebury.

Rosengren A, Orth-Gomer K, Wedel H, Wilhelmsen L (1933) Stressful life events, social support and mortality in men born in 1933. *British Medical Journal* 307:1102–5.

Rowthorn R (2001) Marriage as a signal. In: Dnes AW, Rowthorn R (eds) *The Law and Economics of Marriage and Divorce.* Cambridge: Cambridge University Press, pp.132–56.

Sanders R (2004) *Sibling Relationships: theory and issues for practice.* Hampshire: Palgrave Macmillan.

Sanders RS, Morawska A (2006) Towards a public health approach to parenting. *The Psychologist* 19:476–9.

Sanders MR, Markie Dadds CL (1996) Triple P. A multi-level family intervention programme for children with disruptive behaviour disorders. In: Cotton P, Jackson HE (eds) *Early Intervention and Prevention in Mental Health Application of Clinical Psychology.* Melbourne Australia: Australian Psychological Society, pp.59–87.

Smith R (1997) Parent education: empowerment or control? *Children and Society* 11:108–16.

Speier M (1976) The adult ideological viewpoint in studies of childhood. In: Skolnick A (ed) *Rethinking Childhood: perspective on development and society.* New York: Little Brown, pp.168–86.

Steele H (2002) State of the art: attachment. *The Psychologist* 15:518–22.

Steinberg L, Elmen J, Mounts N (1989) Authoritative parenting, psychosocial maturity, and academic success among adolescents. *Child Development* 60:1424–36.

Steinberg L, Mounts N, Lamborn S, Dornbusch S (1991) Authoritative parenting and adolescent adjustment across varied ecological niches. *Journal of Research on Adolescence* 1:19–36.

Steinberg L, Lamborn S, Dornbusch S, Darling N (1992) Impact of parenting practices on adolescent achievement: authoritative parenting, school involvement and encouragement to succeed. *Child Development* 63:1266–81.

Steinberg L, Lamborn S, Darling N, Mounts N, Dornbusch S (1994) Overtime changes in adjustment and competence among adolescents from authoritative, authoritarian, indulgent and neglectful families. *Child Development* 65:754–70.

Steinberg L, Darling N, Fletcher A, Brown B, Dornbusch S (1995) Authoritative parenting and adolescent adjustment: an ecological journey. In: Moen P, Elder GH Jr, Luscher K (eds) *Examining Lives in Context: perspectives on the ecology of human development.* Washington DC: American Psychological Association, pp.423–66.

Stevenson J, Sonuga-Barke E, Thompson M *et al.* (2004) Effective strategies for parents with young children with behaviour problems. In: Quinton D (ed.) *Supporting Parents*. London: Jessica Kingsley Publishers, pp.218–19.

Stewart M, Reid G, Buckles L, Edgar W, Mangham C (1999) *A Study of Resiliency in Communities.* Ottawa Canada: Ottawa Office of Alcohol, Drug and Dependency Issues, Health Canada.

Thomas A, Chess S (1977) *Temperament and Development.* New York: Brunner/Mazel.

Timmins N (1996) *The Five Giants: a biography of the welfare state.* London: Fontana Press.

United Nations (1989) United Nations Convention on the Rights of the Child. Geneva: UN. www.unhchr.ch/html/menu3/b/k2crc.htm (accessed 19 January 2007).

Utting D, Pugh G (2003) The social context of parenting. In: Hoghughi M, Long N (eds) *The Handbook of Parenting.* London: Sage, pp.19–37.

Utting D, Bright J, Henricson C (1993) *Crime and the Family: improving child rearing and preventing delinquency.* Occasional Paper 16. London: Family Policy Studies Centre.

Warin J, Solomon Y, Lewis C, Langford W (1999) *Fathers' Work and Family Life.* London: Family Policy Studies Centre.

Wallace SA, Crown JM, Cox AD, Berger M (1997) *Child and Adolescent Mental Health.* Abingdon: Radcliffe Medical Press.

Weare K (2000) *Promoting Mental, Emotional and Social Health: a whole school approach.* London: Routledge.

Webster-Stratton C (1999) Researching the impact of parent training programmes on child conduct disorder. In: Lloyd E (ed.) *What Works in Parenting Education?* Barkingside: Barnardo's, pp. 85–114.

Wells L, Rankin J (1991) Families and delinquency: a meta-analysis of the impact of broken homes. *Social Problems* 38:71–89.

Wilkinson RG (1996) *Unhealthy Societies: the afflictions of inequality.* London and New York: Routledge.

Williams R (1999) *Going the Distance: fathers and health visiting.* Reading: The University of Reading in association with the Queen's Nursing Institute.

Williams R, Robertson S (1999) Fathers and health visitors: 'it's a secret agent thing'. *Community Practitioner* 72:56–8.

Acts of Parliament

All these Acts are published by HMSO in London, and all can be accessed from the UK Parliament website (www.publications.parliament.uk).

Education Act 1944
Crime and Disorder Act 1998
Carers and Disabled Children Act 2000
Anti-Social Behaviour Act 2003
Criminal Justice Act 2003
Children Act 2004

Section 3
THE CHILD IN SCHOOL

5

THE SCHOOL AS LOCATION FOR HEALTH PROMOTION

Diane DeBell, Margaret Buttigieg, Sarah Sherwin and Kathryn Lowe

INTRODUCTION

The school as location for health promotion prompts a number of questions. Why the school? What is health promotion? What do we mean by health? In England, the policy context for child health in the school years and in the school environment has become the focus of significant attention during the 21st century. This is echoed in Scotland, Northern Ireland and Wales. Furthermore, cross-government departmental and joint ministerial approaches have become a prominent feature of upstream thinking.

Every Child Matters: change for children (HM Government, 2004) specifies national and local priorities for children's services by articulating five target outcomes for children and young people, and these were given a legal platform in the Children Act 2004, which is applicable across the UK and is the enabling legislation for many of the current developments around services for children and young people. Services include local authority education (state maintained schools) as well as health, social care, youth justice, Connexions, youth workers, and support from the voluntary/charitable sector. The five target outcomes of *Every Child Matters* are a description of what we might think of as a definition for health and well-being amongst children and young people.

• being healthy
• staying safe
• enjoying and achieving
• making a positive contribution
• achieving economic well-being.

The *Every Child Matters* framework dovetails with the Standards set by the *National Service Framework for Children, Young People and Maternity Services* (Department of Health and DfES, 2004) and draws on the work of Hall and Elliman (2003). These upstream policy drivers are behind the work of all four countries of the UK in their planning for services and in their articulation of how to prioritize downstream practices to improve the health of children and young people. This chapter examines the relationship between aspiration and practice, by focusing on the place and meaning of health promotion in the school environment in the UK.

THE SCHOOL AS THE CHILD'S WORKPLACE

One of the determinants of health that has historically made a positive differ- ence to adult health can be found in the developing legislation to improve health and safety in the workplace – safer working conditions; shorter working hours/working week; and legislation to improve the way people treat each other. For children the school is their workplace, but legislation governing the work- place and occupational health does not transfer to the school environment for children – only for teachers and staff. Schools in the UK have historically been the site of endemic child bullying; toilet facilities are often unhygienic, and younger children report menacing behaviours from older children in school toi- lets as well as on playgrounds; food has steadily declined in nutritional value; fresh drinking water has not been freely available; physical activity has declined as a proportion of the time spent at school; and achievement targets for all chil- dren's work in the school environment have been steadily increasing since the Second World War. Mayall *et al.* in 1996 first documented the damaging split between health and education in English schools.

> *Yet education also takes place at home, and health care at school. Children themselves challenge the division of lived life into private and public sec- tors; they take their bodies and emotions as well as their minds, into school each day. For them the maintenance of health there is a key concern.*
> **(Mayall et al., 1996, p.1)**

Yet we also know that individual schools across the UK have created very suc- cessful communities of learning that simultaneously work to improve child health. The reality is that there has been inconsistency of approach, largely because of the executive power of the head teacher within Britain's schools.

The values, ethos and leadership direction of the head teacher have historically had considerable effect on the culture of school life, for example on the question of how the school does or does not relate to its local community and whether or not the school integrates local community resources into school life. It is in this understanding of the school as part of a larger community that we can begin to understand the public health orientation that makes health promotion, its prevention and health-improvement agenda, a part of school life.

Considerable research has begun to focus on establishing evidence of the link between educational attainment and positive emotional and physical health (see, for example, Flynn and Knight, 1998; Prashar, 2003), and the Extended Schools initiative (see p.111) starts from this perspective.

Furthermore, secondary school league tables are now being used to bring pressure on schools to engage in public health practice by indicating a link between schools' levels of success as a correlation with the levels of their work that reflect a public health framework (Department for Education and Skills (DfES) and Department of Health, 2003). And in July 2005, the Office for Standards in Education (Ofsted) published its *Framework for the Inspection of Children's Services* (Ofsted, 2005b), with specifications based on the Children Act 2004 and with principles that align precisely with *Every Child Matters: change for children* (HM Government, 2004) thereby incorporating child health as a basic premise for the inspection of schools.

In other words, the upstream policy pressures to link health and education have been steadily increasing since the turn of the century (e.g. the national Healthy Schools Programme from 1999). And it is in the arena of public health practice that we need to look for evidence of downstream implementation of these national policy directives for the promotion of child health (e.g. see 'Health promotion as targeted interventions', p.122).

Yet, despite considerable pressure to eradicate the historic profile of separation between the child's learning environment and the child's health needs, child health promotion as an explicit curriculum requirement in schools is not driven by legislation apart from the school inclusion agenda, which secures education provision for children with special educational needs (as many as 7 per cent of all children between the ages of 0 and 16 years; and some 18 per cent of children in maintained primary schools in England [Office for National Statistics, 2004]). In other words, the promotion of the child's health in the school environment remains largely a matter of local decisions about how and whether and in what ways to respond to national policy direction.

Thus, thinking about the school as the child's place of work helps us to be clearer about how to conceptualize the school as a location for health promotion, because it also enables us to think about the determinants of health that lie within the social and the physical/emotional context of school life itself as well as the determinants of health that lie within the local community outside the school environment. Attendance at school constitutes the second most important social and physical environment children inhabit outside the family or carer home. It is possible, furthermore, to argue that the school and the home interact with each other as determinants of child health (see Chapter 4).

To think about the school environment in terms of its contribution to, or its potential for harm to child health, necessarily precedes our ability to think of school as a location for health promotion. Whether and how to think about child health at school is a considerable challenge for head teachers and their staff, whose primary function is to deliver teaching that satisfies the requirements of the National Curriculum. It is also a challenge for public health practitioners who work with school-age children: 'Simply going into curriculum-led school lessons is not enough' (DfES and Department of Health, 2006).

THINKING ABOUT HEALTH PROMOTION AND SCHOOL LIFE

Public health practitioners have argued that the school is a key location for health promotion since at least the beginning of the 20th century. For example, a school nurse in New York during 1908 reported that she had identified the four schools in the city with the highest rates of school exclusions. From that specification (a public health assessment), she targeted her subsequent work on the family and school environments of these children in these schools for the purposes of identifying health-improvement strategies that could be conducted by nurses with assistance from schools.

> *After a month's experimental work, made by one nurse as a demonstration, the results were considered so satisfactory that twelve nurses were appointed, and following the report of this month's work with twelve nurses in forty-eight schools (four schools for each nurse), the Board of Health considered that the work . . . had fully demonstrated its practical value as a supplement to the health inspectors. It was seen that the work of the nurses connected the efforts of the Department of Health with the homes of the children, thus supplying the link needed to complete the chain.*
>
> **(Rogers, 1908, p.966)**

This attention to the child's combined school and home environment as a key to health improvement was again repeated in New York in 1941.

> *We called our enterprise 'public health nursing' . . . Our purpose was in no sense to establish an isolated undertaking. We planned to utilize, as well as to be implemented by, all agencies and groups of whatever creed which were working for social betterment, private as well as municipal. Our scheme was to be motivated by a vital sense of the interrelation of all these forces. For this reason we consider ourselves best described by the term 'public health nurses'.*
>
> **(Wales, 1941, p.xi)**

These two early examples contain the principles of the health-promotion concept that would come to be theorized in the late 20th century – interdepartmental work; a social and environmental understanding of child health; and the use of public health-measurement and risk-assessment tools. In both of these pre-war reports, we see the constituent elements of a social model of medicine – the perception that health involves more than a medical model of care, 'All medicine is inescapably social' (Eisenberg, 1999, p.164).

The history of modern medicine and particularly of public health as a medical discipline dates from mid-19th century research and practice. The common thread throughout the public health movement has always been its attention to population health, and the public health pioneers have all been concerned with the social and economic determinants of health alongside questions of infectious and communicable disease control. This has not, however, been uncontested territory. For example, the post-World War Two approach to health improvement in industrialized countries has primarily focused on individual medicine, individualized health care and individualized health risk.

And the recent picture in the UK itself is not entirely consistent either in its conceptual framework. For example, in 2006, the English Department for Education and Skills working with the Department of Health wrote:

> *Schools are particularly important to Every Child Matters because they are the universal service that has the most contact with school-age children and, increasingly, those children accessing the early education offer, as well as frequent and close contact with their families [sic].*
>
> ***(DfES and Department of Health, 2006)***

This quote from the 2006 Extended Schools initiative suggests a policy position that seeks to locate the school in a local community context that is designed to integrate local authority and health services 'in close contact with families' in such a way as to maximize ability to improve child health by changing the very culture of schools and by enlarging their functions (see 'The Extended Schools initiative', p.111)

Yet, in 2004, *Choosing Health* (Department of Health, 2004a) in England had shifted the public health focus away from Acheson's (1998) social model, to a medical model reminiscent of the approach that came to dominance after World War Two in both the US and Britain – a model that gave rise to what we now understand as 'lifestyle medicine', which focuses attention on a model of prevention that primarily seeks to change individual behaviour rather than address the social, economic and structural determinants of health and disease.

> *The school health service should be of such educational value that children learn how to protect their health, to secure medical care when it is needed, and to accept reasonable responsibility for their own health and that of others. Moreover, the parents should be taught how to give their children the care necessary to promote health and maintain efficiency and happiness.*
>
> ***(Department of Health, 2004a)***

In this approach, the school health services (see p.108) were tasked with the goal of improving individual child and individual parental behaviours that affect child health. *Choosing Health* is, in fact, an example of policy shift that moves away from the interpretation of health improvement as a social issue (Acheson, 1998) to a prevention agenda based on increasing individual responsibility for health.

This tension between focusing on individual responsibility for individual health behaviours, on the one hand, and focusing on the social and economic determinants of health on the other hand, is a repeated theme in contemporary government policy on child health (see 'Thinking about the health inequalities agenda', p.104). Public health practitioners tend to respond to these messages by developing practical interventions that focus expertise either on single health issues (e.g. childhood obesity, drug and alcohol abuse, sexual health) or on individual groups of children and young people (e.g. adolescents, children with long-term conditions and/or disabilities, children excluded from school, looked-after children).

In other words, when we think about the school as location for health promotion, we immediately confront a range of questions about the meaning and practice of health promotion itself. In this context, it is helpful to conceptualize our understanding of both the school setting and of what we mean by health promotion, in order to ask ourselves whether and how the school can function as a setting for improving the health of children and young people. *Choosing Health* (Department of Health, 2004a) signalled a focus on individual behaviour, 'lifestyle medicine', rather than on community responsibility, whereas *Extended Schools and Health Services* (DfES and Department of Health, 2006) articulated health improvement as a joint community, family and school responsibility. At best, we can say that there are apparent oscillations in policy approach in the UK, but we can also see that the practice of health promotion itself is not a simple matter of single interventions alone, despite their importance as a platform for practice.

WHAT DO WE MEAN BY HEALTH PROMOTION?

The concept of health promotion first developed out of the discipline of public health in the 1970s. The seminal moment occurred at the Alma Ata, Kazakhstan, International Conference on Primary Health Care in 1978, with commitment to 'an acceptable level of health for all the people of the world by the year 2000' (World Health Organization, 1978). What lay behind this declaration was a conceptual shift away from a primary dependence on vertical healthcare systems (hospital-based and specialist-orientated medicine) to a vision of integrated family- and community-based health care as the lead organizing principle for healthcare systems across the world. In other words, this was a social model of medicine aspiring to the principles of participation, intersectoral collaboration and equity – effectively, an empowerment agenda based within a primary healthcare system.

What made the Alma Ata declaration so radical in 1978 was the shift of focus away from a hospital/medicine-led concept of health and health care, to a vision of services delivered at community level – where people live and work. But Donald Court, in the UK, had already argued for the preventive community agenda by 1976 when he chaired the UK Commission of Enquiry into the Child Health Service.

The connection between health and education is one of the most important aspects of paediatrics. In general our understanding of disorders of learning is still rudimentary, and the problems of intellectual limitation, defective speech, inadequate reading ability, excessive clumsiness, disturbed behaviour, truancy, school phobia and delinquency create a formidable array of disability. These problems will yield only to the combined efforts of doctors, teachers, psychologists, social workers and others. Yet we have found a good deal of evidence that as yet services were not disposed to co-operate in the interests of the child.

(Court, 1976, p.3)

In November 1986, the Alma Ata targets were re-invoked with the signing of the Ottawa Charter for Health Promotion in Canada at the First International Conference on Health Promotion (World Health Organization, 1986). This initial programme was more a checklist than a strategy. Yet the outcome has been the development of what we now refer to as health promotion, a sophisticated way of thinking about the improvement of health across whole populations. In effect, the primary healthcare movement and the health-promotion movement grew up alongside each other.

At the same time, health promotion, as a concept, has been fraught with debate and confusion. And where child health is concerned, health promotion is a concept that is often used when we actually mean health education, which is best described as a subset activity of work within health promotion.

For example, it is helpful to separate formal teaching programmes about health issues (e.g. dental hygiene, puberty, and the subjects within the personal, social and health education (PSHE) curriculum) from health-promotion work *per se*. Only when we have made this discrimination can we begin to talk about the vectors of activities, interventions and responsibilities that make up the work of health promotion in the school environment.

There is inevitably a pressure to define health promotion as a product in terms of interventions and activities (see below) when, in fact, it is part of an emerging pressure toward citizen participation and empowerment. Health promotion might best be thought of in terms of a political communication strategy, and it arises from arguments based in social medicine. And even here it is not without its critics, who argue that health promotion over-emphasizes interventions designed to modify individual behaviour, and neglects the social and economic contexts that determine behaviour (Sidell *et al.*, 1997).

In other words, there is a basic uncertainty about the parameters of health promotion. How, for example, do you build strategies for health improvement if the social, economic or political environment is toxic?

The underpinnings of debate about the meaning of health promotion in the UK also arise from shifts and changes in government policy over the last three decades. For example, the Black Report in 1980 identified the correlation between poor health and low income in modern Britain, but the findings were suppressed by the Conservative government of the time (Black, 1980). Public health practitioners and managers have reported to us that, until 1997, they were instructed by central government not to use the term 'inequalities' in their analyses.

The Acheson Report (1998) signalled a re-focus of attention on the link between socio-economic and health inequalities as explanations for population health profiles (see 'Thinking about the health inequalities agenda', p.104). Yet, by 2004 the policy agenda had shifted attention back again to individual responsibility for health (Department of Health, 2004a). This kind of policy oscillation would return the UK (notably England) to roughly the position that preceded election of the Labour government in 1997. Having said that, there is considerable pressure from both sides of the Atlantic to broaden the analysis of health determinants to a view that encompasses the social, economic and structural factors that influence population-level differences in patterns of health and illness.

In 1993, Labonté designed a model to describe the interaction between three environmental spheres – the community, the natural environment and the economy – in an attempt to visualize the way these factors interact to promote or to inhibit health (see Fig. 5.1).

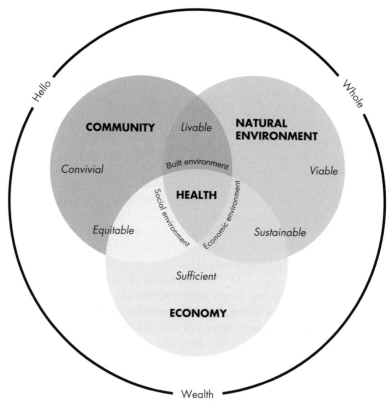

Figure 5.1 Labonté's 1993 holosphere of healthy and sustainable communities. Taken from Butler CD, Friel S (October 2006) Time to Regenerate: Ecosystems and Health Promotion. *PLoS Medicine* 3:10, p.1693, under Creative Commons Attribution License. Derived from Labonté (1993) A holosphere of healthy and sustainable communities. *Australian and New Zealand Journal of Public Health* 17:4–12.

The health inequalities arguments that are proving to have significant effect on both sides of the Atlantic focus on two of Labonté's spheres – the community and the economy. They do not, in fact, attend closely to the natural environment though they invoke the social environment (e.g. roads, housing, safe play areas). The natural environment is a contentious arena for health promotion, but at an international level, it is evident that Labonté's full model is important. Chernobyl (Ukraine) and Bhopal (India), for example, are only two of many longstanding examples of environmental damage that continue to compromise child health. War and civil strife are further examples of 21st century toxic environments.

LOOKING MORE CLOSELY AT HEALTH PROMOTION

At base, health promotion tends toward two areas of activity:

• modifying people's behaviour
• protecting the public through regulatory measures in law.

These two directions often lead to debate about the territory and the purpose of health-promotion work. Which focus should take the lead – behavioural change or regulatory legislation? Government policy continuously oscillates between these two pressures. Reducing smoking and improving nutrition are two useful examples. One could argue that both behaviour change and legislation are necessary to achieve child health improvement in these areas, but they are by no means easy to reconcile.

The questions that arise are about how intrusive the state should be in seeking to improve the health of the public. For example, we are familiar with charges about 'the nanny state' in Britain. If we stay with the examples of nutrition and tobacco use, we find both legislative and resource issues at play. Whether or not to ban tobacco smoking in public areas is only one example of difficult legislation. There are also linked resource issues. Taxes on cigarettes are a benefit to the Treasury; tension between industry regulation and the taxes accrued from the food and drinks industries are always problematic; costs to the Exchequer of providing subsidized school meals raise questions about whether or not to prioritize nutrition within the budget for state education. The list can be long and these are not new arguments.

Contemporary debates about school dinners are a useful example to use when we are thinking about child public health and the role of health promotion in the school in this way. For example, it is rather pointless to promote the 'five a day' fruit and vegetable programme, and then send the child into a lunch that has neither. But the school nutrition landscape began to change significantly from September 2006, including legislation to control food industry advertising directed at children from January 2007.

To take the nutrition issue one step further as an example for exploring what health-promotion work means, it is useful to note that, at base, these are arguments that link into the 21st century public health concern about childhood obesity. In other words, we find an intersection of mixed responsibility when thinking about nutrition, health, the school environment, financial costs to the government of healthy food, and individual child-eating behaviours (the family context and the food industry effect).

This coalescence of factors underpins the theory base for health promotion in the following ways. First, historically, successes in improving health have derived from better housing; improved water supplies and sanitation; safer conditions in the workplace; education; the alleviation of poverty; and the general provision of health and social care services. These agenda items do not remain stable and they require continuous revisiting. For example, Pearson reported findings in 2002 from a health visitor and district nurse seconded to a Newcastle housing department

> *Housing officers often made their decisions about housing in the virtual absence of health information.*
> **(Pearson, 2002, p.59)**

Second, the larger social and economic context in which children live their lives impacts on their health, regardless of individual health behaviours. Furthermore, Benzeval *et al.* were arguing, prior to the change of government in the UK in 1997

> *... since much health-related behaviour itself is socially determined, it is people's circumstances that are the most important determinant of health.*
> **(Benzeval et al., 1997, p.17)**

In 1991, Dahlgren and Whitehead conceptualized health promotion in a model that quickly became the dominant visual representation of the determinants of health (see Fig. 5.2). Their purpose was to seek a way of identifying the factors that affect population health, in order to identify both the policy

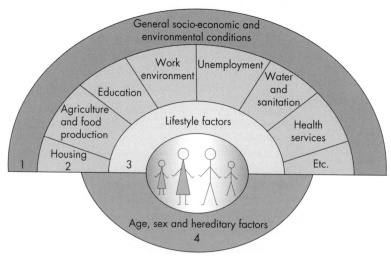

Figure 5.2 Determinants of health. (Reproduced with permission from Dahlgren and Whitehead [1991] *Policies and Strategies to Promote Social Equity in Health*. Stockholm: Institute for Future Studies.)

maker's and the practitioner's place in developing a preventive model of health care that could challenge the dominant curative or medical model. Dahlgren and Whitehead (1991) drew explicit attention to the complexity of social, political, economic, and structural factors that determine health.

This model has been an influential method for conceptualizing the vectors of health-promotion work in the UK for almost two decades. The outer circle refers to the upstream activities of governments at national and international levels, whereas the inner circle draws attention to the personal and the individual. It is at the inner two circles that health-promotion interventions tend to be found. Yet,

> *Effective action to improve people's health co-ordinates activities at all the levels. There is a complex relationship between the worlds in which people live, how they collectively and individually make sense of what happens around them throughout their lives, and how those happenings affect their mental and physical health.*
>
> **(Heer and Woodhead, 2002, p.4)**

It is this co-ordinating activity that is at the heart of repeated calls for cross-departmental and interprofessional collaboration that we find in recent UK policy. It is perhaps the most difficult agenda of all activities for health-promotion work to operationalize, and it is the task of public health practice to do just that.

Furthermore, when we think about child public health, we don't often ask children themselves what their own views are of their health and of their health needs. How, then, do we choose the health issues that we believe we should 'promote'? In other words, what do we know about children's wishes and desires about their own health? And if we did seek the views of children and young people, would we be better able to promote their health?

There exist rarely mentioned and often forgotten human rights protections in Articles 23 to 27 of the 1948 Universal Declaration of Human Rights. Here is Article 25:

> *Everyone has the right to a standard of living adequate for the health and well-being of himself and of his family, including food, clothing, housing and medical care and necessary social services, and the right to security in the event of unemployment, sickness, disability, widow-hood, old age or other lack of livelihood in circumstances beyond his control.*
>
> **(Universal Declaration of Human Rights 1948, Article 25)**

In discussions of children's health within the context of children's rights, we generally refer to Article 12 of the United Nations Convention on the Rights of the Child 1989 (see Chapter 11), but Article 25 of the 1948 agreement provides us with a context for thinking about the rights of the child by specifying our responsibility to the total social context in which the child lives. This is perhaps as good a place as any to position our thinking when we seek to reflect on the meaning of health promotion for children and young people.

THINKING ABOUT THE HEALTH INEQUALITIES AGENDA

How far can people have responsibility for their health if the means to health are outside their control?

(Sidell et al., 1997, p.2)

By the end of the 20th century, the international evidence of the effect of socio-economic inequalities on health had become compelling. Findings from the UK 1991 Census and the 2001 Census both found that families with children were over-represented at the lower end of the income distribution scales, with research providing evidence of a strong association between low income and poor health. Yet in the 1960s, theorists were convinced that social progress would effectively succeed in eliminating the socio-economic gap within the populations of industrialized countries. That has not happened. In fact, we see a widening gap.

Much of the recent evidence linking poor health and low income has derived from research initiated in the UK and in the US. It is not an evidence base without argument and dissent, but it is an evidence base that has influenced government policy in the UK since 1997.

People who live in disadvantaged circumstances have more illnesses, greater distress, more disability and shorter lives than those who are more affluent. Such injustice could be prevented, but this requires political will. The question is: can British policy makers rise to the challenge?

(Benzeval et al., 1997, p.16)

These insights are not new. They were documented in Britain as early as the 1860s. And, notably, Benzeval's argument preceded the change of government in 1997. These insights did, however, immediately become the source of the new government's policy on public health in 1997, and the factors that have directed public health practice since the turn of the new century. Investment in research in the area known as 'health inequalities' has also intensified with a view to proving in repeated studies that the link between socio-economic inequalities and poor health is without question (Wilkinson, 1996; Kawachi *et al.*, 1999; Bartley, 2003; Marmot, 2004; and others). Political economists have been seeking to refine this argument (Hofrichter, 2003), but poverty is at the core of international debates about the determinants of health, notably child health. The question that follows is about how health-promotion activities in the school setting can grapple with the effects of poverty on child health.

Commenting on poor health in Scotland, Macintyre and Hart observed:

There has been a lot of research describing, and attempting to explain, inequalities in health; but much less on effective ways of reducing them.

(Macintyre and Hart, 2000, p.2)

Turn of the century policy in the UK, and differentially in other developed countries, has largely argued the health inequalities premise as the primary determinant of child health. Yet, by 2004, the resource costs to governments of seeking to eradicate socio-economic differences had become increasingly problematic and ideologically uncomfortable, and rather than diminishing, the gap between rich and poor has continued to widen. By 2004, the publication of *Choosing Health* (Department of Health, 2004a) signalled a change in policy direction in England designed to shift responsibility back to the individual and away from the state as the primary vehicle for improving health. And, in late 2006, the UK prime minister announced a review designed to introduce a new social contract setting out what individuals must do in return for receiving services from health, schools and the police.

In effect, this suggests a return to the earlier 'lifestyle behaviours' approach that emerged, though in different forms, in both the UK and the US after World War Two, and it is located within a medical and individual self-care paradigm. It is also at the core of the debate about personal versus state responsibility for the cost of health, education and social care services.

Nevertheless, this shift of investment emphasis has been noticeably uneven. Preschool children in deprived areas of the UK continue to be the focus for resource investment – mainly via Sure Start and Sure Start Plus. The school-age child, however, has come in and out of focus. The Children's Fund for school-age children was launched in 2000 with a generous profile of resources, but was due to cease in 2006 (extended to 2008). Children's trusts, virtual organizations of co-ordinated care and support were first put in position from 2003 (operational from April 2004), and the re-organization of social care and education budgets for children into co-ordinated leadership by single, local authority-based children's services was formalized in England from April 2006.

School-based health services for school-age children, however, remain differentially resourced across all four countries of the UK. And school health services have returned to an uncertain future, as primary healthcare services in the UK adjust simultaneously to structural change and demand for significant cost savings.

In other words, the overall policy picture is one that argues the health inequalities agenda while, at the same time, it often de-prioritizes services that meet the collective or community needs of school-age children compared with the size of resources for preschool children in deprived geographical areas. This is probably the case because of the resource implications and the complexity involved in restructuring public sector provision, the principle resource for child public health practice.

THE HEALTHY SCHOOLS PROGRAMME

A health promoting school is one in which all members of the school community work together to provide children and young people with integrated and positive experiences and structures, which promote and protect their health. This includes both the formal and the informal curriculum in health, the creation of a safe and healthy school environment, the provision of appropriate health services and the involvement of the family and wider community in efforts to promote health.

(Burgher et al., 1999, p.4)

This vision is a fully holistic paradigm of health promotion for school-age children and was agreed by the World Health Organization (WHO) in 1995. However, from its outset, the UK's response to the WHO agenda, the National Healthy Schools Programme (NHSP), has been a voluntary code of practice. Schools are not obliged, though they are strongly encouraged, to participate in the NHSP. The target is to achieve 100 per cent of state-maintained schools participating in England by the end of 2009, with 75 per cent achieving recognized standards. Scotland, Wales and Northern Ireland have also set targets for participation. The programme was first announced in England in 1993 as a response to intended collaboration with the European Network of Health Promoting Schools. It is fair to say that little activity followed until the late 1990s when the NHSP was formally launched in October 1999. By 2005/06, however, the profile of NHSP was demonstrating active cross-departmental collaboration because of its position as a dual responsibility of both the Department of Health and the Department for Education and Skills.

The pressure on schools to participate in the NHSP has been increasing since the turn of the century. At its outset, however, the programme was a teacher-led initiative and this, in itself, slowed initial progress simply because of the absence of the health sector on so many of the key decision-making bodies that led the NHSP in each local authority in the early years.

The Healthy Schools Programme is organized around four themes against which schools are assessed in order to meet specified standards:

• personal, social and health education (PSHE), including sex and relationship education and drug education
• healthy eating
• physical activity
• emotional health and well-being (including bullying) (DfES and Department of Health, 2005).

However, the concept of a whole-school ethos that can promote health relies, inevitably, on the school understanding itself as a resource for children that is located within a broader community framework. It also relies on the school's ability to understand the community from a health perspective by working with other agencies and by combining resources with neighbourhood initiatives that promote child health.

Every school serves a different profile of social, economic and environmental need. For example, the charity Shelter has documented the devastating effects that bad housing alone is having on children's life chances in contemporary England, with more than one million children affected by 2006. Up to 25 per cent of children in England have an increased risk of severe ill-health and disability during childhood and early adulthood as a direct consequence of bad housing (Harker, 2006, p.8). But poor housing is generally clustered in areas of high deprivation and does not affect all school communities equally, thus the need for local school assessments of community-level factors that can affect child health in school (see Mosley and Moorhouse's [2000] example of the Huddersfield profile).

Poor housing alone can impact on a child or young person's ability to learn at school, either because of physical illness, mental health distress or the consequences of accidents[1] directly linked to poor housing. It is, furthermore, an example of the way in which health-promotion work cannot be divorced from the material and cultural environment in which the school is sited. Understanding the community outside the school gates both broadens understanding of child health within the school environment and also deepens understanding of the kinds of health-promotion work that are best designed for any particular school. It is what is meant by a public health approach to health promotion in the school setting.

In other words, child health-promotion work is not simply about lifestyle change. Lifestyle behaviours derive from and are a consequence of social and community cultures. Within a school, for example, the external environment may be such that internal school focus on, for example, obesity or on sexual health may be effectively negated if the child's community and home environment are not factored into the approach. This does not obviate the need for health-promotion interventions focused on lifestyle behaviours (see Chapter 10), but it does demonstrate the need to take the larger social and economic context into consideration.

THINKING ABOUT 'SOCIAL CAPITAL' IN HEALTH-PROMOTION WORK

It was in studies of rural school community centres in the US that the notion of social capital as a factor that affects health first emerged. Hanifan (1916, 1920) introduced the term to describe 'those tangible substances [that] count for most in the daily lives of people' (Hanifan, 1916, p.130), and by this he was referring to the cultivation of good will, fellowship, sympathy and social intercourse, signifiers of a healthy community such as the kind that affects child health in the school environment.

The concept of 'social capital', however, has only recently entered the arena of debates about health and it is used elsewhere in this book. Effectively, it can be used here to talk about the school's ability to work within the local community as a social unit, and as a way of describing the internal school community beyond its articulation as simply a group of individual teachers and individual children. This is where the link between an ethos of healthy schools and a concept of health promotion effectively come together.

In other words, lifestyle behaviours derive from and are a consequence of social and community cultures. They are not simply decisions made by individual children alone. Furthermore, health promotion becomes increasingly difficult in the school-age years as the child develops and grows – particularly during adolescence. As the child gains increasing independence over time, the challenges to 'making a difference' in health outcomes actually mean that successful

[1] Two million children every year are taken to an emergency department as the consequence of accidental injury (Child Accident Prevention Trust, 2006). Accidental injury is the single largest cause of death among children after the age of 1 year in the UK, and the leading cause of disability (Botting, 1995).

outcomes depend more and more on the health-promotion skills of the adults with whom young people come into contact.

The encouragement toward behaviours that are conducive to personal health and well-being is a complex field (see Lister-Sharp *et al.*, 1999). Success relies on the child's or family's motivation and, particularly, success depends on the child's social, cultural and economic environment. Apart from the many environmental factors (safe play areas, healthy food, access to pleasurable physical activity, safe roads, homes and housing), most health-promoting behaviours are also subject to public agencies' abilities to maximize the opportunities to make healthy personal decisions, and are subject to providing access to accurate information (e.g. the information that young people need in order to make decisions about sexual health). Maximizing the circumstances and opportunities in which these enabling factors are available to children and young people is also a part of the health-promotion map in the school environment.

The interaction between individual behaviours and community-level opportunities for improving health is also complex. The English government policy position on the intersection between school and child health is reflected in *Choosing Health* (Department of Health, 2004a) and in *Higher Standards, Better Schools for All* (DfES, 2005a). But these do not go far enough alone.

Lister-Sharp *et al.* (1999) conducted two systematic reviews of the health-promoting schools approach, and these remain the most comprehensive studies achieved by 2007. In their work, they report findings consistent with a concept of social capital,

> *Overall, a multifaceted approach is likely to be most effective, combining a classroom programme with changes to the school ethos and/or environment and/or with family/community involvement.*
> **(Lister-Sharp et al., 1999, p.v)**

THE SCHOOL HEALTH SERVICE

The past decade has witnessed the most radical change in school nurse practice in the whole of its long history, including the virtual disappearance of the school medical officer – a change that has removed 'the doctor's handmaiden' role from the activities and planning of school nursing. Furthermore, 'There has been a paradigm shift in school nurse practice from a medical model to a social model of working' (DeBell and Tomkins, 2006, p.18). Yet, at the same time, the service has not increased in size during the past decade (a maximum of 3000 nurses – most working part-time – for about 11.2 million school-age children in the UK).

The education and training base for the service has been upgraded significantly, and the next decade is also likely to be a critical period in service development, including questions about service redesign. School nursing was first identified as 'child centred public health' in 2002 (Department of Health, 2002) in England. Scotland in 2006 announced plans to introduce community healthcare nursing – school nursing, health visiting and district nursing. In other words, the public health practitioner focus is moving the traditional school nurse service toward the introduction of specialist public health practitioners who can provide the school-age child focus that has always been the rationale behind school nursing.

A provision for health within the school environment has been an issue in the British education system since at least the late 19th century, a point at which the poor health of recruits to the Boer War revealed harm to the health of boys in England's cities and towns, probably originating in the urban working classes because of the Industrial Revolution (Denman *et al.*, 2002). As a consequence, schools were early identified as an ideal setting to promote child health (Harris, 1995). As early as 1882, the Department of Education had issued a policy paper allowing schools to close or to exclude pupils from attending in order to control the spread of infectious disease. These early public health interventions indicated an understanding of the link between the school and a child's health (i.e. the school as a gathering point with potential for targeting infection control and later immunization delivery). However, the perceived link between child health and the school environment was not originally so much about the child as about the consequences of poor child health, mainly boys' health, as a national resource to be protected.

Little, however, was formally accomplished until the Board of Education published a handbook, *Suggestions on Health Education* in 1939 (McNalty, 1939), when a whole-school approach was first argued. This proposal made little headway until 1968 when the Department of Education and Science published its *Handbook for Health Education* (1968). Still, this document fell short of establishing health as a subject within the curriculum.

From small beginnings (one school medical officer in London in 1890 and one school nurse in 1892), the Education (Administrative Provisions) Act of 1907 recognized the school as a location for child health attention by placing a legal obligation on schools to consider the health of the children in their care with a duty placed on school boards

> to provide for the medical inspection of children immediately before, or at the time of, or as soon as possible after, their admission to a public elementary school and on such occasions as the Board of Education direct.
>
> ***(The Education (Administrative Provisions)***
> ***Act 1907, Section 13(1)(b))***

Historically, the repeated impetus of attention to child health was triggered by the need for healthy army recruits. For example, in 1904, as many as 60 per cent of boys were found to be unfit for duty because of poor eyesight, dental caries, heart disease and poor growth arising from poor childhood health (Leff and Leff, 1959). A range of public health reforms designed to improve child health followed – the Open Spaces Act 1906; the Education (Provision of Meals) Act 1906; the Education (Administrative Provisions) Act 1907; the Notification of Births Act 1907; and the Maternity and Child Welfare Act 1918.

Until at least the end of the 20th century, the developing school health services continued to retain as their primary function a screening and surveillance service – the identification of physical health problems, the detection and correction of poor hygiene and malnutrition, and, where possible, the ameliora-tion of the effects of disability. For example, the Education Act 1918 extended the duties of local education authorities by requiring provision of services for the treatment of minor ailments within primary schools and by extending medical inspections to young people in secondary schools. Despite this largely reactive orientation to health provision, Polnay argued in 1995 that school nurses have continuously linked their service back to its original public health roots by means of their historic support for young people's emotional and well-being needs. As far back as the 1950s it was acknowledged that school nurses supported young people in relation to their emotional health and well-being.

In secondary schools adolescent girls often consult her [the school nurse] … and she can do much to help them and relieve their anxiety.

(Leff and Leff, 1959)

In other words, the contemporary school drop-in centres provided by school nurses in order to promote child and adolescent health have a long and surpris-ingly robust history given the uncertainty that has always surrounded the health–education link.

The school health service in the UK has also been problematically situated. Until 1974, school nurses and medical officers were employed by local education authorities. This is the pattern of employment for school nursing in most coun-tries across the world (i.e. school nurses tend to be directly employed by schools or school districts). But in 1974, school nursing transferred to the NHS in the UK. The aim of this new health service for children was to bring together health professionals (e.g. community and hospital paediatricians, clinical medical offi-cers, school nurses, audiologists, speech and language therapists, psychologists and community physiotherapists) in order to provide preschool, school health, hospital and specialist services. The success of this integrated approach to child health has always been patchy, and the consequence for school health services has been to create a profile whereby health has been located outside and separate from the education domain. Furthermore, school nursing as the lead health link has not been universally accepted by schools, despite the fact that most schools do rely heavily on school nurses. Where successful, the development of school nursing has had as much to do with the ingenuity of school nurses as it has had to do with the ability of individual schools to understand the service.

Having said that, it was the Court Report (1976) that caught the sense of radical change in focus to a community-based service, by arguing that child health should be at the centre of planning. Yet, Court drew explicit attention to the inability of services to co-operate across departmental boundaries, 'ser-vices were not disposed to co-operate in the interests of the child' (Court, 1976, p.3). This was a shift of focus, not fully followed up, that understood the community principles that would come to emerge as the health-promotion and primary care movements of the 1980s.

However, what is striking about the school health service in the early years of the 21st century is its commitment to the health of the school-age population rather than its sense of itself as primarily a service for schools. That commitment now takes the form of services delivered at school, in the community, and with families. Scotland, for example, has recognized this with proposals to incorporate health visiting and school nursing as a common service delivering a public health nursing practitioner role for children and young people. Furthermore, Scotland has specified the functional public health role for school nursing as operating within a community as well as a school setting.

> *The national school nursing framework broadens the role of school nursing to include developing health needs assessment for schools, more active involvement in health promotion and supporting schools with the change required to enable mainstreaming of children who require additional support for learning. By 2007, all schools will be expected to become Integrated Community Schools and school nurses will be an integral part of the multi-disciplinary team.*
> **(Scottish Executive, 2003, Summary point 11)**

This is an agenda that matches the aspirations of school nurses themselves (DeBell and Everett, 1997; DeBell and Jackson 2000; DeBell and Tomkins, 2006). How Scotland will actually interpret the functions of school nursing within community nursing is yet to be seen.

THE EXTENDED SCHOOLS INITIATIVE

Firmly based in a long tradition of community development within Britain, the Full Service Extended Schools (FSES) initiative was launched in 2001, became operational in 2003, and is part of a government vision for all schools to offer a core set of additional activities and services in the school environment by 2010.

> *The FSES initiative seeks to support the development in every local authority (LA) area of one or more schools which provide a comprehensive range of services on a single site, including access to health services, adult learning and community activities as well as study support and 8 am to 6 pm wrap-around childcare.*
> **(Cummings et al., 2006, p.ii)**

The location of schools within local communities coupled with their estate value (NB, the buildings themselves are not in use much of the day/year) has always raised questions about how better to maximize use of this resource. The FSES initiative is an imaginative and potentially valuable way of bringing together services that need to be delivered locally, by using the school building itself, its resources, its leadership, and its location. Furthermore, maximizing the use of the schools estate such that schools can become the locus of enhanced services for children and their families makes good community sense.

The first-year rollout of the initiative (2004–05) funded Extended Schools located in Behaviour Improvement Programme (BIP) areas (61 projects in year one). This was a way of focusing services on areas with higher deprivation levels. Year-two rollout (25 additional schools in BIP areas and 20 in non-BIP areas) included clusters of schools working together as single FSES sites. By autumn 2006, more than 3000 schools in England had joined the programme (Training and Development Agency for Schools, 2006).

The initial short-term goals were linked to improving educational achievement levels but the longer-term goals are about the family and community agenda. Project leaders in the first two years sought to embed their work within the framework of the *Every Child Matters: change for children* (HM Government, 2004) agenda. But, significantly, the profile of work is dependent on how well each Extended School is able to develop collaborative, cross-departmental work, and this is at the core of national pressure to find ways to ensure that services work together. This is not an easy agenda. However, there is a long tradition of community-oriented schooling in the UK, and this initiative builds on that by specifying 'full service schools'. The head teachers of the pilot schools have been described as 'enthusiasts' by the Universities of Manchester and Newcastle evaluators (Cummings *et al.*, 2006, p.3). This is unsurprising but it helps to explain the participation rates of schools given the relatively small financial investment in the scheme (£93 000 in year one; £163 000 in year two). However, a question arises about the sustainability of the initiative once funding is reduced and then ceases.

'Reducing health inequalities' is one of many goals within the FSES. In effect, it comes into play by nature of the focus on attending to family and child needs as a whole, whether these are additional learning opportunities (for adults as well as children); school breakfast schemes; or sustained assistance to children who have behavioural problems (i.e. mental health problems – see Chapter 8); or to children who are at risk.

What does this mean for health promotion in the school setting? The FSES has a community empowerment agenda, though this is articulated in a variety of ways. The principle message thus far suggests that Extended Schools tend to (1) make parents feel welcome in the school (open door policy and adult education provision); (2) engage health and social care professionals in the school environment as a way of assisting families in difficulty, including housing difficulties; (3) provide parenting support programmes; (4) resist the quick route of school exclusion by involving child and adolescent mental health specialists in problem solving; (5) participate directly in other community activities.

In effect, these are health-promotion interventions that understand the relationship between the family, the school and the child. Not all schools have been equally successful. Some have reported the familiar difficulty of engaging non-education professionals in their extended work. Others, such as rural schools and special schools have reported difficulties arising from poor transport facilities to the school.

However, the determination to involve non-teacher professionals and voluntary workers in the community-enhancement agenda of the FSES suggests that

> there is some evidence that this configuration around schools maximizes some opportunities for the delivery of services in disadvantaged neighbourhoods.

(Cummings et al., 2006, p.25)

THE CHILD GROWING UP AT SCHOOL

What is particularly noticeable about the FSES initiative is the interpretation of child health and well-being in terms of those factors that are outside the school gates, factors that can make it difficult for a child to function at school because of the social, cultural and/or family environment in which they live. For these children, health-promotion interventions that rely wholly on health-education or health-promotion interventions confined within the school environment can have limited effect.

We have mainly talked about the larger issues, yet it is the child growing up through the school years that is also at issue. Difficulties and needs change during the growing up period. For example, we know that at least one in every ten children and adolescents (The Mental Health Foundation, 1999) or two in every ten children and adolescents (Office for National Statistics 2004) experience mental health distress at some point in the school-age years, and the nature of the presenting problem varies with the child's age. These experience of distress can be brief, prolonged, serious, or time-limited and self-correcting episodes (see Chapter 8). Teachers do not necessarily find this arena of child health easy, and many understandably do not see it as a part of their work profile. In fact, education professionals use a different language. They speak of 'emotional and behavioural problems', not 'mental health problems'.

In addition, consistent reporting over the past decade suggests that about 30 per cent of 16-year-old girls are sexually active. This is a critical health issue because sexual health can affect morbidity, fertility and mental health, and thereby needs to be a target for health promotion and for health education.

We also know that contemporary patterns of childhood nutrition and physical activity are in danger of reducing life expectancy, and we know that an entire generation of parents in the UK has never been taught to cook – school-based food technology was removed from the curriculum in the latter part of the 20th century. Furthermore, we know that too many children arrive at school without breakfast, and that their main meal may well be a school dinner with little nutritional value. The patterns and nature of food consumption, in the home and outside the home, have changed radically in the last decade alone, and the long-term task of improving nutrition and of finding ways to increase physical activity are just that – long-term tasks.

Furthermore, weighing and measuring children at school is effective for collecting epidemiological data (see Box 5.1), but this resource investment does nothing to address the underlying causes of poor nutrition. Indeed, height and weight measurement requires resources that might well be better targeted on health-promotion work in the school, the community and at the national regulatory level. These measurement issues continue to be a source of debate.

We also know that adolescence is a period when risk-taking behaviours increase and, indeed, risk taking is part of growing up. How to help young people think about risk taking is a significant issue for the health-promotion approach (see Chapter 10.)

Box 5.1 The national Childhood Height and Weight data collection programme

---

A key component of both influencing and monitoring obesity prevalence is through the establishment of a national Childhood Height and Weight data collection programme. The programme enables local data on childhood obesity to be collected to inform local planning and targeting of local resources and interventions; to enable tracking of local progress against the Public Service Agreement (PSA) target on obesity, and local performance management; and to improve understanding of the pattern, associated factors and causes of the obesity 'epidemic' among children.

Primary care trusts have now measured all schoolchildren in the reception year (ages 4 to 5 years) and those in year 6 (ages 10 and 11 years). Height and weight data will be used for the calculation of body mass index (BMI) in order to monitor obesity prevalence at a population level (Department of Health, 2006).

We also know that the transition periods in school life are critical moments for child health, notably child mental health. These occur when the child enters school, when the child changes from primary to middle school, and particularly, when the child transfers to secondary school. These are periods of uncertainty and anxiety for every child. Health promotion takes on a particular meaning at such points, if only in terms of assisting children to cope with the stress of being young and vulnerable amongst a new set of peers who are older and who can be frightening. Bullying in UK schools has not decreased, but it can be countered by both the school culture and health and social care professionals if they are integrated within the school itself. It is a factor, for example, when we think about the school as the child's place of work.

Yet we also know that health issues become more, rather than less, difficult to introduce into large secondary schools (from the age of 12 years). This is the critical period of developing independence and it is a critical time for child development (see *Youth Matters*, DfES 2005b). Furthermore, further education colleges now tend to enrol young people from the age of 14 years, but they are the least likely educational environment to take responsibility for adolescent health-promotion work.

And, finally, we have long known that children with disabilities, long-term conditions, and/or complex health needs experience the school years as difficult and problematic (see Chapter 9).

The profile of necessary skills and competencies that practitioners need to have also changes as the child grows and develops from school entry at the age of 4 or 5 years, through the adolescent period and into transition for adulthood. An understanding of the patterns of ill-health and the determinants of health at each stage place singular demands on health-promotion work, and are fundamental for public health practice.

HEALTH EDUCATION IN THE CURRICULUM

Since 2005, schools in England have been encouraged, but not required to use curriculum time for the purpose of developing a more formal role in providing for children's and young people's health. The policy position is that personal, social and health education (the PSHE curriculum) should create a formal structure for the teaching of spiritual, moral and cultural values (Office for Standards in Education (Ofsted), 2005a). The PSHE curriculum, however, is broad, and the concepts within it are open to interpretation by each individual school team. Furthermore, schools face the challenges of finding staff who are sufficiently trained and skilled in order to deliver the curriculum.

To this end, a certification programme (DfES, 2002) has been created to enable joint skills development for teachers and community nurses such that they can work together in delivering the PSHE curriculum. Its purpose is to:

- improve the confidence of teachers and community nurses delivering PSHE in schools and out of schools settings
- provide recognition for individual teachers' and community nurses' experience and skills
- improve the quality and effectiveness of PSHE provided to children and young people
- raise the profile of PSHE
- contribute to the United Kingdom's Teenage Pregnancy Strategy's goal to halve under-18 conception rates by 2010 (Social Exclusion Unit, 1999)
- address issues relating to health inequalities and social inclusion.

The programme was initially devised in response to a report by Ofsted (2002), which highlighted the need for sex and relationship education (SRE) in schools. The SRE curriculum was prompted by the perceived need to establish specialist teams, particularly within secondary schools, that could promote the improvement of young people's sexual health. The certification programme now covers the broader PSHE programme, with a target to achieve at least one trained teacher in every secondary school and one community nurse who can support the school. Again, these are targets – not requirements.

Furthermore, reports from school nurses over the past decade have indicated that teachers often ask healthcare staff to assist them in the classroom when they deliver health education.

This determination to focus joint teacher and community nurse attention on child health is new, and it is underpinned by a range of initiatives that are designed to build into schools a sense of formal responsibility for child health (see 'The Healthy Schools Programme', p.105, and the *Healthy Living Blueprint*, Department of Health, 2004b). Because school constitutes the setting for a very significant proportion of a child's life over many years, and because school is the child's place of work, it is an opportune location for promoting health and delivering health messages and health services. Schools are in a position to reach large numbers of children and young people over the highly formative years from early childhood to adolescence (Naidoo and Wills, 1998).

The purpose of health education within the curriculum is to provide children and young people with a working knowledge about issues that are important to their health (Stewart-Brown, 1998). However, a question immediately arises about the relationship between formal information and its capacity to influence health and health-related behaviours (see Chapter 10).

What children do with the information they receive at school depends on their personal priorities, resources, their attitudes to and understanding of risk, and their self-perception. Ofsted (2005a) reported support for the concept that education about health issues should involve information and knowledge, but also argued that this, in itself, is insufficient and added that children also require skill development. In other words, Ofsted called attention to the need for children and young people to have opportunities at school to formulate, develop and explore their own values and attitudes to health.

There is little argument to suggest that the concept of PSHE as a formal part of the curriculum is other than an appropriate direction of travel for schools. Yet it remains a non-statutory subject within the National Curriculum, and has only recently been introduced as formal guidance. By 2005, a framework developed by the Qualifications and Curriculum Authority (Ofsted 2005b) was in place, with the purpose of assisting schools in planning their PSHE programmes for each age group. There has been considerable debate about whether or not PSHE, like the citizenship curriculum and the sex and relationship curriculum (SRE), should become a statutory subject for all children and young people.

Schools are under pressure to meet government assessment targets, particularly for numeracy, literacy and science. The consequence over recent decades has been steadily to squeeze curriculum time, thereby leaving little latitude during the school day for contextual subjects in the informal curriculum, such as child health. This means that PSHE can, and often does, become marginalized within the curriculum (Naidoo and Wills, 1998). In fact, Ofsted reported in 2005a that some schools do not provide PSHE within the curriculum at all.

Head teachers and their governing bodies are responsible for decisions about the introduction of subjects for study that are additional to core subjects required by statute. There can be a number of reasons for not including formal health-education teaching within the curriculum timetable:

• lack of staff (education and healthcare staff) with appropriate expertise
• history of not perceiving health matters as a school responsibility apart from SEN (under statutory requirement)[2]
• a decision to prioritize other subjects.

[2] SEN is a statutory identifier referring to learning difficulties and disabilities. 'The term learning difficulties and/or disabilities is used to refer to individuals or groups of learners who have either a learning difficulty in relation to acquiring new skills or who learn at a different rate to their peers. The term is used to cross the professional boundaries between education, health and social services and to incorporate a common language from 0–19. The Disability Discrimination Act defines that, "a person has a disability if he or she has a physical or mental impairment that has a substantial and long-term adverse effect on his or her ability to carry out normal day-to-day activities". Physical or mental impairments can include sensory impairments and learning difficulties. The definition also covers medical conditions when they have long-term and substantial effects on pupils' everyday lives. Those designated with special educational needs (SEN) under current legislation (education) all have learning difficulties and/or disabilities that make it harder for them to learn than most learners of the same age' (Ofsted, 2005b, p.3).

However, Ofsted argues that when schools do not play their part in providing for PSHE, they are assuming an untenable position. Policy direction arising from government position papers such as *Every Child Matters: change for children* (HM Government, 2004) and *National Healthy School Status: a guide for schools* (DfES and Department of Health, 2005) also highlight the responsibilities that schools should assume in order to ensure that children and young people achieve better health outcomes. The implicit position is that health status affects ability to learn. The explicit position is evidence of a high correlation between poor health and low educational achievement.

Arguments in the field suggest that within PSHE, children and young people can gain knowledge, develop life skills, and formulate attitudes that are crucial building blocks for living successfully in social environments, and which thus prepare children and young people for the experiences and responsibilities of later life. Such skills include improved communication skills; interpersonal and decision-making skills; abilities in negotiating, formulating and presenting arguments; skills in comparing and contrasting others' views; team and group skills; as well as skills in independent thinking. These are large claims and, if sustainable, they imply that a curriculum-framed input for health-related work would be of considerable value to children and young people during their school years.

The Independent Advisory Group on Sexual Health and Teenage Pregnancy (2005) recommends that PSHE should become a statutory subject for both primary and secondary schools. The outcomes specified in *Every Child Matters: change for children* (HM Government, 2004) are required of all statutory bodies working with children and young people. This includes schools. At present, the only curriculum space, as opposed to other school functions and activities, lies within the PSHE specification.

The arguments for statutory inclusion of PSHE within the curriculum are also posited to be consistent with the larger policy push to improve school inclusion and reduce social inequalities. This is a macro-agenda that affects, in theory, all government departments, including schools. It is, however, a difficult agenda to operationalize, and one that has not been explicitly a school-based responsibility in the past. Some individual schools have always taken these concepts seriously in their work by focusing their attention on the wider community in which the school resides, and by articulating the school itself as an integrated community designed to support the whole of the child's experience at school in an integrated model of learning and health promotion. However, this again is a matter of leadership direction that has historically been left to the discretion of the head teacher.

The profile of expectation about how, and how well the curriculum can improve child health is relatively new (see the discussion of the Healthy Schools Programme, p.105).

The most powerful driver for change in schools' attitudes to child and adolescent health is likely to be the Ofsted (2005b, pp.7–8) *Framework for the Inspection of Children's Services*, which includes schools. The multi-agency inspectors and commissions responsible for implementing the Framework will have the power to specify 'failing schools', and their judgements will be articulations of each school's ability to achieve against the *Every Child Matters* (HM Government, 2004) framework.

The complex relationship between areas of responsibility for child health has beleaguered debates about the function of education since the introduction of compulsory schooling in the late 19th century – now for more than a century – and it continues to produce tension in debates about the function and parameters of responsibility for child health within the school environment. Furthermore, these debates carry a different inflection at different child ages. In other words, primary schools and middle schools tend to have more potential influence over child-health behaviours than do secondary schools. These differences arise from child receptivity to health-education and health-promotion interventions at different ages and stages as the child grows and develops, and they also arise from the very different relationships teachers have with children at each educational stage.

HEALTH-PROMOTION INTERVENTIONS BY PUBLIC HEALTH PRACTITIONERS

Accuracy of information, appropriacy to age and good timing are the three factors that Hall and Elliman (2003) identified as key to good health promotion. This implies that health-promotion work relies on the need to ensure that public health practitioners are cognizant of age-appropriate interventions as well as precisely accurate about the health information that children receive. Furthermore, health promotion is a matter of staged repetition. For example, sexual health promotion needs to be iterative and age appropriate. It also needs to be context specific. This means that location and timing of service delivery is as important for effectiveness as content (DeBell and Tomkins, 2006, p.12).

These are the skills required of those public health practitioners who conduct health-promotion interventions. The health priorities for such interventions arise from public health data and it takes time to gather, validate and analyse such data.

Health promotion is often thought of in terms of interventions. But, before public health practitioners select an issue for intervention for the purpose of improving an aspect of child or adolescent health, a series of steps will have determined the particular priority areas. First, considerable data will have been collected, validated and analysed at the national level in order to identify (1) the determinants of poor health within the total population; (2) the trends in health behaviours amongst the population that are causing poor health outcomes; and (3) the priorities for health-improvement actions.

At local level (regional and local authority levels), similar exercises will be carried out – mainly led by the Public Health Observatories. From these findings (information collection and analysis), priorities for action to improve local health emerge. This, for example, is the way in which childhood obesity emerged as a national priority for health improvement and thus a focus for health-promotion interventions by public health practitioners. *Health Profile of England* (Department of Health, 2006) is a recent example. It provides a picture of the 2004 health status of people in England. Similar exercises are conducted within Wales, Scotland and Northern Ireland.

These data and their analysis are not, however, fully comprehensive. The indicators, nevertheless, are used by healthcare commissioners to determine their investment priorities. The actual interventions by public health practitioners tend to develop over time, by means of close analysis of local population needs and in response to the most pressing need (NB, the alarm generated by increasing levels of obesity amongst children).

An example of sophisticated analysis at the local schools population level was conducted by school nurses Mosley and Moorhouse and published in March 2000 for Huddersfield. This work remains the template for identification of how best to conduct an analysis of the health and health needs of the school-age population, based on both local school and health service data. The work also included information from social care- and local authority-derived data.

However, we still need to ask ourselves the question, 'What are the priorities for child health promotion today?' It is probably fair to say that the areas of health-promotion intervention for children of school age by 2007 have become focused on the following issues (not prioritized):

- nutrition and physical activity
- child and adolescent mental health (emotional health and well-being, including bullying)
- accidental and non-accidental injury (including child protection)
- hygiene and dental health
- immunizations and protection from communicable disease
- sexual health and teenage pregnancy
- risk-taking behaviours, including tobacco, alcohol and illicit substance use
- long-term conditions, complex health needs, and disabilities.

Behind these issues for health promotion interventions lie the key determinants of health: socio-economic inequalities and child poverty; environmental factors such as housing; ethnicity, gender, age and disability profiles; geography; and lifestyle behaviours.

In other words, if we seek to 'improve health' or to 'promote health', we do need to ask ourselves what the baseline for 'health' is. The epidemiological approach begins from measurements of morbidity and mortality and identifies risk factors. This is the starting point for public health practice and for health promotion in the school environment.

PARENTAL VIEWS ON HEALTH PROMOTION IN THE SCHOOL ENVIRONMENT

Some parents rely wholly on the school to inform their children about basic health issues. This is particularly the case at puberty and adolescence with regard to sexual health matters. At the same time, a minority of parents object to the assertion that schools should teach their children about sensitive health matters such as sexual health. Anywhere along this spectrum, the issues of health matters and children's education can become either a collaborative or a dissonant relationship between parents/carers and schools. The repeated policy ideal is that collaborative and consultative approaches between schools and parents, and with other child-orientated agencies, should be the goal. The reality of how to achieve this is challenging.

An initiative to achieve progress toward parent/carer and school collaboration was proposed in the recommendations of *Higher Standards Betters Schools for All: more choice for parents and pupils* (DfES, 2005a). Parent councils are here recommended, in order to assist schools in making decisions relating to health issues such as school meal provision as well as curriculum changes and methods for monitoring parental satisfaction with schools. The policy aspiration is to ensure parental consultation and influence in school decision making. Where child health is concerned, the aspiration is to achieve a collaborative approach whereby parents replicate in the home the health messages provided by the school.

In the 1980s, a parallel approach was attempted with the introduction of parent representation on school governing bodies. The formality of that approach, however, tended inevitably to draw parental involvement from those parents/carers who were most confident and already most involved with their children's education. The new recommendation is for a wider forum of representation that can include the parental voice in decisions about the school curriculum, notably areas that are currently non-statutory elements and that lie within the informal curriculum.

Some parents and carers, for many reasons, require considerably greater levels of practical support in order to improve children's physical health and emotional well-being (see Chapter 4). To meet these needs, the policy aspiration is to put additional activities for parents in place in schools, such as workshops, parenting programmes, behaviour seminars and other related programmes led by health professionals, education staff, Connexions advisers, youth workers and others from the voluntary sector who work with children and young people. In addition, the schools' agenda in England is moving toward transferring greater responsibility for child care and child health to the school environment (see 'The Extended Schools initiative', p.111).

CONSULTING PUPILS

The Education Act 2002 requires all schools to include pupils in the decision-making processes about issues that affect them. Schools are expected to consult children and young people, and to respond to their needs in order to ensure that, for example, a PSHE programme is relevant and effective, and that the potential for learning is maximized fully (National Children's Bureau, 2003). This is in line with the UN Convention on the Rights of the Child 1989 (see Chapter 11).

A survey published by Ofsted (2002) found that few schools engaged pupils in planning or evaluating sex and relationship education (SRE) programmes or policies. (SRE is a tandem aspect of the informal curriculum focused on child health.) However, the report also highlighted areas where consultations do take place and, where this does occur, children and young people reported that they value such discussions and that the school gains fresh insights into the curriculum that can assist in longer-term development. It needs, however, to be emphasized that such consultations vary considerably in quality and depth. (See Kirk [Chapter 9] on the failure of schools to consult with children who have disabilities, long-term conditions or complex health needs.)

The introduction of school councils and the initiation of young people's focus groups have proved to be useful vehicles in gathering such information, including views about personal health and health-related priorities. The Welsh Assembly has taken this approach to a national level in its use of the Funky Dragon initiative, a national approach to consultation focused on participation of all school-age children.

THINKING ABOUT HEALTH-PROMOTION INTERVENTIONS

On the whole, public health practitioners begin to think about health promotion in the school setting from either the perspective of health risk to children (e.g. road safety, reductions in risk taking) or from the perspective of health improvement (e.g. nutrition, sexual health, hand washing and hygiene). However, there is a pre-step that Billingham captured in 1997. She sought to describe public health practice as a way of 'seeing' health problems.

> *Essentially public health is a distinctive way of seeing health problems: public health nurses and doctors ask different questions about their practice, requiring them to look beyond individuals to populations, such as:*
>
> - *why is this happening?*
> - *how often?*
> - *what is the social context?*
> - *who else should be involved?*
> - *what works and what doesn't?*
>
> *They also make different connections: between one individual and another, between individuals and communities, between individuals and social structures, between the stories that people tell them and the epidemiological evidence, between health services and other agencies, between medical and social models of health, and between health and social policies. Public health nurses, moreover, tend to have a commitment to a set of values based on equity, justice and work for social change at local and national levels.*
>
> **(Billingham, 1997, 271)**

Blair *et al.* (2003) take this further:

> *In practice, many child health workers combine the individual and population perspectives in their day-to-day work and share a similar aim – that of optimizing the health and well-being of all children and young people. Defining common ground, and understanding what those with*

> *different backgrounds can contribute to the common cause, is an import-
> ant objective of child public health.*
>
> **(Blair et al., 2003, p.3)**

These writers emphasize the point that 'common understanding and co-operation' goes beyond the health sector, thus including teachers, social workers, educational psychologists, school nurses, youth justice teams, youth workers and others who work with children and young people. In other words, public health practitioners do not work alone nor do they work to single-issue agendas.

HEALTH PROMOTION AS TARGETED INTERVENTIONS

We have cautioned against the over-simplification inherent in focusing on individual behaviour change and on a definition of health promotion that con-fines this work to categories of individual interventions. Nevertheless, public health practitioners need to see their work grounded in activities that do link into practical tasks.

To put it another way, the practitioner needs to focus his or her work with children and young people in approaches to health improvement that can make a difference – that produce evidence of change for the better. The school is a location for such work because it is where children gather. In effect, it is an opportunistic location. It is also the child's workplace, and learning to take care of personal health is as critically important to the child's future as is learning to read. Furthermore, the younger the child the more open he/she is to health information, education and health-promotion interventions.

The challenges in the intervention approach, however, are twofold. Individual health risks as a focus for health-promotion activities are themselves susceptible to fashion and change in terms of the attention they demand from public health practitioners. In the 1990s, young people's sexual health was the major public health preoccupation. By the mid-point of the first decade of the 21st century, obesity had moved to centre-stage. Sexual health had not been resolved, but it had begun to lose sustained media attention. In fact, we do not have sufficient national evidence to know whether or not sexual health among young people has continued to worsen. For example, full national coverage for chlamydia screening is scheduled for rollout by March 2007, which means that results should be clearer by 2009. The challenge, of course, is how to capture such information such that it gives us reliable data about young people of school age.

Blair *et al.* (2003) caught this 'feel' for the way public health practice responds to shifts both in policy pressure and in the relative profiles of health issues, when they included a chapter of practical examples (scenarios) for pub-lic health practitioners in child public health (Blair *et al.*, 2003, pp.192–243).

It is probably fair to say that most health-promotion interventions arise from experimental approaches by public health practitioners. This is the case, for example, with many school nurse initiatives. The 'sharing of good practice' that we see in journals, in public policy documents and at conferences is of this kind and is generally under-evaluated or poorly evaluated. The question that arises is how can we know which preventive strategies do work and in what contexts and with what population groups?

For example, a recently published *BMJ Online* study in Scotland (Henderson *et al.*, 2007) reported research that measured the relative effectiveness of conventional school sex education compared with a theoretically based sex education programme (SHARE) by using a follow-up of cluster randomized trial. The SHARE (sexual health and relationships) programme was experimental and considerably more expensive than the conventional school sex education programme because it involved different approaches, more expensive materials and higher levels of investment in staff training by health-promotion departments. Yet, 4.5 years after the two interventions (girls followed up at age 20 years), no significant difference was found between the two programmes in the numbers of conceptions and terminations.

The single finding of significance was that

> *...effective programmes have to address fundamental socio-economic divisions in society, while the influence of parenting factors on sexual experience points to strategies involving parents.*
>
> *(Henderson et al., 2007)*

Neither the school sex education programme nor the SHARE programme had focused on parental involvement or on socio-economic population profiles as a factor in teenage sexual health, yet these were identified as the highest correlation factors in rates of teenage pregnancy.

In other words, sexual risk taking is closely linked to the socio-economic profile of the particular child population within the school, not merely linked to the school-based health-promotion interventions. This means that family, community and cultural attitudes to early sexual experience and to conception and terminations of conceptions are powerful influences on teenage decision making about sexual behaviour and about teenage pregnancy.

Tabberer *et al.* (2000) found this to be the case in their study of teenage girls' attitudes to early pregnancy. Their qualitative study of 41 young women in Doncaster found that teenage pregnancy was not planned but was relatively common in the locality under study, and they also found that families, especially the young women's mothers, often played a crucial part in supporting teenagers who gave birth. The health-promotion need was for early advice and counselling and early information about abortion. Later studies have found that early access to emergency contraception and to information about and access to condoms that is also linked to informal access to information about sexual health is a critical need for young people.

Across the UK, a range of health-promotion interventions by school nurses, health-promotion specialists, and youth workers have together developed precisely these kinds of resources, including access to emergency contraception (DeBell and Tomkins, 2006).

Successive studies have consistently reported that about one-third of 16-year-old girls across the UK are sexually active. This population group needs access to sexual health services that are designed such that young people will find them easy to use and easily accessible.

But it is fair to say that we need far more evidence of the effects of health-promotion interventions than we currently have. The health-related choices children and young people make are not merely a consequence of good or poor health education and health-promotion interventions, though these may be a factor for individual children and young people. Choices are powerfully linked to the social environment in which the child lives. This is important for understanding how to select health-promotion interventions during the school-age years. The need is for investment in research that can measure the effects of existing health-promotion interventions.

A task force in the US was established in the early 1990s to do just this (Zara *et al.*, 2005). In 1996, the Department of Health and Human Services (HHS) established the Task Force on Community Preventive Services with a 15-member panel of experts working with the Centres for Disease Control and Prevention. By 2005, dozens of health specialists and scientists, by working together, had produced *The Guide to Community Preventive Services: what works to promote health?* and this work continues. Its purpose is to answer three key questions about health-promotion interventions that all public health practitioners need to answer:

- *what has worked for others and how well?*
- *how can I select among interventions with proven effectiveness?*
- *what might this intervention cost, and what am I likely to achieve through my investment?*

(Zara **et al.,** *2005, p.xxv)*

These are the primary questions that all public health practitioners need to ask when planning health-promotion interventions for children and young people and for making decisions about such interventions in the school setting.

CONCLUSION

The school is an opportune location for health-promotion work because it is where children and young people gather; where they spend the greatest part of their growing up years outside the home environment; and it is, effectively, their workplace. Historically in the UK, there has always been a damaging split between education and health, despite periodic attempts to integrate the two. The 21st century, however, has seen a systematic attempt to shift policy and practice to an integrated approach to child health and education, and to do so in terms of a community/neighbourhood perspective. As a social paradigm for health rather than a medical model, this is recognizable and welcoming for the work of public health practitioners.

Every Child Matters: change for children (HM Government, 2004), which is legally underpinned by the Children Act 2004, is the framework that has been designed to define positive child and adolescent health and to specify expected outcomes from services. It is an ambitious direction of travel. It is not, however, an easy agenda because it requires cross-government departmental co-operation and interprofessional working. Particularly since the World War Two, departmental boundaries (e.g. education, health, social care, the police, housing) have produced, across all four countries of the UK, diverse ways of working and thinking that are powerfully affected by training cultures. Each professional group articulates its work in its own language and to its own service objectives. Teachers and public health practitioners present us with a useful example of such diversity in working practices and service objectives. Partnership working can be difficult to negotiate for both professions. Having said that, the 'legal duty on local authorities is now to co-operate to improve the well-being of children and young people living in their area' (Evans and Halliday, 2006, p.2).

Health promotion is also a complex field. At base, it tends to be articulated in terms of either interventions or changes in regulatory measures designed to improve health and to prevent ill-health. Health-promotion work developed, and began to be theorized in the 1980s, out of public health roots. It focuses attention on the determinants of health. These are not merely lifestyle behaviours but also involve attention to those socio-economic, environmental and cultural factors that determine how individual children and young people respond to efforts designed to improve their health or to prevent poor health.

With health-promotion work, the public health practitioner finds himself/ herself engaged in an activity that demands analysis of the community in which the child lives; attention to the family circumstances; and appropriate response to the individual child. It is this way of 'seeing' the whole of the health-improvement agenda and the whole of the child's circumstances that is demanded of public health practitioners when they think about working with children and young people in the school environment. And where their work is most effective it understands the school as part of a larger community while, at the same time, it involves working with diverse agencies as well as with families themselves.

KEY POINTS

- The history of child health in the school setting in the UK is not a heartening picture, but policy shift in the 21st century across all four countries has provided both the framework (*Every Child Matters: change for children*, HM Government, 2004) and the legal pressure (the Children Act 2004) that could enable significant change in this profile.
- A paradigm shift to a social model of health across all departments, agencies, and professions is needed in order to improve child and adolescent health.
- Health promotion, as theorized since the 1980s, can be a powerful tool for public health practitioners. It includes analysis of the determinants of health – the socio-economic, environmental, psychosocial and cultural factors that affect child health – and it includes practical interventions.
- Health-promotion interventions require, and do not at present have, a firm evidence base for practice, but public health practitioners tend to think of health promotion, first, in terms of practical interventions.

- Health education is a subset of activities within the health-promotion portfolio. Health education is not a legal curriculum requirement at 2007, but there is considerable pressure from the schools standards authority (Ofsted) for schools to demonstrate that health-improvement measures are integrated into schools' work.
- The National Healthy Schools Programme is not a legal requirement but it does represent a pressure on schools to demonstrate their commitment to child and adolescent health.
- Public health practitioners working to health-promotion agendas in the school environment 'see' their work in terms of the child, the family, the school and the local community outside the school gates.

REFERENCES

Acheson D (1998) *Independent Inquiry into Inequalities in Health.* London: Department of Health.

Bartley M (2003) *Health Inequality: an introduction to concepts, theories and methods.* London: Blackwell.

Benzeval M, Judge K, Whitehead M (1997) Tackling inequalities in health: extracts from the summary. Kings Fund. In: Sidell M, Jones L, Katz J, Peberdy A (eds) *Debates and Dilemmas in Promoting Health: a reader.* Basingstoke: Macmillan, pp. 16–23.

Billingham K (1997) Public health nursing in primary care. *British Journal of Community Health Nursing* 2:270–4.

Black D (1980) *Report of the Working Group on Inequalities in Health. Department of Health.* London: HMSO.

Blair M, Stewart-Brown S, Waterston T, Crowther R (2003) *Child Public Health.* Oxford: Oxford University Press.

Botting (1995) *The Health of Our Children: a review of the mid 1990s.* London: Office of Population Census.

Burgher MS, Rasmussen VB, Rivett D (1999) *The European Network of Health Promoting Schools: the alliance of education and health.* Copenhagen: WHO Regional Office for Europe.

Child Accident Prevention Trust (2006) www.capt.org.uk/allaboutcapt/main.htm (accessed 24 January 2007).

Court D (1976) *Fit for the Future.* London: UK Commission of Enquiry into the Child Health Services.

Cummings C, Dyson A, Papps I *et al.* (2006) *Evaluation of the Full Service Extended Schools Initiative, Second Year: thematic papers.* London: Department for Education and Skills and Universities of Manchester and Newcastle.

Dahlgren G, Whitehead M (1991) *Policies and Strategies to Promote Social Equity in Health.* Stockholm: Institute for Future Studies.

DeBell D, Everett G (1997) *In a Class Apart: a study of school nursing.* Norwich: Norfolk Health Authority.

DeBell D, Jackson P (2000) *School Nursing within the Public Health Agenda: a strategy for practice*. London: McMillan Scott.

DeBell D, Tomkins A (2006) *Discovering the Future of School Nursing: the evidence base*. London: McMillan-Scott.

Denman S, Moon A, Parsons C, Stears D (2002) *The Healthy Promoting School: policy, research and practice*. London: Routledge.

Department of Education and Science (1968) *Handbook for Health Education*. London: HMSO.

Department for Education and Skills (2002) *PSHE Certification Programme for Teachers*. Nottingham: DfES Publications. www.wiredforhealth.gov.uk (accessed 24 January 2007).

Department for Education and Skills (2005a) *Higher Standards Better Schools for All: more choice for parents and pupils*. Nottingham: DfES Publications.

Department for Education and Skills (2005b) *Youth Matters: next steps – something to do, somewhere to go, someone to talk to*. Nottingham: DfES Publications. www.dfes.gov.uk/publications/youth/ (accessed 24 January 2007).

Department for Education and Skills and Department of Health (2003) *How the National Healthy School Standard Contributes to School Improvement*. London: Department of Health.

Department for Education and Skills and Department of Health (2005) *National Healthy Schools Status: A guide for schools*. Nottingham: DfES.

Department for Education and Skills and Department of Health (2006) *Extended Schools and Health Services – working together for better outcomes for children and families*. London: CSIP.

Department of Health (1999) *Healthy Schools Programme*. London: HMSO.

Department of Health (2002) *School Nurse Practice Development Pack*. London: Department of Health.

Department of Health (2004a) *Choosing Health: making healthy choices easier*. London: Department of Health.

Department of Health (2004b) *Healthy Living Blueprint*. London: Department of Health.

Department of Health (2006) *Health Profile of England*. London: Department of Health.

Department of Health and Department for Education and Skills (2004) *National Service Framework for Children, Young People and Maternity Services*. London: Department of Health. www.dh.gov.uk/PolicyAndGuidance/HealthAndSocialCareTopics/ChildrenServices/ChildrenServicesInformation/ChildrenServicesInformationArticle/fs/en?CONTENT_ID=4089111&chk=U8Ecln (accessed 5 February 2007).

Eisenberg (1999) Does social medicine still matter in an era of molecular medicine? *Journal of Urban Health* 76:164–75.

Evans S, Halliday S (2006) *Indications of Child Health in the East of England: No. 1: introduction and overview*. Inpho Briefing Papers on topical public health issues. Issue 20. Cambridge: Eastern Region Public Health Observatory. www.erpho.org.uk (accessed 24 January 2007).

Flynn P, Knight D (1998) *Inequalities in Health in the North West.* Warrington: NHS Executive North West. www.nwph.net/nwpho/Publications/inequalities.pdf (accessed 31 January 2007).

Grant AH (1942) *Nursing: a community health service.* Philadelphia: WB Saunders Company.

Hall D, Elliman D (2003) *Health for all Children* (4e). Oxford: Oxford University Press.

Hanifan LJ (1916) The rural school community center. *Annals of the American Academy of Political and Social Science* 67:130–8.

Hanifan LJ (1920) *The Community Center.* Boston: Silver Burdett.

Harker L (2006) *Chance of a Lifetime: the impact of bad housing on children's lives.* Edinburgh: Shelter.

Harris B (1995) *The Health of the School Child: a history of the school medical service in England and Wales.* Buckingham: Open University Press.

Henderson M, Wight D, Raab GM *et al.* (2007) Impact of a theoretically based sex education programme (share) delivered by teachers on NHS registered conceptions and terminations: final results of cluster randomised trial. *BMJ* 334:133.

Heer B, Woodhead D (December 2002) *Promoting Health, Preventing Illness: Public health perspectives on London's mental health.* London: The King's Fund.

HM Government (2004) *Every Child Matters: change for children.* Nottingham: DfES Publications. www.everychildmatters.gov.uk/_content/documents/Every%20Child%20Matinserts.pdf (accessed 21 January 2007).

Hofrichter R (ed.) (2003) *Health and Social Justice: Politics, Ideology, and Inequity in the Distribution of Disease: a public health reader.* San Francisco: Jossey Bass Publication.

Independent Advisory Group on Sexual Health and Teenage Pregnancy (2005) *Personal, Social and Health Education in Schools: time for action.* www.dfes.gov.uk/teenagepregnancy (accessed 24 January 2007).

Kawachi I, Kennedy B, Wilkinson RG (eds) (1999) *Income Inequality and Health: the society and population health reader.* Vol 1. New York: The New Press.

Labonté R (1993) A holosphere of healthy and sustainable communities. *Australian and New Zealand Journal of Public Health* 17:4–12.

Leff S, Leff V (1959) *The School Health Service.* London: Lewis.

Lister-Sharp D, Chapman S, Stewart-Brown S, Sowden A (1999) Health promoting schools and health promotion in schools: two systematic reviews. *Health Technology Assessment NHS R&D HTA Programme* 3:22. www.ncchta.org/fullmono/mon322.pdf (accessed 24 January 2007).

Macintyre S, Hart G (2000) *Synergy No 3. Tackling Health Inequalities in Scotland: a policy relevant research agenda.* Glasgow: Universities of Glasgow and Strathclyde. www.strath.gla.ac.uk/synergy/policy/3.html (accessed 24 January 2007).

Marmot M (2004) *Status Syndrome.* London: Bloomsbury.

Mayall B, Bendelow G, Barker S, Storey P, Veltman M (1996) *Children's Health in Primary Schools.* London: The Falmer Press.

McNalty A (1939) *Suggestions on Health Education. Board of Education for England.* London: HMSO.

Mental Health Foundation (1999) *Bright Futures: promoting children and young people's mental health.* London: Mental Health Foundation.

Mosley H, Moorhouse J (2000) *A Profile of the Health and Health Needs of School Age Children in Huddersfield.* Huddersfield: Huddersfield NHS Trust.

Naidoo J, Wills J (1998) *Health Promotion Foundations for Practice.* London: Baillière Tindal.

National Children's Bureau (2003) *Developing a whole school approach to PSHE and Citizenship.* London: National Children's Bureau. www.ncb.org.uk (accessed 24 January 2007).

Office for National Statistics (2004) *The Health of People and Young People.* London: Office for National Statistics.

Office for Standards in Education (2002) *Sex and Relationship Education.* London: HMSO.

Office for Standards in Education (2005a) *Personal, Social and Health Education in Secondary Schools.* London: HMSO.

Office for Standards in Education (2005b) *Every Child Matters: framework for the inspection of children's services.* London: Adult Learning Inspectorate, Healthcare Commission, HMcpsi, Audit Commission, HMIC, HMiP, csci, HM Inspectorate of Prisons, HMiCA.

Pearson P (2002) Public health and health promotion. In: Cowley S *Public Health in Policy and Practice.* London: Ballière Tindall, pp.44–62.

Polnay L (1995) *Report of a Joint Working Party on Health Needs of School Age Children.* London: British Paediatric Association.

Prashar A (2003) *Key Themes in Supporting Children and Young People in the North West: public health policy and practice.* Salford: Institute for Public Health Research and Policy.

Rogers LL (1908) Some Phases of School Nursing. *American Journal of Nursing* 8:966–74. Reprinted (October 2002) *Journal of School Nursing* 18:253–6.

Scottish Executive (2003) *A Scottish Framework for Nursing in Schools.* Edinburgh: Scottish Executive.

Sidell M, Jones L, Katz J, Peberdy A (1997) *Debates and Dilemmas in Promoting Health: a reader.* Basingstoke: Macmillan.

Social Exclusion Unit (1999) *Teenage Pregnancy Strategy.* London: Social Exclusion Unit.

Stewart-Brown S (1998) New approaches to school health. In: Spencer N (ed.) *Progress in Community Health.* Vol 2. Edinburgh: Churchill Livingstone, 137–58.

Tabberer S, Hall C, Prendergast S, Webster A (2000) *Teenage Pregnancy and Choice: abortion or motherhood: influences on the decision.* York: Joseph Rowntree Foundation.

Training and Development Agency for Schools (2006) *DfES Announcement – 19 September 2006.* www.tda.gov.uk/remodelling/extendedschools/research-sep06. aspx (accessed 24 January 2007).

Wales M (1941) *The Public Health Nurse in Action.* New York: Macmillan.

Wilkinson RG (1996) *Unhealthy Societies: the afflictions of inequality.* London: Routledge.

World Health Organization (1978) *International Conference on Primary Health Care (1978) Declaration of Alma-Ata.* www.who.dk/AboutWho/Policy/20010827_1 (accessed 24 January 2007).

World Health Organization (1986) *First International Conference on Health Promotion. Ottawa Charter for Health Promotion: the move towards a new public health.* Geneva: World Health Organization. www.who.int/hpr/NPH/docs/ottawa_charter_hp.pdf (accessed 24 January 2007).

Zara S, Briss PA, Harris KW (ed.) (2005) *The Guide to Community Preventive Services: what works to promote health?* Oxford and New York: Oxford University Press.

Acts of Parliament

All these Acts are published by HMSO in London, and all can be accessed from the UK Parliament website (www.publications.parliament.uk).

Education (Provision of Meals) Act 1906
Open Spaces Act 1906
Education (Administration Provisions) Act 1907
Notification of Births Act 1907
Education Act 1918
Maternity and Child Welfare Act 1918
Children Act 2004

Section 4
THE CHILD IN THE COMMUNITY

6

YOUNG PEOPLE, LEISURE CAPITAL AND HEALTH

Simon Bradford and Yvonne McNamara

INTRODUCTION

European industrialization and changing family forms in the 19th century demarcated childhood from adulthood, creating a space – *leisure* – where young people were neither in school, at home or working. Activities in emergent leisure organizations during this period were designed to discipline and train working class young people for good citizenship. Regulation of leisure also became more overt, a common pattern during times of social change, but especially prior to and during periods of war when concerns for the physical condition of young men and the domestic health of young women were at their highest (Bradford, 2006, p.132). Similarly, in the UK at present, leisure is one site where the exigencies of childhood and youth are managed in order to secure young people's responsible citizenship (Department for Education and Skills [DfES], 2006).

This chapter explores young people's leisure and particularly its potential as a location for health interventions. We use the term 'young people' to include all children of school age, roughly 4 to 18 years. Leisure is a complex concept, not least because of the diversity of definitions of leisure activities in societies where leisure, like all else, is increasingly individualized (Beck, 2004). However, the exponential rise of leisure opportunities and experiences is mirrored by increasing inequality in the UK. Young people's leisure experiences are radically shaped by social difference, principally, we argue, by social class, gender and race. In Western knowledge societies, leisure is no longer exclusively a domain of *pleasure*, but a setting in which indispensable skills and capacities are transmitted and developed. As leisure has also become significant as a site for health interventions aimed at young people (for example, in relation to diet or sexuality), unequal access to leisure opportunities may be reflected in differential consequences for young people's health (Department of Health, 2005; Shaw *et al.*, 2005; National Statistics, 2006).

Leisure has at least four important dimensions for young people. First, it is an institution where they acquire social and cultural capital. Social capital refers to the networks of interpersonal relationships in which young people are situated, and in public health terms constitutes social well-being through 'the capacity to function as a social being, to form healthy supportive relationships, and to participate positively in community affairs' (Blair *et al.*, 2003, p.112). Health depends on positive social networks and the individual's ability to contribute to them. This is particularly relevant when considering young people's health. Cultural capital resides in the forms of knowledge and skill that enable people to become competent members of a society, is acquired initially from parents, and its acquisition is gendered, racialized and classed.

Second, leisure provides psychosocial benefits for young people in terms of developing self-esteem, psychological well-being and health.

Third, leisure defines the symbolic and material spaces ('leisure and pleasure') in which young people engage in the construction of identity, an important component of good health, and when they are, in theory, relatively free from adult intervention. Although all leisure activities seem to have a non-compulsory dimension in common, this does not mean that they are necessarily 'freely chosen'. Patterns of leisure activity are shaped by dispositions and capacities; are based on social difference; and are inculcated through experience over time.

Finally, in the UK, leisure has been both 'managed' via organized attempts to influence young people, and simultaneously neglected in circumstances where young people are left to themselves. Youth leisure has been the location of a range adult 'care and control' interventions, whether through the 19th century ideology of 'rational recreation' or in the contemporary concept of the 'preventive state' (Parton, 2006, p.164) of *Every Child Matters* (Chief Secretary to the Treasury, 2003) and *Youth Matters* (DfES, 2005). Health initiatives targeted on young people have increasingly been conducted in leisure space, and leisure is now central to public health policy.

PUBLIC HEALTH, POLICY AND YOUNG PEOPLE'S LEISURE

Public health as policy and practice is concerned with identifying and managing social, cultural, institutional and environmental factors that contribute to the health of given populations (Cowley, 2002, p.7). There is debate, however, about what counts as health – a fluid, contested and socially constructed concept. But there is even greater debate about *public* health, because the concept is multifaceted with complex intersecting psychological, physiological, cultural and social dimensions.

Child public health focuses on the promotion of the 'health and well being of young people in the widest sense' (Blair *et al.*, 2003. p.1). This encourages a holistic view of young people in the context of their communities, and reflects the social, political and economic factors that contribute to health rather than focusing on individualized medical issues. As such, child public health moves beyond issues of mortality, morbidity and the absence of disease, towards a broader concern with communities, patterns of social interaction within them and the impact these may have on health. This places young people's leisure, as a site of social interaction, centre-stage in any consideration of public health.

However, there are tensions here in policy terms. Although in the UK, New Labour has been influenced by the work of social capital theorists (Etzioni, 1997; Putnam, 2000), it has been suggested that constraints on expenditure mean that *individualizing* health responses has offered government an easier option (Goodwin and Armstrong-Esther, 2004). Indeed, 'health' has become a 'badge' of responsible citizenship in, for example, the obesity debate, where slimness is emblematic of 'embodied social fitness'. As Monaghan writes in relation to the individualization of obesity, 'more expansive and intimately connected problems associated with social injustice get hidden' (Monaghan, 2005, p.308). Indeed, social policy in the UK, as in other liberal democracies, continues to privilege individual responsibility in the attempt to manage the health of the population as a whole (Petersen, 1997, p.197).

We depart from a view of policy making as a linear practice in which problems are identified, responses formulated, and strategies subsequently implemented. This approach is sometimes referred to as a 'policy cycle' (e.g. Parsons, 1995, p.77), but fails to acknowledge the complexity and the contested nature of policy making and implementation. Policy should be understood as 'discourse', thus acknowledging the power practices that are entailed in policy making actions (Ball, 1993). Kingdon's (1995) model of the 'policy window' was developed to explain central government *policy action* in which 'policy windows' open and close by the articulation of three figures: '*problems*', '*politics*' and '*policies*'. In relation to young people's health, we take the view that there is currently a policy window framed by *political* definitions of health *problems*.

'Problems', 'politics' and 'policies' in young people's health

Young people's health in the UK is shaped by the shifting relationships between problems, politics and policies. Historically, young people have been viewed as an essentially problematic social category (as a source of social disorder and disruption), and their health 'problems' have been variously defined in a range of legislation and concerns that are continually shifting in the light of wider political developments. For example, concerns about morbidity and mortality from infectious disease have been replaced by the 'morbidities of modern living', and are reflected in the current moral panic about 'healthy childhoods' and healthy leisure.

Current challenges to young people's health – defined as *problems* – include a rise in mental ill-health, eating disorders, suicide and self-harm; obesity; substance use (alcohol and drugs); teenage pregnancy; and the health effects of poverty (Blair *et al.*, 2003, p.27). In England, Scotland and Wales these concerns form key *policy* strands (Scottish Executive, 2003; Welsh Assembly, 2003; Department of Health, 2004). The politics of these initiatives are complex but the dominant *political* strategy in the UK is articulated as 'partnership' (including young people as partners) and is centred on a range of 'auditable' outcomes (based on 'evidence') and targeted on 'at-risk' groups. However, 'what works' is often contested. Policy in Wales, for example, asserts that school-based health initiatives are successful (Welsh Assembly, 2003, p.7). Yet recent work indicates that in relation to drug education, for example, there is apparently little evidence of the success of school-based approaches (Advisory Council on the Misuse of Drugs, 2006, p.9). We take the view that such disparities reflect the political nature of health policy.

All child public health strategies in the UK acknowledge, implicitly or explicitly, the importance of leisure. This is a space in which young people can acquire *leisure capital* (knowledge, skills and capacities that have the potential to contribute to well-being and, in this context, to health) and that anticipate future life experiences and life chances (Zeijl *et al.*, 2002, p.381). Like other forms of capital, leisure capital is differentially distributed; therefore *some* young people acquire good knowledge of sexual health, drug and alcohol use and mental health support. Such knowledge or skill (as a form of capital) can be transformed into resilience and the dispositions needed to be able to cope with the exigencies of contemporary life. Other young people's acquisition of leisure capital, such as 'looked after' young people (Department of Health, 2002a, p.1), is more problematic, and these young people are less likely to develop the necessary capacities to deal effectively with challenges arising in their lives.

Social difference, leisure and young people

One of the characteristic features of contemporary societies like the UK is that the logic and certainty of social solidarity fostered by class identity has been supplanted by the much less certain, yet seductive, power of (individualized) consumption, which confers a sense of identity and status. As a consumed commodity, leisure (activities, fashions, clothes, mobile phones, MP3 players, and so on) may have real significance as a source of, albeit temporary, stability, identity and a sense of well-being. However, the 2001 UK census identified a growing divide between rich and poor, with large concentrations of poverty in the post-industrial towns, especially in the North. This fact alone raises questions about inequitable access to leisure as consumption.

Recent research has demonstrated that societies in which the difference between rich and poor is greatest also have the poorest health indices (Goodwin and Armstrong-Esther, 2004, p.50). The Millennium Survey of poverty and social exclusion in Britain found a bias towards the well-off in leisure service provision, noting that poverty affects children and young people's access to leisure more than any other section of the community (Pantazis *et al.*, 2006, p.464). This matters because sociability and leisure participation partially define social inclusion and 'normality' (Hey and Bradford, 2006), and poverty is a significant risk factor in becoming socially excluded, with all the implications this has for health and well-being. Children and young people are particularly caught up in this scenario because they are targeted by the producers of leisure experiences, yet their capacity to consume leisure is shaped by deepening social inequality. Insofar as leisure offers opportunity for the realization of public health policy, this is clearly important.

Young people's leisure choices and practices are influenced by at least four significant factors. First, parents shape young people's leisure choices. Government takes the view that this should be encouraged in the interests of children being helped to make good 'lifestyle decisions that impact on their health' (Department of Health, 2004, p.6). Parents act as role models and support, for example, by encouraging children to engage in physical exercise and other such activities. Their support consists of a range of cultural and financial resources but these are invariably differentiated by social class (Department for Work and Pensions, 2005, p.207). Such resources include time, energy, money, transport and parental presence at leisure activities. There is contradictory evidence about whether these resources are important for the social reproduction of leisure behaviour and, therefore, to some extent health. UK studies suggest that a relationship between class and leisure participation can be reproduced over generations (Biddle *et al.*, 2004, p.686).

Second, access to physical and social environments matters in shaping children's participation in leisure activities. Urban, rural and suburban locations have different implications for young people's access across a range of potential opportunities. Furthermore, the understanding of built environments, specifically crystallized in parental fears about safety and traffic, appears to have resulted in what Biddle *et al.* (2004, p.687) refer to as 'activity toxic environments', where levels of physical activity have diminished. In England and Wales, for example, the Department for Transport estimates a significant decline in the numbers of children walking to school (Department for Transport, 2005, p.47).

Parental perceptions of risk may be important here. More broadly, gender and race also mediate perceptions of what constitutes safe leisure spaces. Watt and Stenson's research (1998) in south-east England, for example, demonstrates the extent to which young people see some settings as unsafe at particular times of the day or week because of the risk of physical and sexual violence. For some children and young people, this perception of risk can result in a sense of alienation from their own neighbourhoods (Morrow, 2000, p.147). Such perceptions, often perpetuated through peer and friendship groups, mean that some leisure activities become impossible to access, and this can be further compounded by physical distance or poor public transport.

Third, the child's age is important in shaping approaches to leisure and the extent to which leisure can be a vehicle for effective public health interventions. Clearly, there are very significant differences in the leisure practices of, say, 5-year-olds and those of 16-year-olds. Their personal needs, interests and interface with health issues are quite different. For younger school-age children, though not exclusively, *play* as a principal leisure form has enormous significance for health and well-being. The literature identifies the specific health benefits that play provides for younger children in terms of physical and mental health. There is evidence that the earlier children engage in physical leisure activity through play, the more likely it is that they will become routinely socialized into such activities, thus increasing the potential health benefits to them (Meltzer *et al.*, 2000). Some evidence indicates that the transition from primary to secondary school in the UK is particularly influential in children's leisure choices. For example, increased demands from coursework and homework, and growing corporeal self-consciousness (particularly for young women) appear to become barriers to some physical activities (Mulvihill *et al.*, 2000). Interestingly, there is evidence from Canada suggesting that following the transition to secondary school young people see themselves as 'too old' to begin learning new activity skills (Thompson *et al.*, 2005, p.435), although there is no specific UK evidence to support this.

Hendry *et al.* (1993) developed a useful age-based framework for understanding the leisure transitions of children and young people through the school-age years to adolescence. The young people he studied moved from participation in *organized leisure*, predominantly led by adults and typified by the leisure activities of younger children, to *casual leisure* in early adolescence (hanging out with friends) and finally, during later adolescence, to participation in *commercial leisure* (going to pubs, clubs and other commercial sites). Age is suggested as the primary determinant here, although Hendry acknowledges gender differences in the way that boys and girls use leisure opportunities. This work suggests a degree of universalism in leisure patterns and transitions. However, more recent work suggests that leisure has become much more commodified and 'individualized', and less attached to or determined by earlier class solidarities (Hendry *et al.*, 2002, p.12). This does not mean that social class is no longer a contributing factor and, clearly, some young people have much greater capacity to consume leisure opportunities than do others.

Finally, friendship and other peer group relationships are significant in shaping leisure practices because of their impact on the development of personal identity. Indeed, many leisure activities are tied to peer and friendship groups: these groups are constituted in leisure spaces and leisure time. Indeed, peer groups appear to provide a basis for 'peer education', to which we refer below.

YOUNG PEOPLE, LEISURE AND HEALTH INTERVENTIONS

We consider three settings in which young people engage in leisure and in which leisure capital may be acquired. Importantly, these are contexts where health policy interventions in the lives of young people in the UK have been developed and/or are argued by policy makers and practitioners as suitable for intervention.

Public autonomous space

The 'street' may be *the* symbol of young people's potential for autonomy, yet young people have always been subjected to surveillance on 'the street' through the institutions of the adult gaze (police, street wardens, youth workers, residents and so on). Arguably, the street (as a metaphor for public space more generally) has always been *adult* space despite its contested nature. Nevertheless, it provides an important leisure space for the young, and this remains the case despite a recurrent historical concern about the imagined relationship between the street, as a 'dangerous' place, and youth and children as either vulnerable or dangerous social categories (Muncie, 2004, p.232).

Meeting and being with friends, on the street, in the park, in shopping centres and malls is an alternative to commercial leisure provision and is an important leisure activity for many young people. In a recent UK survey, 60 per cent of 14- to 16-year-olds agreed that 'I often hang about with my friends doing nothing in particular' (Children's Society, 2006, p.14). Research in London (Bradford *et al.*, 2003, pp.32–3) confirms this is its main appeal, freedom from adult supervision. The problem for young people is that adults often interpret 'hanging out' as being threatening, dangerous or sinister. In a culture defined by standard attainment tests (SATs), accredited learning and certificated outcomes, just 'hanging out' seems aimless and unproductive, almost crying out for adult intervention.

Under the rubric of 'community safety' (Squires, 2006), the panoptic surveillance of CCTV has become ubiquitous in streets, shopping centres, public and private buildings, pubs, clubs, leisure and youth centres. Furthermore, antisocial behaviour orders (ASBOs), introduced in the Crime and Disorder Act 1998, and now applied to children under 10 years, have criminalized what were, in many instances, civil offences 'committed' by young people in leisure space. Dispersal orders (preventing young people under 16 years of age from being on the streets unaccompanied by an adult after 9 pm) are a further constraint on young people's leisure. The underlying message is that young people constitute a problem and that they are increasingly unwelcome in public space.

Despite this authoritarian and problematizing approach to young people, public spaces have become settings for some health-related work. A recent national study noted the significant growth in the number of street-based youth work projects (564 projects in England and Wales that had contact with 65 325 young people) with high-risk groups and working on particular issues. For example, the youth workers interviewed reported that 30 per cent of the young people they were in contact with had health-related problems (Crimmens *et al.*, 2004). Street-based or 'detached' youth work appears to offer some potential as a means of working with young people who do not come into contact with other agencies. Its strength seems to lie in youth workers' acceptance of young people as active participants in informal education work.

Proponents argue that detached work has the capacity to contact disaffected or excluded young people and offer information and advice on a range of health-related behaviours. There are many local projects of this kind in the UK, but hard evidence of long-term effectiveness is difficult to capture. One Scottish report suggests that, although this work has potential for helping young people with health issues, for example, evaluation mechanisms are frequently underdeveloped (Furlong *et al.*, 1997). More recent work in Northern Ireland indicates that there is evidence of detached youth workers' positive impact on young people's sexual and mental health (Harland, *et al.*, 2005, p.26). In England, some evidence suggests the effectiveness of informal work on health issues in street settings (Merton *et al.*, 2004, p.10) and others engaged in street-based work report successful engagement with young people in discussing sexual health (Baraitser *et al.*, 2002, p.21).

There seem to be three points here. First, this informal or detached work is based on the assumption that interventions in spaces that young people see as 'theirs', and that are made on 'their terms', are likely to be effective. Second, however, there has been little or no rigorous, large scale and long-term research on the effectiveness of street-based work on health issues with young people. Third, because of the often brief, informal, 'person-centred' and fluid practices in this work, hard evidence of long-term success in this work is difficult to adduce.

Organized leisure space

The boundary between leisure and non-leisure is increasingly permeable, and distinctions between the two are becoming less meaningful. As part of the *Every Child Matters* agenda (Chief Secretary to the Treasury, 2003) and its five outcomes, developments in 'extended schools' mean that increased opportunities for leisure activities focusing on health and well-being and, linked to the five outcomes, may become available to those who are able to take advantage of them. Broadly, this means that young people's leisure time has become more structured and more likely to be subject to adult control. There are social class variations to this, but as leisure has become increasingly perceived to be a source of social and cultural capital, middle class parents, for example, tend to invest time and personal resources in 'leisure as life-chance'.

Fears about young people's safety have also led to increased supervision of leisure space and activity, particularly for girls and young women (Aapola *et al.*, 2005, p.115). Increasing parental labour market participation has also led to some children and young people being enrolled in an increasing variety of 'after-school' clubs and groups that provide adult supervision.

Some general patterns of participation in out-of-school sporting activities, an area of focus for a range of health-related interventions, are evident, and social class and gender difference are both very significant here. More boys than girls participate in sports activities across the age ranges, and participation in physical activities diminishes with age (British Heart Foundation, 2004, p.6). A survey of the 16- to 19-year age group indicated that 72 per cent of those studied had participated in sports, games or physical activities during the survey reference period (Fox and Rickards, 2004, p.3). There is also evidence that girls are increasingly likely to participate in sports that, hitherto, have been associated with young men, for example, football and basketball (Sport England, 2003, p.41).

There are complex relationships between other forms of social difference (class, disability and ethnicity) and physical activity. It is clear that social class shapes access to leisure opportunities. Young people from the most deprived areas of the country are less likely to be members of sports clubs, youth clubs and other similar organizations. The participation rates of disabled young people are lower than for other young people. Young people from Indian, Pakistani, Bangladeshi and Chinese backgrounds have lower participation rates than do white young people (British Heart Foundation, 2004, p.7). Insofar as these opportunities have the potential to confer leisure capital on young people, evidence suggests that this is differentially distributed throughout the population.

The most recent and reliable figures suggest that at any given time, 20 per cent of 13- to 19-year-olds are participating in youth service activities: clubs, projects and centres (Department for Education, 1995). Youth clubs have been the primary focus of youth work, providing a place where young people meet 'that is safe and warm, where they can associate, try out new activities and learn new skills, relate to adults, obtain advice and information, and run things for themselves' (Robertson, 2005, p.3) and they often appeal to younger teenagers. As a 15-year-old young woman in West London said 'when you get to, like, 14 or 15, you're not going to go down a youth club and get told what to do, you get me? They don't like it' (Bradford *et al.*, 2003, p.35). Despite this, subsequent research (Bradford *et al.*, 2004, p.34) has found that older teenagers can also be committed to club membership. In this work, one young person identified their youth club as 'a place to have fun, to meet friends, talk with your mates and just mellow out, to get away from schoolwork and parents, a place where you are given a chance'.

In the London-based research, 31 per cent of the total number of young people interviewed belonged to a youth organization; more females than males belonged; 14 years was the peak age; and there was a significant drop in membership at age 16 years. The main reason given for belonging to a club was that it provided 'somewhere to meet my friends' but young people value their experiences in youth clubs for a variety of reasons. Informal access to health information and to informal support is one aspect of this as the following narrative (Bradford *et al.*, 2004, p.38) suggests.

> Interviewer: *What do you learn at this club?*
> Sara: *Sex education …*
> Chloe: *Drugs …*
> Kelly: *Yeah, about drugs, safety, sanitary and hygiene …*
> Interviewer: *Periods and stuff? (Kelly nods)*

This echoes Baraitser *et al.* (2002), who point to the value of informal and flexible health-oriented work in leisure settings. In the wider discussion above, the young women identified learning opportunities that fulfilled many of the PSHE (personal social and health education) and citizenship elements of the school curriculum. They also acknowledged a growth in self-esteem and self-worth, as well as important elements of what we understand as social and cultural capital that they acquired through their youth club membership. Broadly, young people value four aspects of belonging to a leisure time youth organization that may have an important bearing on informal health education:

- the provision of accessible and safe leisure space
- a balanced combination of relevant 'leisure' and 'educational' opportunities
- relationships between youth workers and young people that emphasize young people as 'active participants' rather than 'passive consumers' of services, and work that emphasizes the person-centred *process* element of youth work
- the provision of relevant information, advice and informal support or counselling.

It is provision of this kind that is most likely to articulate with young people's own understanding and interpretation of their health needs. Indeed, this recognition of young people as active agents in the processes involved resonates with current government policy about incorporating user perspectives in public health initiatives (Department of Health and Department for Education and Skills, 2004).

Ironically, in the context of New Labour's modernization of services, this generic, flexible and specifically *leisure-based* youth club work has appeared to diminish. Targeted work with young people deemed to be at risk, as well as work designed to achieve the outcomes specified by *Every Child Matters* (Chief Secretary to the Treasury, 2003) dominate the current agenda.

The last few years have seen the development of a range of government initiatives designed to improve young people's health, often established as *partnerships* that involve various stakeholders and that are aimed at increasing the *inclusion* of *at-risk* groups, and intended to boost *personal responsibility*. Much of this work focuses on problems that have achieved a high political profile: notably drug use, sexuality and teenage pregnancy, but some effective informal work may be lost in the highly prescriptive approaches that now lead the agenda. Programmes like *Positive Futures* (10- to 19-year-olds) and *Positive Activities for Young People* (8- to 19-year-olds) have been established to work on health issues with marginalized young people during their leisure time. Typically, as the interim evaluation report for *Positive Futures* puts it, there is a need to engage in longer-term work before effectiveness can be identified (Crabbe, 2005, p.119).

Sure Start Plus, another initiative exemplifying this approach, worked with pregnant teenagers and teenage parents through the use of mentoring, personal advisers and other forms of intensive work in leisure time. The national evaluation of Sure Start Plus acknowledged innovative work but suggested that the scheme had 'less apparent impact on specific health objectives' (Wiggins, *et al.*, 2005, p.2).

Peer-based education projects have proliferated across the UK but evidence of effectiveness appears ambiguous (sometimes because of poor evaluation strategies and insufficient resources devoted to evaluation) and is contested (Mellanby *et al.*, 2000, p.543; Swann *et al.*, 2003, p.42). Indeed, qualitative evidence from peer mentor schemes, 'buddy schemes' and other peer-based initiatives that were part of the National Healthy Schools Standard suggests that young people often do not use or trust them (Blenkinsop *et al.*, 2004, pp.11–12). The appeal of peer-based strategies, sometimes stronger for adults than for young people, apparently lies in their claim to empower individuals by encouraging the development of knowledge, skill and individual responsibility.

Private domestic space as leisure space

Parental fears about their children's vulnerability to traffic, drug abuse, alcohol consumption, violence or paedophiles have become particularly acute in contemporary Britain and reflect a generalized culture of social anxiety in developed countries. These dangers are not necessarily imaginary, but the disquiet they provoke is invariably disproportionate to the extant risks (Furedi,

2005). This is a culture in which children and young people are thought to be specifically vulnerable. The perceived risks they encounter in public space has, arguably, led to some young people's leisure becoming increasingly privatized in a growing 'bedroom culture' (Lincoln, 2005, p.400).

Some UK organizations actively promote safe public play space for young people as a response to the growth of bedroom culture and concern about health issues, in the widest sense, are at the forefront of this. The Groundwork Trust is a good example of this and the Supergrounds campaign exemplifies this commitment to outside play (www.teachernet.gov.uk/growingschools/news/detail.cfm?id=31). Growing adult unease alongside potential for moral panic about the perceived risk of web-based predatory paedophiles; arguments about the electronic dissipation of children's creativity; and the potential for social isolation through the development of increasingly personalized digital technologies (Lewis, 2006; Stutz, 1996) is already evident. Although the possible risks entailed in bedroom activities should be acknowledged, these can be overestimated, and domestic space is *one* important space in which there appears to be some potential for positive health interventions and where leisure capital may be acquired. Addressing inherent anxieties and taking a broader view of health, the Child Exploitation and Online Protection Centre has established a website designed to enable children and young people to report potential and real online abuse (http://thinkuknow.co.uk).

For many children and young people, private domestic space, where this exists, is an important feature of growing autonomy. For income-poor children, for looked after children, and for other disadvantaged young people, this may present difficulties (Department of Health, 2002b, p.38). Bedroom culture is based principally on the use of electronic media, which confers cultural capital on participants. Evidence suggests that large numbers of children are engaged in leisure-based media practices almost from birth (Marsh *et al.*, 2005, pp.24–5). Young people with internet connections have developed on-line *virtual* game spaces that provide settings for interactions that contribute to autonomy and agency (Crowe and Bradford, 2006), and such access is growing: currently about 70 per cent of UK families. An estimated 5 per cent of children in the 9- to 19-year age range have personal computers or laptops in their bedrooms. Ownership is powerfully shaped by social difference, not only by socio-economic status.

Levels of family *cultural* capital (e.g. parental post-school educational background) are also important. Middle class young people have higher internet access, and young people in families with less cultural capital tend to own more screen entertainment media. Marsh *et al.* calculated in 2005 that, typically, the young people in their study engaged in screen use (TV, computer games, watching videos, and playing hand-held games) for 2 hours and 6 minutes every day. Although a relatively unexplored setting for public health policy makers, initiatives exist that draw on young people's ICT competences.

'Wired for Health' (www.wiredforhealth.gov.uk/home.php?catid=872), operating under the National Healthy School Standard, comprises four age-graded health-focused websites. The site for younger children (Key Stage 1, ages 4–7 years) provides a mixture of familiar narrative stories based on family life, that are designed to encourage reflection on health issues (e.g. smoking, personal hygiene, dental health, safety at home) alongside basic information designed to enhance healthy choices. The site for 14- to 16-year-olds (Key Stage 4) is sophisticated and includes health issues through advice, information, tips, links to other websites and help-lines. The common link between these initiatives is an aim of empowering young people to make good, individual decisions on the basis of accurate information, and to provide links to further help and advice. It is difficult to know how effective this initiative has been; it is not specifically referred to in the evaluation of the National Healthy School Standard under whose aegis it operates.

Initiatives aimed at older young people are accessible through the online Connexions Direct website (www.connexions-direct.com/). Health quizzes, comprehensive information on health matters, and the opportunity to post 'my story' online for others to read are all offered in a familiar and accessible teenage magazine format and designed in language for this age group. The website provides email, phone, text and online access to advisers, and is intended to be able to deal with any of the issues referred to on the website. A similar site focusing on drug use for young people, parents and carers is FRANK, supported by the Department of Health, the Home Office and the DfES (www.talktofrank.com/), provides phone and email contacts, a range of health information, and advice in similar format to Connexions Direct.

'Blogging' has grown as a familiar cultural form, and may have educational potential for young people and health through its capacity to establish online communities, to provide easy access and participation in discourse (Nardi, 2004). The increasing popularity of 'you tube'; 'my space'; and 'vampire freaks.com' suggests that these media are enormously attractive to young people. Whether the incorporation of this format into health initiatives would be quite as engaging, remains an open question. These technologies are very new and substantially unresearched. However, as social interaction has important health benefits, the outcomes of 'virtual' sociability framed in the context of bedroom cultures is an important area for further research and potential practice.

CONCLUSION

Leisure is a complex and, primarily, *paradoxical* concept. It designates an inexhaustible range of practices, activities, material and temporal spaces whose sole commonality is constituted by being defined and – freely – chosen by participants as 'leisure'. The paradox lies in leisure's potential for, and claim to 'freedom'. Yet, it has a simultaneous designation as a setting in which young people and children, who are often construed as risky social categories, find that they are subjected to increasingly invasive adult surveillance. Leisure, it seems, will always be a vehicle for other interventions. Clearly, leisure spaces exist in which young people can, and should, engage in critical dialogue about health and well-being – perhaps as part of a wider discussion of citizenship – with sympathetic professionals. In other material and virtual settings young people can be left to their own devices away from the perpetual adult gaze.

Health, particularly public health, is also a problematic concept. Should health be regarded as a right or a responsibility (or both), *whose* responsibility is health and *who* is entitled to health as a right? To what extent should states be charged with intervening in the private domain (e.g. leisure) in order to encourage happy, productive and healthy citizens?

We have suggested that the effectiveness of interventions in young people's leisure time and space is invariably difficult to establish because the nature of the evidence base (its epistemological status) is always in question. This is the case because either the existing evidence is not sufficiently robust or because of the political nature of policy making itself. It is well to remember that the absence of evidence does not necessarily signal the ineffectiveness of a given intervention, despite the difficulties that managerialized cultures have in acknowledging this.

Although central to the lives of young people in providing relative autonomy, psychosocial well-being, and the acquisition of forms of capital (for example, social and cultural capital), leisure has also become thoroughly commodified as part of consumer culture. In a society characterized by growing inequality, this has led to the differential distribution of young people's leisure opportunities, determined by social class position and by social difference more widely (by gender and race particularly). Insofar as leisure provides opportunities for young people to develop *leisure capital* (knowledge, skills and dispositions that may be transformed into resilience and the means for coping with life challenges such as health concerns), inequality is of primary significance. The question of *who* acquires leisure capital, and who does not, needs to be addressed. Conceivably, the development of Young People's Services, signalled under *Every Child Matters* (Chief Secretary to the Treasury, 2003) and *Youth Matters* (Department for Education and Skills, 2005) will enhance the voice of young people in advocating their own health interests and challenging the inequalities that continue to compromise their well-being.

KEY POINTS

- Leisure is a space of choice and freedom but is simultaneously designated as a setting for informal health interventions in young people's lives.
- The boundary between leisure and non-leisure is permeable: activities in 'extended schools', for example, can be seen as bridging the two.
- Fears about young people's safety have meant that leisure is increasingly supervised by adults.
- Young people's access to leisure opportunities is shaped by social difference: class, gender and race in particular.
- Leisure is the setting for a range of informal health interventions in young people's lives, focused on healthy eating, exercise, drug use and abuse, suicide and self-harm, sexuality, and so on.
- Reflecting patterns of social difference, young people differentially acquire leisure capital: knowledge, skills and disposition in relation to health that can be transformed into resilience and coping strategies.

- Different leisure settings (public space, organized leisure spaces and private domestic space) can provide a range of opportunities for health interventions.
- Evidence for effective health interventions in young people's leisure space is incomplete and evaluation strategies have often been insufficiently robust.
- New policy initiatives – *Every Child Matters* and *Youth Matters*, for example – introduce possibilities for addressing inequalities in leisure provision, the unequal acquisition of leisure capital and, therefore, health inequalities among young people.

REFERENCES

Aapola S, Gonick M, Harris A (2005), *Young Femininity, Girlhood, Power and Social Change*. Basingstoke: Palgrave Macmillan.

Advisory Council on the Misuse of Drugs (2006), *Pathways to Problems, Hazardous use of Tobacco, Alcohol and other Drugs by Young People in the UK and its Implications for Policy*. London: Home Office.

Ball SJ (1993), What is policy? Texts, trajectories and toolboxes. *Discourse* 13:9–17.

Baraitser P, Dolan F, Feldman R, Cowley S (2002) Sexual health work in a playground: lessons learnt from the evaluation of a small-scale sexual health project. *Journal of Family Planning and Reproductive Health Care* 2002:28:18–22.

Beck U (2004) *Risk Society Towards a New Modernity*. London: Sage Publications.

Biddle SJH, Gorely T and Stensel DJ (2004) Health-enhancing physical activity and sedentary behaviour in children and adolescents. *Journal of Sports Sciences* 22:679–701.

Blair M, Stewart-Brown S, Waterston T, Crowther R (2003) *Child Public Health*. Oxford: Oxford University Press.

Blenkinsop S, Eggers M, Schagen I *et al.* (2004) *Evaluation of the Impact of the National Healthy School Standard. Final report*. www.wiredforhealth.gov.uk/PDF/Full_report_2004.pdf (accessed 10 January 2007).

Bradford S (2006) Practising the double doctrine of freedom: managing young people in the context of war. In: Gilchrist R, Jeffs T, Spence J (eds) *Drawing on the Past: studies in the history of community and youth work*, Leicester: National Youth Agency, pp.132–49.

Bradford S, Kindness L, Hey V, Cullen F (2003) '*You're either in or you're out or you're a Saddo . . .*' Report of the Young Agenda Survey completed in the London Borough of Richmond upon Thames. London: Richmond Parish Lands Carity in association with Brunel University.

Bradford S, Hey V, Cullen F (2004) *What Works? An exploration of the value of informal education work with young people*, London: Clubs for Young People in association with Brunel University.

British Heart Foundation (2004) *Couch Kids: the continuing epidemic*. London: British Heart Foundation.

Chief Secretary to the Treasury (2003) *Every Child Matters* (Cm 5860). London: Stationery Office. www.everychildmatters.gov.uk/_content/documents/EveryChildMatters.pdf (accessed 17 January 2007).

Children's Society (2006) *Good Childhood? A question for our times*. London: Children's Society.

Cowley S (2002) Public health practice in nursing and health visiting. In: Cowley S (ed.) *Public Health in Policy and Practice, a Sourcebook for Health Visitors and Nurses*. Edinburgh: Balliere Tindall, pp.5–24.

Crabbe T (2005) *'Getting to Know You': engagement and relationship building first interim national positive futures case study research report*. London: Positive Futures.

Crimmens D, Factor F, Jeffs T *et al.* (2004) *Reaching Socially Excluded Young People. A national study of street-based youth work*. London: Joseph Rowntree Foundation and The National Youth Agency.

Crowe N, Bradford S (2006) 'Hanging out in RuneScape': identity, work and leisure in the virtual playground. *Children's Geographies* 4:331–46.

Department for Education (1995) *OPCS Survey of Youth Service Participation*, London: HMSO.

Department for Education and Skills (2005) *Youth Matters*. Nottingham: DfES Publications.

Department for Education and Skills (2006) *Youth Matters: next steps. Something to do, somewhere to go, someone to talk to*. Nottingham: DfES Publications.

Department of Health (2002a) *Promoting the Health of Looked After Children*. London: Department of Health Publications.

Department of Health (2002b) *Children's Homes, National Minimum Standards*. London: The Stationery Office.

Department of Health (2004) *Choosing Health, making Healthy Choices Easier*. London: The Stationery Office.

Department of Health (2005) *Tackling Health Inequalities: status report on the programme for action*. London: The Stationery Office.

Department of Health and Department for Education and Skills (2004) *National Service Framework for Children, Young People and Maternity Services*. London: Department of Health.

Department for Transport (2005) *Focus on Personal Travel*. London: Stationery Office.

Department for Work and Pensions (2005) *Family Life in Britain: findings from the 2003 Families and Children Study (FACS)*. Leeds: Corporate Document Services.

Etzioni A (1997) *The New Golden Rule: community and morality in a democratic society*. London: Profile Books.

Fox K, Rickards L (2004) *Sport and Leisure, Results from the Sport and Leisure Module of the 2002 General Household Survey*. London: The Stationery Office

Furedi F (2005) *Culture of Fear: risk taking and the morality of low expectations*, London: Continuum.

Furlong A, Cartmel F, Powney J, Hall S (1997) *Evaluating Youth work with Vulnerable Young People*. Glasgow: Scottish Council for Research in Education.

Goodwin M, Armstrong-Esther D (2004) Children, social capital and health. Increasing the well being of young people in rural Wales. *Children's Geographies* 2:49–63.

Harland K, Morgan T, Muldoon O (2005) *The Nature of Youth Work in Northern Ireland: purpose, contribution and challenges*. Belfast: Department of Education.

Hendry LB, Shucksmith J, Love JG, Glendinning A (1993) *Young People's Leisure and Lifestyles*. London: Routledge.

Hendry L, Kloep M, Espnes G *et al.* (2002) Leisure transitions – a rural perspective. *Leisure Studies* 21:1–14.

Hey V, Bradford S (2006) Re-engineering Motherhood? Surestart in the Community. *Contemporary Issues in Early Childhood* 7:53–67.

Kingdon J (1995) *Agendas, Alternatives, and Public Policies* (2e). New York: Longman.

Lewis P (2006) *Teenage Networking Websites Face anti-paedophile Investigation*. www.guardian.co.uk/uk_news/story/0,,1811159,00.html (accessed 10 January 2007).

Lincoln S (2005) Feeling the noise: teenagers, bedrooms and music. *Leisure Studies* 24:399–414.

Marsh J, Brooks G, Hughes J *et al.* (2005) *Digital Beginnings: young children's use of popular culture, media and new technologies*. Sheffield: Literacy Research Centre.

Mellanby A, Rees J, Tripp J (2000) Peer-led and adult-led school health education: a critical review of available comparative research. *Health Education Research Theory and Practice* 15:533–45.

Meltzer H, Gatward R, with Goodman R, Ford T (2000) *The Mental Health of Children and Adolescents in Great Britain, Summary Report,* London: National Statistics.

Merton B, Payne M, Smith D; Youth Affairs Unit, De Montfort University (2004) *An Evaluation of the Impact of Youth Work in England, Research Report RR606*. Nottingham: DfES Publications.

Monaghan LF (2005) Discussion piece: a critical take on the obesity debate. *Social Theory and Health* 3:302–14.

Morrow VM (2000) 'Dirty looks' and 'trampy places' in young people's accounts of community and neighbourhood: implications for health inequalities. *Critical Public Health* 10:141–52.

Mulvihill C, Rivers K, Aggleton P (2000) *Physical Activity 'At Our Time': qualitative research among young people aged 5 to 15 years and parents*. London: Health Education Authority.

Muncie J (2004) *Youth and Crime* (2e). London: Sage Publications.

Nardi B (2004) *Learning and Web Technologies in Evolution: creativity and catharsis in blogging*. www.ilrt.bris.ac.uk/news/conferences/colston2004/programme/nardi.pdf (accessed 10 January 2007).

National Statistics (2006) *The Health of Children and Young People*. www. statistics.gov.uk/children/default.asp (accessed 10 January 2007).

Pantazis C, Gordon D, Levitas R (2006) *Poverty and Social Exclusion in Britain: the Millennium Survey*. Bristol: Policy Press.

Parsons W (1995) *Public Policy. An introduction to the theory and practice of policy analysis*. Aldershot: Edward Elgar.

Parton N (2006) *Safeguarding Childhood: early intervention and surveillance in late modern society*, Basingstoke: Palgrave Macmillan.

Petersen A (1997) Risk, governance and the new public health. In: Petersen A, Bunton R (eds) *Foucault, Health and Medicine*. London: Routledge, pp.189–206.

Putnam RD (2000) *Bowling Alone, the Collapse and Revival of American Community* . New York: Touchstone Books.

Robertson S (2005) *Youth Clubs Association, Partnership, Friendship and Fun*. Lyme Regis: Russell House Publishing.

Scottish Executive (2003) *Improving Health in Scotland, the Challenge*. Edinburgh: The Stationery Office.

Shaw M, Davey Smith G, Dorling D (2005) Health inequalities and New Labour: how the promises compare with real progress. *British Medical Journal* 330:1016–21.

Sport England (2003) *Young people and Sport in England Trends in Participation 1994–2002, Research study conducted for Sport England by MORI*. London: Sport England.

Squires P (ed.) (2006) *Community Safety. Critical perspectives on policy and practice,* Bristol: Policy Press.

Stutz E (1996) Is electronic entertainment hindering children's play and social development? In: Gill T (ed.) *Electronic Children: how children are responding to the information revolution*. London: National Children's Bureau, pp.59–70.

Swann C, Bowe K, McCormick G, Kosmin M (2003) *Teenage Pregnancy and Parenthood: a review of reviews, evidence briefing*. London: Health Development Agency.

Thompson AM, Rehman LA, Humbert ML (2005) Factors influencing the physically active leisure of children and youth: a qualitative study. *Leisure Sciences* 27:421–38.

Watt P, Stenson K (1998) The Street: 'It's a bit dodgy around there', safety, danger, ethnicity and young people's use of public space. In: Skelton T, Valentine G (eds) *Cool Places, Geographies of Youth Cultures* London: Routledge.

Welsh Assembly (2003) *Health and Wellbeing for Children and Young People: action in response to the issues raised in the Health Behaviour in School-aged Children (HBSC) Study, 1986–2000*. Cardiff: Welsh Assembly Government.

Wiggins M, Rosato M, Austerberry H, Sawtell M, Oliver S (2005) *Supporting Teenagers who are Pregnant or Parents. Sure Start Plus National Evaluation*: *Executive Summary*. London: Social Science Research Unit Report, Institute of Education. www.ioe.ac.uk/ssru/reports/ssplusexecutivesummary2005.pdf (accessed 10 January 2007).

Zeijl E, Du Bois-Reymond M, Te Poel Y (2002) Young adolescents' leisure patterns. *Society and Leisure* 24:379–402.

Act of Parliament

This Act is published by HMSO in London, and can be accessed from the UK Parliament website (www.publications.parliament.uk).

Crime and Disorder Act 1998

7 VULNERABLE CHILDREN

Jane V Appleton

INTRODUCTION

The public inquiry into the death of Victoria Climbié drew significant national and international attention to the failings of public agencies to protect a vulnerable child.

> *When Victoria was admitted to the North Middlesex Hospital on the evening of 24 February 2000 she was desperately ill. She was bruised, deformed and malnourished. Her temperature was so low it could not be recorded on the hospital's standard thermometer. Dr Lesley Alsford, the consultant responsible for Victoria's care on that occasion, said, 'I had never seen a case like it before. It is the worst case of child abuse and neglect that I have ever seen'.*
> **(Department of Health and Home Office, 2003, Para 1.5)**

Victoria was 8 years and 3 months old when she died on the afternoon of 25 February 2000, 'the victim of almost unimaginable cruelty' (Department of Health and Home Office, 2003, Para 1.1). Lord Laming's Inquiry into her death (Department of Health and Home Office, 2003) identified many occasions when agencies had the chance to intervene and protect Victoria, but they failed to do so. His damming report highlighted significant problems in both single-agency and multi-agency work and cited 'widespread organisational malaise' (Para 1.21) as the main reason for failure to protect Victoria. The inquiry report resulted in a series of 108 basic good-practice recommendations, and was closely followed by the publication *Keeping Children Safe* (Department for Education and Skills [DfES], Department of Health and Home Office,

2003) the government's response to the Victoria Climbié Inquiry Report and the Green Paper *Every Child Matters* (Chief Secretary to the Treasury, 2003).

In the light of continuing failures to safeguard vulnerable children, subsequent policy developments have reiterated the need to prioritize preventive work and strengthen services for children, young people and their families (HM Government, 2004). Policy has shifted from dealing with the consequences of disadvantage and deprivation, to early identification and the provision of greater support to children living in vulnerable circumstances. It is therefore important to consider the needs of the vulnerable school-age child, when addressing public health practice with the school-age population.

This chapter examines the concept of vulnerability and presents key evidence as to why vulnerable school-age children present a significant public health concern. It explores how the adoption of a public health approach is crucial in ensuring that vulnerable school-age children are identified at an early stage and offered the services and support that they need to maximize their health and well-being and potentially to prevent child abuse and neglect.

VULNERABLE CHILDREN AND YOUNG PEOPLE – WHO ARE THEY?

There are many groups of school-age children who may be vulnerable and in need. The phrase 'vulnerable child' is used frequently in health and social care practice and has been used interchangeably with 'disadvantaged child', 'cause for concern', 'high dependency', 'high risk' or 'child in need'. Vulnerable children have been defined as 'those disadvantaged children who would benefit from extra help from public agencies in order to make the best of their life chances' (Department of Health, 1999, p.4). They include:

• children looked after by local authorities
• children in public care, i.e. hospital or residential care
• children and young people with disabilities
• children with mental health problems
• children with poor school attendance or who are excluded from school
• children and young people with behaviour problems
• young carers
• homeless young people
• young offenders
• young substance misusers
• teenage parents
• children of refugees or asylum seekers
• children and young people who are separated (Blair *et al.*, 2003; De Bell and Tomkins, 2006).

From a policy perspective, 'vulnerable children and young people' also include 'children in need' and those suffering 'significant harm'.

Terminology is often used interchangeably and in some policy guidance, such as the *Common Assessment Framework* (CAF) documentation (HM

Government, 2006a, 2006b) and *Lead Professional Good Practice Guidance* (DfES, 2005a), vulnerable children are referred to as 'children with additional needs' or 'complex needs'. Vulnerable children include those at risk of suffering poor outcomes in relation to the five outcomes identified in *Every Child Matters* (Chief Secretary to the Treasury, 2003, p.14):

• being healthy
• staying safe
• enjoying and achieving
• making a positive contribution
• achieving economic well-being.

The term also refers to those children with 'more significant or complex needs which meet the threshold for statutory involvement' (HM Government, 2006b, p.2) and are in need of protection.

THE CONCEPT OF VULNERABILITY

The origins of the concept of vulnerability

The conceptual basis of much research on vulnerability is seldom clearly specified, but links can often be traced to origins in psychology or sociology. Psychologists in particular have examined the links between vulnerability, stress and health (Selye, 1973). Lazarus's (1976) transactional model regards stress as a process in which the person is an active agent who can influence the impact of stress through behavioural, cognitive and emotional strategies. The adoption of such coping mechanisms can be important in reducing the effects of stress and can have a positive influence on health. Sociologists report vulnerability factors leading to ill-health, low self-esteem or an inability to cope, particularly when triggered by distressing life events or major difficulties and when protective factors are weakened or absent.

Several authors regard vulnerability as a continuum that is dynamic and constantly changing (Rose and Killien, 1983; Rose, 1984; Copp, 1986; Lessick *et al.*, 1992; Appleton, 1994; Rogers, 1997). Individuals move in and out of vulnerability at various stages of the life trajectory. This appears to be dependent on a complex interplay of internal and external stress factors and coping ability (Rose and Killien, 1983; Appleton, 1994), with children and young people becoming more vulnerable at times of biological, psychological or social transition, such as during adolescence, school transition, teenage pregnancy and teenage parenthood (Rose and Killien, 1983; Wells, 1986; Rich, 1992; Rogers, 1997). It is widely recognized that there are different levels or degrees of vulnerability. Early assessment of a child or young person's needs is essential to ensure that sources of stress for children within families are identified, and appropriate interventions offered (HM Government, 2006c). Some children are more susceptible to the negative effects of stress than others, and are therefore more likely to be vulnerable and suffer health and/or social problems.

Vulnerability is often described in terms of, or used interchangeably with the concept of risk. This is a trend that is particularly evident in the mental health, child protection and social work research literature. Rose and Killien (1983, p.61) have usefully differentiated between the concepts of vulnerability and risk, describing vulnerability as 'personal factors that interact with the environment to influence health' and risk as 'the presence of potentially stressful factors in a person's environment' hazardous to health. Risk factors 'are influences, occurring at any systemic level (i.e. individual, family, community, society), that threaten positive adaptational outcomes' (Waller, 2001, p.292). Rose and Killien (1983, p.67) suggest that risk and vulnerability are interrelated, 'that one affects the other in a dynamic way' and that characteristics of both the individual and environment may contribute to health, illness and vulnerability (Phillips, 1992; Rogers, 1997).

Research evidence continually illustrates that vulnerability is a complex concept. It is widely acknowledged that a range of predisposing factors can contribute to vulnerability amongst school-age children (Aggleton, 1996; Stewart-Brown, 1998; Mental Health Foundation, 1999a; Hall and Elliman, 2003). It is often not difficult to explain the causes of or describe the circumstances of a child or young persons' vulnerability. Lists of vulnerability risk factors abound, particularly in relation to child abuse, yet accurately predicting from a research perspective as to which parents are at risk of abusing their children is fraught with difficulty and potential inaccuracies (Goddard *et al.*, 1999).

However, lists of vulnerability risk factors can be useful in assisting public health professionals to determine whether a child or young person *is* vulnerable, in need or in need of protection. For example, in Chapter 8, Rees and Morley highlight risk factors for children suffering mental health problems. Likewise Hall and Elliman (2003, p.269) describe the following risk factors for the development of psychological and mental health problems amongst children :

- poor/inadequate parenting
- families who are socially deprived
- living in an inner-city area
- being a boy
- having learning difficulties and, in young children, delayed language development or other communication difficulties
- having other health problems or development problems
- adolescence rather than earlier childhood
- being 'looked after'.

Risk factors associated with the wider family and family relationships are also regarded as contributors to children's and young people's emotional and mental health problems (Aggleton, 1996; NHS Executive, 1996, pp.269–70; Mental Health Foundation, 1999b; Hall and Elliman, 2003). These include:

- marital discord/parental divorce/volatile relationships
- family breakdown
- family violence
- physical, sexual and/or emotional abuse

- parental mental health problems
- lack of warmth/affection/parental coldness or irritability towards the child
- poor parental supervision/neglect of the child.

There is also evidence that a number of resilience factors can enable some vulnerable children to thrive in difficult circumstances and reduce the effects of any risk factors. These are sometimes referred to as a child's 'resources' or 'protective factors'. For example, many separated children, such as unaccompanied young asylum seekers, demonstrate considerable resilience and determination to succeed. There is growing evidence that the act of becoming a young asylum seeker requires great capability and strength of character (Kohli and Mather, 2003).

The Mental Health Foundation (1999a) has outlined resilience factors for children suffering mental health problems in terms of child, family and environmental characteristics and these are summarized in Table 7.1.

There is clearly a diverse range of adverse life experiences that may result in a child or young person being vulnerable. Vulnerability itself is a complex phenomenon, although it is well recognized that there are particular sets of circumstances that may result in a child being more susceptible to vulnerability. In practice each child's and young person's needs should be assessed on an individual basis, using tools such as the *Framework for the Assessment of Children in Need and their Families* (Department of Health *et al.*, 2000) or the *Common Assessment Framework for Children and Young People* (CAF) (HM Government, 2006a). While it may not be difficult to explain the causes of or describe the circumstances of a child's or young person's vulnerability, what remains the key challenge is identifying ways to prevent or reduce that vulnerability (DeBell and Tomkins, 2006).

TABLE 7.1   *Resilience factors*

In the child	In the family	In the environment
Being female	At least one good parent–child	Wider supportive network
Higher intelligence	relationship	Good housing
Easy temperament	Affection	High standard of living
when an infant	Supervision, authoritative	High school morale and
Secure attachment	discipline	positive attitudes
Positive attitude,	Support for education	Schools with strong academic
problem-solving	Supportive marriage/absence	and non-academic
approach	of severe discord	opportunities
Good communication		Range of positive sport/
skills		leisure activities
Planner, belief in control		
Humour, religious faith		
Capacity to reflect		

Reproduced with permission from: Mental Health Foundation (1999) *Bright Futures – Promoting Children and Young People's Mental Health*. London: The Mental Health Foundation.

VULNERABLE CHILDREN AND THE WIDER SAFEGUARDING AGENDA

So, where does the vulnerable school-age child fit into the wider safeguarding agenda? Put simply, safeguarding is 'an umbrella term incorporating all aspects of work with vulnerable children, children in need and children who are suffering, or at risk of significant harm' (Appleton and Clemerson-Trew, 2007). Safeguarding mirrors the conceptual basis of vulnerability highlighted earlier in this chapter, and can be used to illustrate the continuum of needs and children's potential vulnerability. Figure 7.1 illustrates the continuum of needs and services for all children and young people outlined in the CAF documentation. This continuum reflects the different levels of children's needs and vulnerability ranging from children with no additional needs to those with complex difficulties. In the case of Victoria Climbié, who was at the acute end of the spectrum, at very high risk and in need of protection, the continuum illustrates the potential for such acute vulnerability to end tragically in death.

Vulnerable children and, in particular, the concept of 'children in need' has often been conceptualized as a continuum. This perspective emerged from *Child Protection: messages from research* (Department of Health/Dartington Social Research Unit, 1995), and the subsequent 'refocusing debate'. This debate drew attention to the need to identify ways in which more multi-agency work can be undertaken preventatively with children in need, to prevent problems and family breakdown rather than focusing the majority of services on assessment and inquiry into child protection concerns. Viewing vulnerability as a continuum embraces a focus on early needs identification through holistic assessment and an increasing focus on agencies working together to meet the needs of the school-age child.

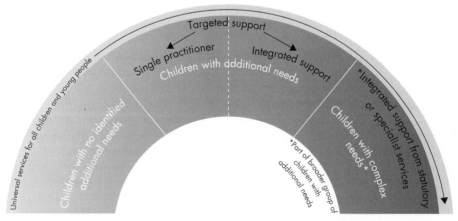

Figure 7.1 The continuum of needs and services for all children and young people outlined in *The Common Assessment Framework for Children and Young People*. From HM Government (2006b) *Common Assessment Framework for Children and Young People: managers' guide. Integrated working to improve outcomes for children and young people*. Nottingham: DfES Publications, p.7. Crown Copyright material is reproduced with the permission of the Controller of HMSO and the Queen's Printer for Scotland.

Safeguarding children

It was the Children Act 1989 that first placed a duty on local authorities 'to safeguard and promote the welfare' of vulnerable children (Section 17) (Department of Health, 1989). At its simplest, safeguarding is about 'keeping children safe from harm, such as illness, abuse or injury' (Children's Rights Director, 2004, p.3). This view was extended in the *Framework for the Assessment of Children in Need and their Families* (Department of Health, 1999) to incorporate two elements: 'a duty to safeguard children from maltreatment' and a 'duty to prevent impairment'. The Assessment Framework, developed as part of the Quality Protects Programme provides a systematic approach to assessing children and families' needs. It incorporates three key areas:

- the child or young person's developmental needs
- the capacity of parents to respond appropriately to those needs
- the impact of wider family and environmental factors on parenting capacity and the child (Department of Health *et al.*, 2000).

Widespread use of the Assessment Framework across several agencies, not just social work, has helped to support the broad shift in policy, from one where the central focus has been the identification of child abuse, to the adoption of a broader and more holistic view of children's well-being, with impairment identified in the context of a child's development and their current and long-term health and well-being (Department of Health *et al.*, 2000; Gray, 2002; Cleaver *et al.*, 2004; Parton, 2006).

This point is illustrated further in the most recent *Working Together to Safeguard Children* (HM Government, 2006c) guidance, which defines 'safeguarding and promoting the welfare of children' as:

> - *protecting children from maltreatment;*
> - *preventing impairment of children's health or development; and*
> - *ensuring that they are growing up in circumstances consistent with the provision of safe and effective care;*
> - *and undertaking that role so as to enable those children to have optimum life chances and to enter adulthood successfully.*

> **(HM Government, 2006c, p.5)**

Working Together to Safeguard Children (HM Government, 2006c) acknowledges that these elements of safeguarding and promoting children's welfare are cumulative and contribute to the *Every Child Matters* (Chief Secretary to the Treasury, 2003) outcomes.

Thus, vulnerable school-age children are increasingly defined as those children where there are concerns about their welfare. Safeguarding includes the need for early interventions to identify such children proactively, who, with their families, could benefit from professional input and support. In schools and further education (FE) institutions, 'safeguarding responsibilities extend to pupil health and safety, bullying, fulfilling specific statutory requirements together with other issues, for example, arrangements for meeting the medical needs of children with medical conditions, providing first aid, school security, drugs and substance misuse' (Department of Health and DfES, 2004). The continuum of needs recognizes that there is a potential for any child to be vulnerable and in need of additional support.

Child welfare concerns, children in need and significant harm

Since the mid-1990s there has been a change of focus for much of the work that in the late 1980s and early 1990s would have been considered to be child protection work. Since the publication of *Child Protection: messages from research* (Department of Health/Dartington Social Research Unit, 1995) and the subsequent 're-focusing debate', it has been widely accepted that child protection must be viewed as a broad concept including all elements of children in need and significant harm. This is further substantiated by the recent policy move to focus on safeguarding children. Local Safeguarding Children Boards largely agree that initial responses to referrals to children's social services should be viewed as being about child welfare concerns. Following an initial assessment, this may indicate that a child is a 'child in need' as defined by Section 17 of the Children Act 1989.

A child is in need (Children Act 1989, Part III Section 17(10)) if his/her vulnerability is such that:

- '. . . he [or she] is unlikely to achieve or maintain, or have the opportunity of achieving or maintaining a reasonable standard of health or development without the provision for him [or her] of services by the local authority'
- '. . . his [or her] health or development is likely to be significantly impaired, or further impaired without the provision of such services', or
- '. . . he [or she] is disabled'.

The important factors to be considered in deciding whether a child is in need under the Children Act 1989 are 'What will happen to a child's health or development without services being provided, and the likely effect the services will have on the child's standard of health and development' (HM Government, 2006c, Section 1(22), p.5).

Working Together to Safeguard Children (HM Government, 2006c) outlines the role that the local authority children's social care has in co-ordinating multi-agency children in need assessments in order to provide welfare support to the child and family. The joint agency care plan agreed with the parents and school-age child should include practical steps that the parents agree to carry out to achieve change in their parenting and the nature of the support to be provided by appropriate professionals to the young person. Some work may be carried out jointly, for example a school nurse and a child and adolescent mental health service (CAMHS) therapist might work with a teenager and their parents on dealing with disruptive school behaviour (Buckland *et al.*, 2005). Such joint working has been outlined as part of the refocusing debate and falls within children in need legislation in The Children Act 1989 (Section 17). The types of interventions and services that may help school-age children and their families will vary significantly depending on their particular needs and individual circumstances (HM Government, 2006c).

At the acute end of the continuum, child protection is a key aspect of safeguarding and promoting welfare (HM Government, 2006c). In serious or chronic cases where it is suspected that a child is suffering or is likely to suffer significant harm as result of abuse or neglect, child protection procedures and a core assessment under Section 47 of The Children Act 1989 will be needed (HM Government, 2006c). When a child protection conference is convened, the conference members should consider if a child is at continuing risk of significant harm when determining whether the child should be the subject of a child protection plan. 'The test should be that either:

- the child can be shown to have suffered ill-treatment or impairment of health or development as a result of physical, emotional, or sexual abuse or neglect, and professional judgement is that further ill-treatment or impairment are likely; *or*
- professional judgement, substantiated by the findings of enquiries in this individual case or by research evidence, is that the child is likely to suffer ill-treatment or the impairment of health or development as a result of physical, emotional, or sexual abuse or neglect' (HM Government, 2006c, Section 5(102–103), p. 101).

Significant harm is the threshold beyond which children in need are regarded as children needing protection, and child protection procedures are instigated. A child is in need of protection where there is likely or actual significant harm, or he/she is at risk. Yet neither the Children Act 1989 nor *Working Together to Safeguard Children* (HM Government, 2006c) give a definitive interpretation of the concept of significant harm. In fact *Working Together to Safeguard Children* states that 'there are no absolute criteria on which to rely when judging' this. It says 'sometimes a single traumatic event may constitute significant harm, e.g. a violent assault, suffocation or poisoning. More often, significant harm is a compilation of significant events, both acute and longstanding which interrupt, change or damage the child's physical and psychological development' (HM Government, 2006c, Section 1(25), p.6). The guidance highlights research on sources of stress for children and families that may have an adverse effect on a child's health, development, and well-being, and that should be taken in to account when children's and families' needs are assessed. These sources of stress include social exclusion, mental illness of a parent or carer, parental learning disability, domestic violence and drug and alcohol misuse (HM Government, 2006c, Section 9(11–25), pp.158–62).

WHY VULNERABLE CHILDREN AND YOUNG PEOPLE ARE A SIGNIFICANT PUBLIC HEALTH ISSUE

The evidence base

The key argument for viewing vulnerable school-age children as a public health issue is the negative impact that unidentified or unresolved vulnerability has on the individual child, school community and society (Department of Health,

2004a). While at one level the government has acknowledged the impact on children's public health of wider social influences such as poverty, unemployment, homelessness and social exclusion (Acheson, 1998), the publication of *Choosing Health* (Department of Health, 2004b) has produced tensions by focusing attention on a model of prevention that seeks to focus on individual responsibility for health behaviour. Identifying problems early, or intervening to reduce their initial occurrence or subsequent escalation is central to the government's agenda outlined in the *Every Child Matters: change for children* (HM Government, 2004) programme. This view is reiterated in *Youth Matters: next steps* (DfES, 2006a) and the Social Exclusion Action Plan *Reaching Out* (HM Government, 2006d), which reinforce the government's commitment to support children and young people with poor life chances who are especially vulnerable to social exclusion. It is also a central theme of the Treasury document *Policy Review of Children and Young People. A discussion paper* (HM Treasury and DfES, 2007) prepared for the government's 2007 Comprehensive Spending Review.

There is an increasing body of evidence illustrating the adverse consequences for children of a failure to address their needs effectively, linked to negative outcomes in terms of their later social and emotional development (Macdonald, 2001). Children living in poverty are more likely to suffer disadvantage including emotional and behavioural problems than those children from more affluent backgrounds (Seccombe, 2000). These children and young people are more likely to experience peer relationship difficulties, suffer depression, or social withdrawal, have low self-esteem and self-confidence and do badly at school (Seccombe, 2000). The inter-generational cycle of disadvantage is well reported, with children born into disadvantaged or at-risk families having a greater chance of experiencing similar difficulties to their parents (Social Exclusion Unit, 2004).

In terms of child protection, the relationship between child-rearing problems such as harsh discipline and subsequent childhood behaviour problems, later delinquency, conduct disorders and criminality is well recognized (Farrington, 1995; Buchannan, 1996; Hosking and Walsh, 2005). Farrington (1995) and Silverman *et al.* (1996) have highlighted the potential long-term mental health difficulties and behavioural problems associated with physical abuse and neglect in childhood. Research evidence suggests that there may be a correlation between adult mental health problems, a history of past child abuse or neglect, and subsequent ability to parent successfully (Gibbons *et al.*, 1995). Child abuse can result in poor self-esteem or an inability to form social relationships (Mullen *et al.*, 1996; Bifulco and Moran, 1998). In chronic situations this may result in childhood behaviour and conduct disorders, antisocial behaviour, substance misuse and later delinquency, violence and imprisonment (Farrington, 1995).

The influential report *Child Protection: messages from research* (Department of Health/Dartington Social Research Unit, 1995) described the long-term negative impacts on children of living in low-warmth/high-criticism environments as far more damaging than a single incident of over-chastisement. Roberts (1996) and Hagell (1998) have also reported the negative effects of children growing up in such environments. An absence of family support mechanisms during childhood may result in high levels of aggression and risk-taking behaviour in later adulthood

(Roberts, 1996). Reder and Duncan (1999) suggest that a further effect of child-hood distress can be seen in family life-cycles, particularly at times of transition such as birth, unemployment or during bereavement. Unresolved childhood vulnerability might affect an adult so their ability to adjust to changes may be prolonged, or result in relationship difficulties or psychological symptoms.

Domestic violence can also have a damaging effect on childhood outcomes (Osofsky, 2003; Hosking and Walsh, 2005; Smith Stover, 2005; Department of Health, 2006) and, in particular, children and young people's socio-emotional and behavioural development (Edleson, 1999). Of children on the child protection register 'nearly three-quarters live in households where domes-tic violence occurs' (Department of Health, 2002a, p.16). The risks to children are further increased when domestic violence occurs alongside parental mental illness or drug and alcohol misuse (Cleaver *et al.*, 1999). Violent childhood experiences have also been linked with intimate partner violence in later adult-hood relationships (Coid *et al.*, 2001; Whitfield *et al.*, 2003).

There is also considerable evidence that certain groups of vulnerable chil-dren are more likely to suffer negative outcomes. For example, looked after children and young people are at increased risk of mental health problems (Meltzer *et al.*, 2003; Stanley *et al.*, 2005), they often have poor access to health services and are in greater need of effective health-promotion interventions, particularly in relation to emotional well-being (Department of Health, 2002b; Scottish Executive, 2004; Fleming *et al.*, 2005; Simpson, 2006). Likewise there are strong links between being a young carer who lacks adequate professional support and experiencing impaired psychosocial development (Hall and Elliman, 2003) and low school achievement (DfES, 2006b; Hall and Elliman, 2003). 'Almost one-third of young carers have serious educational problems or have dropped out of school, with nearly all reporting missing school when the person they care for is having difficulties' (DfES, 2006b).

While it is clearly well documented that chronic poverty and social disadvantage do increase the likelihood of negative outcomes for children and young people, it is important to stress that not all children growing up in such vulnerable family households will experience poor outcomes (Seccombe, 2000, 2002; Barrett, 2003). In spite of considerable adversity, young people can and do rise above past abuse, poverty, loss and relationship problems to become mature and well-balanced indi-viduals (Bifulco and Moran, 1998; Heller *et al.*, 1999; Matsen *et al.*, 1999). Waller (2001, p.292) has argued that 'resilience is not the absence of vulnerability' but the presence of protective factors and a 'positive adaptation in response to adver-sity'. While there is considerable interest in the concept of resilience (Waller, 2001), as yet there is little understanding of the factors that make some children more resilient than others to child abuse and neglect (Macdonald, 2001).

Statistics

Statistical evidence pertaining to the health needs of the school-age population provides further evidence that vulnerable school-age children are a significant public health issue.

Vulnerable children

In 2005 the DfES estimated that of 11 million children in England, 3 million are vulnerable and living in disadvantaged circumstances, with between 300 000 and 400 000 being 'children in need' and known to social services at any one time (HM Government, 2006d). This is only the second time that the government has offered an official estimate of the numbers of vulnerable children in England, and this is likely to be a significant underestimate of the actual numbers of vulnerable children in society. However, regular statistics are collated in the UK on the numbers of children in need, children looked after and the children referred to social services and subject to child protection procedures.

Children in need

Since February 2000, the Office for National Statistics has collected data from local authorities on the numbers of children in need through the Children in Need (CiN) census. The CiN census is 'a biennial census of all children receiving a service from a social services department during the nominated census week' (National Statistics and DfES, 2006a, p. 6). This census organizes children's social services activity into three areas of work:

• intake and referral
• initial assessment work
• ongoing work (National Statistics and DfES, 2006a).

In February 2005 it was calculated that there were 385 300 children in need in England (National Statistics and DfES, 2006a).

Children looked after

Some children and young people who are referred to social services go on to be 'looked after'. Children 'looked after' are a subgroup of children in need and include:

• children accommodated under a voluntary agreement with their parents
• children who are the subject of an interim or full care order
• children compulsorily accommodated, including children on remand, those detained or committed for trial and children subject to short-term emergency orders or police protection (Department of Health, 1997a; National Statistics and DfES, 2006b).

In England on 31 March 2005, it was estimated that 60 900 children were being looked after by local authorities, with 3000 of these on child protection registers (National Statistics and DfES 2006a, 2006b). Table 7.2 illustrates the numbers of children looked after by local authorities from 2001 to 2005, by age, gender, legal status and placement. However, it excludes those looked after children who were the subject of an agreed series of short-term placements under Section 20 of the Children Act 1989. This table illustrates the increasing numbers of children looked after by local authorities, with only a slight fall in 2005. 'The largest category of placement for children looked after on 31 March

TABLE 7.2 Children looked after at 31 March in England, by age, sex, legal status and placement, 2001–2005.[1] Figures have been rounded to the nearest 1000, and to the nearest 10 otherwise. From National Statistics and DfES (2005) Children Looked After in England (Including Adoptions and Care Leavers), 2004–05. First release. Nottingham: DfES Publications, p.6. Crown Copyright material is reproduced with the permission of the Controller of HMSO and the Queen's Printer for Scotland.

		England					Numbers, percentages, and rates per 10000 children under 18				
		2001[2]	2002[2]	2003[2]	2004[3]	2005[3]	2001[2]	2002[2]	2003[2]	2004[3]	2005[3]
All children[1]		58 900	59 700	60 800	61 100	60 900	100	100	100	100	100
Rates per 10 000 children under 18		53	54	55	55	55				55	55
Sex	Male	32 600	33 200	33 200	33 900	33 700	55	56	55	55	55
	Female	26 300	26 500	27 200	27 200	27 700	45	44	45	45	45
Age	Under 1	2 300	2 300	2 600	2 600	2 800	4	4	4	4	5
	1–4	9 300	9 200	9 200	8 900	8 700	16	15	15	15	14
	5–9	13 400	13 300	13 300	12 700	12 100	23	22	22	21	20
	10–15	24 600	25 300	26 100	26 500	26 500	42	42	43	43	44
	16 and over	9 300	9 500	9 600	10 300	10 800	16	16	16	17	18
Legal status	Care orders	37 600	38 400	39 600	39 600	39 400	64	64	65	65	65
	Interim	7 900	8 800	10 200	9 000	9 500	13	15	17	15	16
	Full	29 800	29 600	29 300	30 600	29 900	51	50	48	50	49
	S20 CA 1989	19 100	19 000	18 900	18 800	18 800	32	32	31	31	31
	Freed for adoption[4]	1 600	1 800	1 900	2 400	2 300	3	3	3	4	4
	Other[4]	570	540	460	270	270	1	1	1	0	0
Placement	Foster	38 300	39 200	41 100	41 200	41 700	65	66	68	67	68
	Children's homes[5]	6 800	6 800	6 600	7 000	7 000	11	11	11	11	11
	With parents	6 900	6 700	6 400	5 900	5 700	12	11	10	10	9
	Placed for adoption	3 400	3 600	3 400	3 600	3 100	6	6	6	6	5
	Other[6]	3 400	3 400	3 300	3 500	3 300	6	6	5	6	5

1. Figures exclude children looked after under an agreed series of short-term placements
2. Figures are taken from the CLA100 return
3. Figures are taken from the SSDA903 return
4. Includes children who are on remand, committed for trial or detained, and children subject to emergency orders or police protection
5. Includes secure units, homes and hostels but excludes residential schools
6. Includes residential schools, lodgings and other residential settings

TABLE 7.3   *Unaccompanied asylum-seeking children looked after at 31 March in England by sex and region, 2002–2005.[1] Figures have been rounded to the nearest 100 if they exceed 1000, and to the nearest 10 otherwise. From National Statistics and DfES (2005) Children Looked After in England (Including Adoptions and Care Leavers), 2004–05. First release. Nottingham: DfES Publications, p.7. Crown Copyright material is reproduced with the permission of the Controller of HMSO and the Queen's Printer for Scotland.*

		England				Numbers and percentages			
		2002	2003	2004	2005	2002	2003	2004	2005
All children[1]		2 200	2 400	2 900	2 900	100	100	100	100
	Male	1 700	1 900	2 100	2 000	78	76	70	70
	Female	490	580	870	880	22	24	30	30
Region	North[2]	50	100	140	170	2	4	5	6
	Midlands[3]	160	230	270	280	7	9	9	10
	London	1 600	1 700	2 000	2 000	72	71	70	69
	South East (excl. London)	410	390	470	460	19	16	16	16

1. Figures exclude children looked after under an agreed series of short-term agreements
2. Includes North East, North West, Merseyside and Yorks & Humber
3. Includes East Midlands, West Midlands, South West and Eastern

2005 was foster care, accounting for 68 per cent of all placements', with the numbers of children in foster care placements having increased by 9 per cent since 2001 (National Statistics and DfES, 2005, p.1).

Statistics are also collated on vulnerable unaccompanied asylum-seeking children. These statistics illustrate that in England at 31 March 2005, there were 2900 unaccompanied asylum-seeking children looked after by local authorities (see Table 7.3), with 69 per cent of these being accommodated in London (National Statistics and DfES, 2005).

Child protection statistics

Annual child protection statistics have been collated in England since 1998 on the numbers of children registered on local authority child protection registers, and those subsequently de-registered. These statistics are based on the responses from all local authorities with children's social care service responsibilities. Annual figures are also maintained on the numbers of children referred to social services departments, the numbers of initial and core assessments conducted and the numbers of Section 47 enquires. 'At 31 March 2005 there were 25 900 children and young people on child protection registers in England, 1 per cent fewer than a year earlier. This represents a rate of 23 children per 10 000 in the population aged under 18' (National Statistics and DfES, 2006a, p.10). Fifty-nine per cent of these children were aged 5 years and over (National Statistics and DfES, 2006a).

While these statistics do go some way to demonstrating that vulnerable children are a significant public health issue, caution needs to be maintained when interpreting these figures as they are not a record of all vulnerable children (Department of Health, 1997b), only of vulnerable children who have been officially recognized (Corby, 1990). Furthermore, in terms of child protection statistics, the 1999

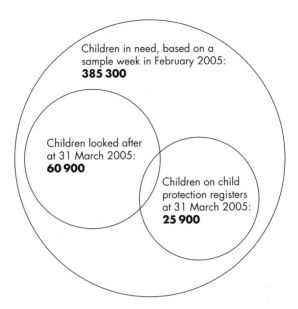

Figure 7.2 Numbers of children in need, children who are looked after and children who are on child protection registers in England, and the relationship between them. From National Statistics and DfES (2006a) *Statistics of Education: referrals, assessments and children and young people on child protection registers: year ending 31 March 2005*. London: National Statistics, p.7. *Crown Copyright material is reproduced with the permission of the Controller of HMSO and the Queen's Printer for Scotland.*

Working Together to Safeguard Children guidance (Department of Health *et al.*, 1999) 'raised the threshold for [child protection] registration by changing the criteria' from having suffered or was likely to suffer significant harm, to being at 'continuing risk of harm' and the requirement to have a child protection plan put in place (National Statistics and DfES, 2006a p. 10). Unsurprisingly this has resulted in a fall in the numbers of children on child protection registers. Indeed a recent NSPCC report (Cawson, 2002) estimated that as many as 16 per cent of children may have experienced serious maltreatment by their parents.

Links between children in need, children looked after and children registered on child protection registers

Figure 7.2 illustrates the relationship between children in need, children on the child protection register and children looked after. 'There is a small overlap between children who are looked after and children who are on child protection registers (3000 [12 per cent] as at 31 March 2005)' (National Statistics and DfES, 2006a, p.6).

Serious case reviews

Serious case reviews (SCRs) conducted by Local Safeguarding Children Boards (LSCBs) provide further evidence of children's vulnerability and the extent of serious injury and death. These reviews are conducted, 'when a child dies (including death by suicide), and abuse or neglect is known or suspected to be a factor in the child's death' (HM Government, 2006c, p.143). The SCR process examines the involvement of agencies and professionals in the child's case, to determine if lessons can be learned about the ways in which professionals and organizations work together to safeguard and promote children's welfare (HM Government, 2006c). However, no data are currently collated on the numbers of SCRs conducted across the UK. A recent Department of Health study estimated that there are about 90 child deaths each year that are the subject of an SCR (Sinclair and Bullock, 2002), while the National Society for the Prevention of Cruelty to Children (NSPCC) (2000) reports that there may be as many as 100–200 case reviews in the UK each year involving the death or serious injury of a child as a result of abuse or neglect.

In addition, acquiring accurate child homicide figures for the UK is problematic (Creighton, 1995, 2000) as data are not currently recorded for all fatal child abuse. A conservative estimate by the NSPCC suggests that at least 1–2 children die each week as a result of abuse and neglect (NSPCC, 2000), while WAVE (Worldwide Alternatives to ViolencE) Trust (Hosking and Walsh, 2005, p.91) highlights the large numbers of public inquiries that follow child abuse deaths '24 in the 1970s, 25 in the 1980s, and 22 in the 1990s', with 'no visible reduction in levels of child abuse'.

While these figures do not offer a complete picture of the numbers of vulnerable children, they do go some way towards demonstrating that the care of vulnerable children is a significant public health issue affecting the child population. There is a clearly need for more accurate and reliable official government statistics, in particular around child homicide and serious case reviews, to provide a more effective picture of child protection trends (NSPCC, 2000). Recent *Working Together to Safeguard Children* guidance (HM Government, 2006c) has laid down requirements for LSCBs to provide a copy of the overview report, action plan and individual management reports for each SCR to the Commission for Social Care Inspection (CSCI) and DfES, for collation on a national basis. It is planned that national overview reports will be commissioned by the DfES every two years. In addition LSCBs are now required to establish Child Death Review Panels (which will become compulsory on 1 April 2008) to collect and analyse information on the deaths of any children (under 18 years) resident in the LSCB area.

What existing figures do highlight though is the importance of identifying and working with the vulnerable school-age population.

WORKING WITH VULNERABLE CHILDREN – ADOPTING A PUBLIC HEALTH APPROACH

A whole-population approach

The need for improved identification of vulnerable children, through services that are developed from sound public health principles and a whole-population approach is outlined in the *Every Child Matters: change for children* programme (HM Government, 2004), the *National Service Framework for Children, Young People and Maternity Services* (Department of Health and DfES, 2004) and reinforced in *Reaching Out* (HM Government, 2006d). In the UK, the Child Health Promotion Programme implemented in schools primarily through the work of school nurses working in conjunction with teachers and other professionals, is important because it provides the gateway to identifying school-age children who are experiencing health difficulties (Hall and Elliman, 2003; Department of Health and DfES, 2004). Such collective approaches are required, at least initially, to ensure those vulnerable children who are in need (and their families) are reached and offered appropriate services. Individual work with a child and family would only take place once a health, development or learning need has been identified, and this individual focus is not reached unless the whole population has access to such universal provision.

The identification of vulnerable school-age children must therefore be addressed through public health values and concepts, principally universal access to public health professionals through the Child Health Promotion Programme (Hall and Elliman, 2003; Department of Health and DfES, 2004), which includes the whole population and should ensure targeted follow-up of children who are missing from school and who (potentially with their families) do not initially take up interventions or services offered.

Safeguarding is everyone's responsibility

Section 11 of the Children Act 2004 emphasized that 'safeguarding children is everyone's responsibility' (HM Government, 2005a, p.9) and placed a statutory duty on key agencies to safeguard and promote the welfare of children. All public health practitioners working with school-age children and their families have an important public health role in the identification of vulnerable children and children at risk of significant harm. All staff working with school-age children must be trained and knowledgeable about the signs of child abuse and neglect. *Every Child Matters* (Chief Secretary to the Treasury, 2003) recommended that everyone working with children, young people and their families should have a common core of skills and knowledge. Subsequently, and in recognition of the increasingly multidisciplinary workforce, the DfES has published the *Common Core of Skills and Knowledge for the Children's Workforce* (HM Government, 2005b). This guidance sets out the knowledge and skills required to work at a basic level in the following six areas of expertise:

- effective communication and engagement
- child and young person development
- safeguarding and promoting the welfare of the child
- supporting transitions
- multi-agency working
- sharing information (HM Government, 2005c).

Section 175 of the Education Act 2002 placed a duty on local education authorities and governing bodies of schools and FE institutions to safeguard and promote children's welfare. Core Standard C2 of *National Standards, Local Action* (Department of Health, 2004c, p.28) set out the responsibilities of healthcare organizations in safeguarding work. This stated that 'Health care organisations protect children by following national child protection guidance within their own activities and in their dealings with other organisations'. Eight markers of good practice for agencies in safeguarding and promoting the welfare of children and young people have been outlined in Standard 5 of the *National Service Framework for Children, Young People and Maternity Services* (Department of Health and DfES, 2004). All organizations providing children's services must ensure that they have clear policies and procedures for employees about how to safeguard and promote the welfare of children (HM Government, 2006c). In addition, many public health professionals will have access to training, practice guidance and child protection supervision, which will aid in the identification of vulnerable children and young people. Public health professionals will also be supported by named and designated child protection professionals, and by designated 'looked after professionals'.

Working Together to Safeguard Children (HM Government, 2006c) has detailed the role of all health professionals who work with children in terms of safeguarding and promoting their welfare. Staff are encouraged to adhere to the Department of Health (2003) guidance *What to do if you're Worried a Child is being Abused*, LSCB procedures and *Responding to Domestic Abuse: a handbook for health professionals* (Department of Health, 2006). Furthermore, public health practitioners should be using the *Framework for the Assessment of Children in Need and their Families* (Department of Health *et al.*, 2000, p.3) for assessing vulnerable school-age children and their families. Indeed many primary care trusts have adapted their health records to incorporate this framework and are planning implementation of the CAF locally to avoid duplication and repeated assessments of children and families. It is also likely that many public health practitioners will take on the 'lead professional role' with some children who have significant or complex needs, to avoid overlap of and reduce inconsistency of services (DfES, 2005a).

Public health activity

If we think back to the continuum discussed earlier in the chapter (see Fig. 7.1), a public health professional may be involved in reviewing health needs across the school age population as part of baseline preventative work or early intervention work to identify vulnerable children. For example, a school nurse should review each school-age child's record at school entry to review the health status of all children. This is important in order to identify health needs, particularly physical, emotional and social needs, so that appropriate interventions can be delivered, and so that children are better able to reach their potential (DfES and Department of Health, 2006).

Public health professionals may, following an initial or targeted school-age child and family health assessment, identify one or more health needs that require short-term targeted support/intervention. For example, if a child has been bullied, a school nurse could work with the teacher, child and parents to increase the child's self-esteem and ability to socialize appropriately with his/her peers. The school nurse or other professional may also be responsible for referring a school child and their family for specialist assessment and input, depending on the nature of the needs identified. Further along the continuum, programmes promoting the development of parenting skills may be offered through 'extended school' projects or children's centres, perhaps involving psychologists, for parents whose children have additional needs such as behavioural issues.

Still further along the continuum, day or respite care for children might be offered and the provision of services for 'looked after children' (Children Act 1989, Part III Section 22(1), p.17). At the far end of the continuum, high-level intervention will include children who are at continuing risk of significant harm and are the subject of a formal child protection plan and receiving integrated support from statutory and specialist services, with a minority of cases culminating in court proceedings (HM Government, 2006c). It is important to recognize that multi-agency assessment and care planning could occur at any point along the vulnerability continuum, reinforced through the implementation of the *Framework for the Assessment of Children in Need and their Families* (Department of Health *et al.*, 2000) and the Common Assessment Framework (HM Government, 2006a, 2006b).

Shared and joint assessment is a central feature of public health working. Research evidence indicates that inter-agency collaboration during the assessment process of a child referred to local authority social care departments has improved since the implementation of the National Assessment Framework (Cleaver *et al.*, 2004), and may continue to improve joint working as the Common Assessment Framework is implemented throughout the country. This is important in the area of safeguarding and the care of vulnerable children, as Lord Laming's Inquiry Report (Department of Health and Home Office, 2003) continually exposed the danger to children's health of poor assessments and recording, inadequate information-sharing systems amongst professionals, and a lack of inter-agency working (Department of Health and Home Office, 2003). In England, it is planned that the Information Sharing (IS) Index will enable practitioners working with children to find and contact each other easily and to share information when vulnerable children go missing from school and/or need services and support (DfES, 2006c).

Government policy increasingly recognizes the importance of supporting school-age children and their families, while emphasizing the need for professionals and their organizations, families, schools, local communities and the voluntary sector to work more closely together to improve outcomes for children and young people (HM Government, 2005a; DfES, 2005b). Effective partnership working with both children and their parents, and between professionals and their agencies, is an essential part of public health working to ensure the needs of vulnerable children are met (Department of Health *et al.*, 1999; HM Government 2005a, 2006a). It is generally recognized that improved outcomes are more likely to be achieved if the child or young person is focused on as a whole, if services are child-centred and if people work together (Department of Health and DfES, 2004; HM Government, 2006c). This latter point was a critical finding of Lord Laming's Inquiry Report:

> *I am in no doubt that effective support for children and families cannot be achieved by a single agency acting alone. It depends on a number of agencies working well together. It is a multi-disciplinary task.*
> **(Department of Health and Home Office, 2003,**
> **Paragraph 1.30)**

This theme of partnership is continually emphasized in recent policy, with calls for better linkages across health services, more effective inter-agency strategies and professionals to work openly together and with children, young people and their families (HM Government, 2005a, 2006c). Furthermore, through each area's Children and Young People's Plan (CYPP), there is an increasing emphasis on integrated planning and commissioning to deliver needs-based services relevant to vulnerable children in the local community (HM Government, 2005c).

CONCLUSION

This chapter has explored the concept of vulnerability, its conceptual origins and its relevance to children and young people's health. It has examined how vulnerable children and young people fit into the UK's wider safeguarding policy agenda, and has presented key research evidence as to why vulnerable school-age children present a significant public health concern. Public health practitioners must be knowledgeable about the new legislative and multi-agency practice issues surrounding safeguarding children work and the implications this has for their practice.

The key argument for viewing vulnerable school-age children as a public health issue is the negative impact that unidentified or unresolved vulnerability has on the individual child, their family, school community and society (Department of Health, 2004a). Adopting a public health approach is crucial in ensuring that vulnerable school-age children are identified early and offered the services and support that they and their families need to promote their health and well-being. This is important to enable these children to reach their full potential and to prevent child abuse and neglect.

It is also worth considering whether 'vulnerable' is really an appropriate term to be using when assessing children's needs, bearing in mind many children and young people will not identify themselves in this way. Finally, while the Victoria Climbié Inquiry Report (Department of Health and Home Office, 2003) has had a major impact on children and young people's services in the UK, it remains to be seen whether the subsequent legislative changes and service developments really do improve the health outcomes for all children and young people.

KEY POINTS

- The care of vulnerable children is a significant public health issue affecting the child population.
- The term 'vulnerable child' is used to describe children with additional health and social care needs, who would benefit from additional support and services.
- Vulnerability in childhood is inextricably linked to disadvantage and health inequalities.
- A diverse range of adverse life experiences may result in a child or young person being vulnerable. Yet there is also evidence that a number of resilience factors can enable some vulnerable children to thrive in difficult circumstances and reduce the effects of risk factors on health.
- The key argument for viewing vulnerable school-age children as a public health issue is the negative impact that unidentified or unresolved vulnerability has on the individual child, school community and society.
- A public health approach ensures that potentially vulnerable children and young people are identified early and secure the support that they and their families need to promote their health and well-being, to enable them to reach their full potential and to prevent child abuse and neglect.

REFERENCES

Acheson D (1998) *Independent Inquiry into Inequalities in Health Report.* London: The Stationery Office.

Aggleton P (1996) *Health Promotion and Young People.* London: Health Education Authority.

Appleton JV (1994) The concept of vulnerability in relation to child protection: health visitors' perceptions. *Journal of Advanced Nursing* 20:1132–40.

Appleton JV, Clemerson-Trew J (2007) Safeguarding children: a public health imperative. In: Cowley S (ed.) *Public Health in Policy and Practice. A sourcebook for health visitors and community nurses* (2e). London: Baillière Tindall Limited (in press).

Barrett H (2003) *Parenting Programmes for Families at Risk. A source book.* London: National Family and Parenting Institute.

Bifulco A, Moran P (1998) *Wednesday's Child.* London: Routledge.

Blair M, Stewart-Brown S, Waterston T, Crowther R (2003) *Child Public Health.* Oxford: Oxford University Press.

Buchannan A (1996) *Cycles of Child Maltreatment: facts, fallacies and interventions.* Chichester: Wiley.

Buckland L, Rose J, Greaves C (2005) New roles for school nurses: preventing exclusion. *Community Practitioner* 78:16–19.

Cawson P (2002) *Child Maltreatment on the Family: the experience of national sample of young people.* London: NSPCC.

Chief Secretary to the Treasury (2003) *Every Child Matters* (Cm 5860). London: Stationery Office. www.everychildmatters.gov.uk/_content/documents/EveryChildMatters.pdf (accessed 17 January 2007).

Children's Rights Director (2004) *Safe From Harm: children's views report.* London: Commission for Social Care Inspection.

Cleaver H, Unell I, Aldgate J (1999) *Children's Needs – Parental Capacity: the impact of parental mental illness, problem alcohol and drug use, and domestic violence on children's development.* London: The Stationery Office.

Cleaver H, Walker S, Meadows P (2004) *Assessing Children's Needs and Circumstances. The impact of the assessment framework.* London: Jessica Kingsley Publishers.

Coid J, Petruckevitch A, Feder G *et al.* (2001) Relation between childhood sexual and physical abuse and risk of revictimization in women: a cross-sectional survey. *Lancet* 358:450–4.

Copp LA (1986) The nurse as advocate for vulnerable persons. *Journal of Advanced Nursing* 11:255–63.

Corby B (1990) Making use of child protection statistics. *Children and Society* 4:304–14.

Creighton SJ (1995) Fatal child abuse – how preventable is it? *Child Abuse Review* 4:318–28.

Creighton SJ (2000) Government statistics on child deaths where abuse or neglect may be implicated. In: NSPCC (2000) *NSPCC Out of Sight.* London: NSPCC, pp.31–3.

DeBell D, Tomkins A (2006) *Discovering the Future of School Nursing: the evidence base.* London: McMillan-Scott.

Department for Education and Skills (2005a) *Lead Professional Good Practice Guidance.* London: Department for Education and Skills.

Department for Education and Skills (2005b) *Engaging the Voluntary and Community Sectors in Children's Trusts.* Nottingham: DfES Publications.

Department for Education and Skills (2006a) *Youth Matters: next steps.* London: Department for Education and Skills.

Department for Education and Skills (2006b) *Targeted Youth Support: young carers' after school club.* www.everychildmatters.gov.uk/search/EP00224/ (accessed 22 January 2007).

Department for Education and Skills (2006c) *Fact Sheet Information Sharing (IS) Index.* www.ecm.gov.uk/index.

Department for Education and Skills and Department of Health (2006) *Looking for a School Nurse?* Nottingham: DfES Publications.

Department for Education and Skills, Department of Health and Home Office (2003) *Keeping Children Safe. The Government's response to The Victoria Climbié Inquiry Report and Joint Chief Inspectors' Report Safeguarding Children.* London: The Stationery Office.

Department of Health (1989) *An Introduction to the Children Act 1989.* London: HMSO.

Department of Health (1997a) *Children Looked After by Local Authorities. Year ending 31 March 1996, England.* London: Government Statistical Service.

Department of Health (1997b) *Statistics of Children and Young People on Child Protection Registers. Year ending 31 March 1997, England.* London: Government Statistical Service.

Department of Health (1999) *Framework for the Assessment of Children in Need and their Families. Consultation Draft.* London: Department of Health.

Department of Health (2002a) *Women's Mental Health: into the mainstream. Strategic development of mental health care for women.* London: Department of Health.

Department of Health (2002b) *Promoting the Health of Looked after Children.* London: The Stationery Office.

Department of Health (2003) *What To Do If You're Worried a Child is being Abused.* London: Department of Health.

Department of Health (2004a) *The Chief Nursing Officer's Review of the Nursing, Midwifery and Health Visiting Contribution to Vulnerable Children and Young People.* London: Department of Health.

Department of Health (2004b) *Choosing Health. Making healthier choices easier.* London: Department of Health.

Department of Health (2004c) *National Standards, Local Action.* London: Department of Health.

Department of Health (2006) *Responding to Domestic Abuse. A handbook for health professionals.* London: Department of Health.

Department of Health/Dartington Social Research Unit (1995) *Child Protection: messages from research.* London: HMSO.

Department of Health and DfES (2004) *National Service Framework for Children Young People and Maternity Services. Core standards.* London: Department of Health.

Department of Health and Home Office (2003) *The Victoria Climbié Inquiry. Report of an Inquiry by Lord Laming.* London: HMSO.

Department of Health, Home Office and Department for Education and Employment (1999) *Working Together to Safeguard Children: a guide for inter-agency working to safeguard and promote the welfare of children.* London: Department of Health.

Department of Health, Department for Education and Employment and the Home Office (2000) *Framework for the Assessment of Children in Need and their Families.* London: HMSO.

Edleson JL (1999) Children's witnessing of adult domestic violence. *Journal of Interpersonal Violence* 14:839–70.

Farrington D (1995) Intensive health visiting and the prevention of juvenile crime. *Health Visitor* 68:100–2.

Fleming P, Bamford DR, McCaughley N (2005) An exploration of the health and social wellbeing needs of looked after young people – a multi-method approach. *Journal of Interprofessional Care* 19:35–49.

Gibbons J, Conroy S, Bell C (1995) *Operating the Child Protection System: a study of child protection practices in English local authorities.* London: HMSO.

Goddard CR, Saunders BJ, Stanley JR (1999) Structured risk assessment procedures: instruments of abuse? *Child Abuse Review* 8:251–63.

Gray J (2002) National policy on the assessment of children in need and their families. In: Ward H, Rose W. *Approaches to Needs Assessment in Children's Services*. London: Jessica Kingsley Publishers, pp.169–94.

Hagell A (1998) *Dangerous Care. Reviewing the risks to children from their carers*. London: Policy Studies Institute and The Bridge Child Care Development Service.

Hall DMB, Elliman D (2003) *Health for all Children* (4e). Oxford: Oxford University Press.

Heller SS, Larrieu JA, D'Imperio R, Boris NW (1999) Research on resilience to child maltreatment: empirical considerations. *Child Abuse and Neglect* 23:321–38.

HM Government (2004) *Every Child Matters: change for children*. Nottingham: DfES Publications. www.everychildmatters.gov.uk/_content/documents/Every%20Child%20Matinserts.pdf (accessed 21 January, 2007).

HM Government (2005a) *Statutory Guidance on Making Arrangements to Safeguard and Promote the Welfare of Children under Section 11 of the Children Act 2004*. Nottingham: DfES Publications.

HM Government (2005b) *Common Core of Skills and Knowledge for the Children's Workforce*. Nottingham: DfES Publications.

HM Government (2005c) *Guidance on the Children and Young People's Plan*. Nottingham: DfES Publications.

HM Government (2006a) *The Common Assessment Framework for Children and Young People: practitioners' guide. Integrated working to improve outcomes for children and young people*. Nottingham: DfES Publications.

HM Government (2006b) *Common Assessment Framework for Children and Young People: managers' guide. Integrated working to improve outcomes for children and young people*. Nottingham: DfES Publications.

HM Government (2006c) *Working Together to Safeguard Children. A guide to inter-agency working to safeguard and promote the welfare of children*. www.everychildmatters.gov.uk/socialcare/safeguarding/workingtogether/ (accessed 10 January 2007).

HM Government (2006d) *Reaching Out: an action plan on social exclusion*. London: Cabinet Office.

HM Treasury and Department for Education and Skills (2007) *Policy Review of Children and Young People. A discussion paper*. London: HM Treasury.

Hosking G, Walsh I (2005) *The WAVE Report 2005. Violence and what to do about it*. Croydon: Wave Trust.

Kohli R, Mather R (2003) Promoting psychosocial well-being in unaccompanied asylum seeking young people in the United Kingdom. *Child and Family Social Work* 8:201–12.

Lazarus R (1976) *Patterns of Adjustment*. New York: McGraw-Hill.

Lessick M, Woodring BC, Naber S, Halstead L (1992) Vulnerability: a conceptual model applied to perinatal and neonatal nursing. *Journal of Perinatal Nursing* 6:1–14.

Matsen A, Hubbard J, Gest S *et al.* (1999) Competence in the context of adversity: pathways to resilience and maladaptation from childhood to late adolescence. *Development and Psychopathology* 11:143–69.

Macdonald G (2001) *Effective Interventions for Child Abuse and Neglect. An evidence-based approach to planning and evaluating interventions.* Chichester: John Wiley and Sons Ltd.

Meltzer H, Gatward R, Corbin T, Goodman R, Ford T (2003) *The Mental Health of Young People Looked After by Local Authorities in England.* London: The Stationery Office.

Mental Health Foundation (1999a) *Bright Futures – Promoting Children and Young People's Mental Health.* London: The Mental Health Foundation.

Mental Health Foundation (1999b) *The Big Picture – Promoting Children and Young People's Mental Health.* London: The Mental Health Foundation.

Mullen PE, Martin JL, Anderson JC, Romans SE, Herbison GP (1996) The long term impact of the physical, emotional and sexual abuse of children: a community study. *Child Abuse and Neglect* 20:7–21.

National Statistics and DfES (2005) *Children Looked After in England (Including Adoptions and Care Leavers), 2004–05. First release.* Nottingham: DfES Publications.

National Statistics and DfES (2006a) *Statistics of Education: referrals, assessments and children and young people on child protection registers: year ending 31 March 2005.* London: National Statistics.

National Statistics and DfES (2006b) *Statistics of Education: children looked after by local authorities year ending 31 March 2005 Volume 1: national tables March.* London: National Statistics.

NHS Executive (1996) *Child Health in the Community: a guide to good practice.* London: Department of Health.

NSPCC (2000) *Out of Sight.* London: NSPCC.

Osofsky J (2003) Prevalence of children's exposure to domestic violence and child maltreatment: implications for prevention and intervention. *Clinical Child and Family Psychology Review* 6:161–70.

Parton N (2006) *Safeguarding Childhood: early intervention and surveillance in a late modern society.* Basingstoke: Palgrave Macmillan.

Phillips CA (1992) Vulnerability in family systems: application to antepartum. *Journal of Perinatal and Neonatal Nursing* 6:26–36.

Reder P, Duncan S (1999) *Lost Innocents. A follow-up study of fatal child abuse.* London: Routledge.

Rich OJ (1992) Vulnerability of homeless pregnant and parenting adolescents. *Journal of Perinatal and Neo-natal Nursing* 6:37–46.

Roberts I (1996) Family support and the health of children. *Children and Society* 10:217–24.

Rogers AC (1997) Vulnerability, health and health care. *Journal of Advanced Nursing* 26:65–72.

Rose MH (1984) The concepts of coping and vulnerability as applied to children with chronic conditions. *Issues in Comprehensive Pediatric Nursing* 7:177–86.

Rose MH, Killien M (1983) Risk and vulnerability: a case for differentiation . . . between personal and environmental factors that influence health and development. *Advances in Nursing Science* 5:60–73.

Scottish Executive (2004) *Forgotten Children*. Edinburgh: The Stationery Office.

Seccombe K (2000) Families in poverty in the 1990s: trends, causes, consequences, and lessons learned. *Journal of Marriage and the Family* 62:1094–113.

Seccombe K (2002) 'Beating the odds' versus 'changing the odds': poverty, resilience and family policy. *Journal of Marriage and the Family* 64:384–94.

Selye H (1973) The evolution of the stress concept. *American Scientist* 61:692–9.

Silverman A, Reinherz HZ, Giaconia RM (1996) The long-term sequelae of child and adolescent abuse: a longitudinal study. *Child Abuse and Neglect* 20:709–23.

Simpson A (2006) Promoting the health of looked after children in Scotland. *Community Practitioner* 79:217–20.

Sinclair R, Bullock R (2002) *Learning from Past Experience – A Review of Serious Case Reviews*. London: Department of Health.

Smith Stover C (2005) Domestic violence research what have we learned and where do we go from here? *Journal Of Interpersonal Violence* 20:448–54.

Social Exclusion Unit (2004) *Breaking the Cycle – Taking Stock of Progress and Priorities for the Future*. London: Social Exclusion Unit.

Stanley N, Riordan D, Alaszewki H (2005) The mental health of looked after children: matching response to need. *Health and Social Care in the Community* 13:239–48.

Stewart-Brown S (1998) New approaches to school health. In: Spencer N (ed.) *Progress in Community Child Health*. Edinburgh: Churchill Livingstone, pp.137–58.

Waller MA (2001) Resilience in the ecosystemic context: evolution of the concept. American *Journal of Orthopsychiatry* 71:290–7.

Wells DL (1986) Vulnerability in elderly patients in the acute-care hospital. *Perspectives* 10:9–10.

Whitfield CL, Anda RF, Dube SR, Felitti VJ (2003) Violent childhood experiences and the risk of intimate partner violence in adults: assessment in a large health maintenance organization. *Journal of Interpersonal Violence* 18:166–85.

Acts of Parliament

All these Acts are published by HMSO in London, and all can be accessed from the UK Parliament website (www.publications.parliament.uk).

Children Act 1989
Education Act 2002
Children Act 2004

Section 5
CORE HEALTH ISSUES

Dawn Rees and Dinah Morley

INTRODUCTION

> *Children are living beings – more living than grown-up people who have built shells of habit around themselves. Therefore it is absolutely necessary for their mental health and development that they should not have mere schools for their lessons, but a world whose guiding spirit is personal love.*
> **(Rabindranath Tagore (1933), Calcutta India, Nobel Literature Laureate 1914)**

Why does mental health and emotional well-being matter? It is because our children are the adults of the future. That might imply that childhood is merely a necessary pathway to adulthood. It is much more than that. Children are people in their own right and exist in their own time. They make an enormous contribution to the development of the culture and meaning of their own generation and the meaning that parents and society attribute to them (Reder *et al.*, 1993). They have a right to positive advantage, which should enhance every aspect of their childhood.

Childhood disadvantage is inextricably linked with parental disadvantage which is 'represented as the enduring context in which the child is conceived, born and grows up. Physical and emotional health in childhood, together with healthy behaviour are seen to directly affect health in adulthood' and, as a result, society at large (Graham and Power, 2004, p.26).

Positive parent–child relationships scaffold the child's experience of life; they enhance the sense of self, and over time and in the early years are a metaphor for the world in a child's eyes. Developing and maintaining positive mental health, enhanced by a sense of belonging, helps the individual construct a mature and sophisticated range of responses and behaviours. A mix of positive and negative experiences, mediated by good relationships, makes it more likely that they will understand themselves and others, and positively manage the inevitable disappointments and discontinuities in life as well as experiencing fun and enjoyment. Thus being 'mentally healthy' can be said to be a key prerequisite for health and success in all aspects of life.

> *Children's mental health is the strength and capacity of children's minds to grow and develop with confidence and enjoyment. It consists of the capacity to learn from experience and to overcome difficulty and adversity. It's about physical and emotional well-being, the ability to live a full and creative life and the flexibility to give and take in friendships and relationships. Children who are mentally healthy are not saints or models of perfection but ordinary children making the most of their abilities and opportunities.*
> **(YoungMinds, 2006)**

Achieving positive mental health and well-being is enhanced by genetic, family, social and educational conditions. The enhancement of childhood experience through positive conditions, as a place where adults nurture and allow the child to take reasonable risks; where friends are made and social relationships are maintained; where making mistakes is acceptable and learning from them encouraged; where there is no bullying or suffering from discrimination; achievement at school and moving into adulthood with the ability to live autonomously and to earn a living. These are all factors that are underpinned by the delicate set of interrelated factors and relationships that support the growing child's sense of self, development of empathy for others, and physical and emotional resilience.

Being unhappy, isolated or unable to understand what is happening in your life, and experiencing this from a base where adults in the world do not appreciate your stage of development and/or the reasons why you are feeling that way, sets a child on an uncertain trajectory into adulthood and at greater risk of mental health problems (Health Advisory Service, 1995; Audit Commission, 1999; Meltzer *et al.*, 2005).

The *tabula rasa* of infancy and childhood is profoundly affected by influences on neurological, emotional and cognitive development. Healthy and uninterrupted development is crucial in terms of positive future outcomes. For this reason, the combined impact of social and economic disadvantage can have a profound impact on the developing child, but what appears to mediate these potentially negative factors is the child's self-esteem.

Rutter (2001) argues that poverty makes parenting more difficult, and McLoyd (2001) observes that poverty and economic loss affect parental ability to provide the consistent support and involvement children need.

THE EVIDENCE BASE

Recent research has built on that of earlier attachment theorists such as Rutter (1975), Ainsworth *et al.* (1978), Cicchetti and Barnett (1991), Fonagy *et al.* (1991), Murray (1992) and Lyons-Ruth (1996), and reinforces the importance of positive nurturing relationships in infancy and their effect on the development of neurological pathways in the brain (Schaffer, 1996; Elliot, 1999; Balbernie, 2001).

> *There is increasing evidence that social interactive experiences affect cognitive growth and entail mutual cooperation of a participant child and a sensitive adult.*
>
> **(Schaffer, 1996, p.99)**

Infancy sees the most rapid rate of brain growth and hardwiring of neurons, and this process is significantly affected by the child's experience of emotional and physical environments.

Childhood is characterized by periods of transition and reorganization, and living in a positive environment (not necessarily a financially rich one) makes all the difference to children's perceptions of themselves. This in turn impacts upon their ability to understand others (Vygotski, 1978; Fonagy *et al.*, 1991; Schaffer, 1996; Balbernie, 2001) and to develop sharing and reciprocal relationships with peers.

During adolescence we see a further period of significant brain activity. As the frontal cortex develops, there is increased myelination (development of the neuronal sheaths) which speeds up cognitive abilities (Blakemore and Frith, 2005). During this period the young person can feel very confused and may behave irrationally as the process unfolds.

Achieving the mental health of all children is a key component in the future health of the population and a key factor in the cohesion of families, communities and cultures. This principle has been reinforced at policy level in England through initiatives such as Sure Start, the development of children's centres, and programmes such as *Birth to Three Matters* (Department for Education and Skills [DfES], 2005a). Sure Start aims to increase the proportion of young children from birth to age 5 years with normal levels of personal, social and emotional development, and to increase the proportion of young children with satisfactory speech and language development at age 2. The *Birth to Three Matters* framework supports children in their earliest years, and reinforces the importance of positive early experiences.

It is important therefore to make reference to early childhood development in a book about school-age children, because it directly informs some of the components of child and adolescent mental health that are discussed in this and other chapters.

DEFINITIONS OF MENTAL HEALTH IN CHILDREN AND YOUNG PEOPLE

We tend to think, almost automatically, that when we talk about *mental health* we mean *mental illness*. But, as we shall see below, only about 10 per cent of the child population has a mental disorder or illness (Meltzer *et al.*, 2005). We all have mental health, in the same way that we have physical health. Sometimes our physical health is not so good, but it does not necessarily mean that we are seriously ill. Usually we recover quickly with a little love and care from friends and family. So it is with mental health. Sometimes we may suffer from low mood, mild depression and sometimes mild agitation. With a little support, and – usually – a listening ear, we are soon feeling fine again.

So what are the components of mental health, and what helps us to have it? The following definition is used in much of the literature, sometimes articulated in different words but basically saying the same thing.

Mental health is:

• the ability to develop psychologically, emotionally, intellectually and spiritually
• the ability to initiate, develop and sustain mutually satisfying personal relationships
• the ability to become aware of others and to empathize with them
• the ability to use psychological distress as a developmental process so that it does not hinder or impair further development (Health Advisory Service, 1995).

To attain good mental health, every child needs an environment where he/she can develop as a rounded, secure person with personal resources that will allow the child to recover safely from bad and sad experiences and to learn and mature from those experiences. Again it is possible to see the similarities between mental and physical health.

The ability to initiate and sustain good relationships is essential to a fulfilling life, and this includes the capacity to be aware of what is going on in the minds and lives of others – as Fonagy (Hartley-Brewer, 2005, p.7) puts it, to be able to mentalize or to empathize with others. Failure to acquire this capacity seems to have serious consequences for actions later in life. This is generally referred to as a 'theory of mind' (Vygotski, 1978; Astington *et al.*, 1988; Schaffer, 1996). Put very simply – if you cannot imagine the impact that you have on someone and how they feel, you are unlikely to be able to modify your own behaviour appropriately in relation to the other person.

It is in all our interests to ensure that the children and young people with whom we come in contact and for whom we have responsibilities are supported to achieve optimum mental health. It is a well-used phrase, but *children's mental health is everybody's business and everyone's responsibility.*

It has only been comparatively recently that mental health problems, disorders and illnesses in children have been recognized and thought worthy of consideration and remediation (Kurtz, 1996). Much of the pathological behaviour in children has, in the past, been attributed to inherited defect or lack of control and framed in terms of bad behaviour, illness, madness or social aberration, and sometimes described as irredeemable or requiring punishment. It is only more recently that more flexible levels of public and independent service have been developed across agencies working with children and their families in response to the range of possible presentations and the acknowledged importance of co-ordinated approaches to assessment and treatment for mental disorders in childhood and adolescence.

The specialist mental health services for children are part of what is referred to as the comprehensive child and adolescent mental health service (CAMHS). This comprehensive service is usually described as being in four tiers (see p.195) from tier 1, which encompasses all those practitioners who work with children but who are not mental health specialists, through to tier 4, which describes the highly specialized, usually inpatient, provision. This four-tier model is used in the four countries of the UK, although there are local differences in delivery, which depend on the country's government and local health service configuration.

It is still true to say that many people would not subscribe to the possibility that children can have mental disorders. For example the Office for National Statistics (ONS) data (Meltzer *et al.*, 2003) that 1 in 10 children between the ages of 5 and 16 years have mental disorders surprised and shocked the public. This public reaction contrasts starkly with other data which show that many adults with mental disorders had their problems diagnosed in childhood and often failed to receive appropriate treatment. Young people with mental health problems, even when those difficulties are marked, are often not recognized as being in difficulty. In two separate studies in Scotland, teachers and general practitioners (GPs) only identified a minority of such young people (Blair, 2001; Potts *et al.*, 2001).

Opinions are divided as to whether use of the terms mental health and mental disorder in relation to children and young people is stigmatizing and can marginalize young people's experience. Some argue that an alternative and less specific description should be used – such as emotional health and psychological well-being – to encompass the broad psychosocial spectrum of both presentation and disorder.

Others argue that using the term 'mental health' should not be avoided as it is only through accurate assessment, diagnosis and naming, which in turn leads to evidence-based intervention, that the prejudice against mental illness can be challenged and the resources to provide appropriate local levels of service for the most vulnerable young people can be agreed. In other words, not naming mental illness diminishes the significance of a diagnosable condition and has the potential to restrict treatment options. This is inevitably a simplification of the complex paradigms of medical and psychosocial models of categorization and public perception.

The politics of naming is fraught with difficulty. Even 'diagnosis' sometimes seems to be a movable feast, given that medical diagnosis is based upon a clear manualized framework. The language developed by different professions to describe similar sets of presentations further adds to the confusion when we approach the concept of child and adolescent mental health in a multi-agency context. A child with 'behaviour problems' in school might be diagnosed with a 'conduct disorder'; within CAMHS the diagnosis may be an associated 'developmental disorder' in paediatric and/or learning terms; for other agencies, this may be articulated as 'misusing' substances and/or 'involved' in the criminal justice system. But it becomes even more complicated when co-morbidity (i.e. having more than one condition at the same time) is present.

So what is the difference between a 'problem', a disorder and an illness? A mental health *problem* is something that many of us experience. A young person may be sad or anxious for a short period and can be comforted and helped through this time with the support of family, friends and others who are not specialist CAMH professionals. A *disorder* is when mental health problems become severe and persistent, significantly interfering with the child's ability to function in the world; and the term '*illness*' is used to describe the most severe symptoms such as severe depression, psychoses and severe eating disorder.

When disorder and illness are thought to be present there is need for a more clinical approach to formulating a diagnosis and subsequent treatment plans within the health system. The health classification system most often used is the 10th International Classification of Diseases (ICD-10; World Health Organization, 1992). Less frequently in the UK, and usually for specific reasons, which allow a more diverse set of symptoms to be considered during diagnosis, the *Diagnostic and Statistical Manual of Mental Disorders* (DSM IV; American Psychiatric Association, 1994) will be used. These are the classifications that doctors and clinical psychologists are trained to use in formulating a diagnosis in order to match the most appropriate treatment to the problem. In a similar way, one would consider the range, pattern and impact of a number of symptoms that would differentiate a diagnosis of chickenpox from meningitis, or a torn ligament from a broken leg.

IDENTIFYING MENTAL HEALTH PROBLEMS, DISORDERS AND ILLNESSES

Mental health exists along a continuum of presentation, description and understanding, and is recognized, categorized, named, diagnosed and treated in a variety of settings in the UK and through a range of assessment and treatment modalities. These are undertaken by different professionals who are, in the main, trained to work with young people and who understand normal and abnormal child development.

Some young people are significantly affected by relatively small changes and challenges in their lives, and use various strategies to deal with these difficulties. At the same time, and perversely, other young people appear to defy life-shattering events and sail through, seemingly unscathed.

Children and young people may present with behavioural, developmental, attachment, conduct and/or clinical problems that sometimes exist in the absence of an obvious cause, as we have seen. The presentation of the problem will be influenced by family, environmental and genetic factors, along with variations in levels of personal adjustment and function, and social as well as clinical factors may predispose, precipitate or prolong symptoms. Symptoms may be transitory, ever present and manageable, or they might interrupt a young person's ability to get on with daily life to such a degree that they are both noticed by others and referred to a range of professionals.

Sometimes symptoms exist but go unnoticed. Young people may then deal with them, with or without informal interventions by others, and grow through them with minimal disruption. In other cases, the ways in which young people function in the world may be profoundly affected, causing them to require intensive support and treatment.

It is important therefore to be able to distinguish between the understandable distress and short-term worries that all children experience, and other problems and disorders that significantly impact upon a child's everyday life and relationships. In such cases, the child may need treatment and/or a range of other supports alongside treatment.

Because the young person's adaptive mechanisms may be more visible in family, social, education or community settings, their problems are frequently dealt with through a variety of means before the young person is referred to a CAMHS team or other professional.

With mental disorder and illness, the child might present in more complicated ways. This presentation must be assessed in the context of the child within the whole family. The family will have attempted to deal with the symptoms for a significant period of time and will have adapted to the behaviour/presentation but with little understanding of what is wrong, why and how to deal with it. It is the interrelationship between symptoms and their intensity, functional impairment, and the system in which the child lives that, through assessment, a CAMHS team approach will seek to unpick in order to formulate a treatment plan. CAMHS teams use a variety of assessment tools and statistical manuals including the ICD-10 and DSM IV in order to develop a consistent approach to description and categorization.

> *A disorder is classed as present if the diagnostic criteria are met as defined by these manuals (ICD-10 and DSM IV).*
>
> **(Dogra et al., 2003, p.23)**

The classification of mental disorder and illness presents significant challenges to professionals because of the impact of a child's cognitive and physical development, language skill and level of ability to verbalize feelings. Age and authority; gender and ethnicity; culture and environment all impact on the ability to formulate an accurate diagnosis. Also, the description of the problem is often mediated through parents, teachers, social workers and other professionals. The young person might, therefore, be referred to a specialist CAMHS team where there is a concern about the child but in the absence of an identifiable mental disorder.

There has been an historical tendency *not* to 'diagnose' mental illness in young people, and former diagnosis manuals were based on adult mental illness. Nevertheless, the diagnosis of mental illness in young people is formulated by the level and type of symptoms; the intensity of the symptoms; and the impact of the symptoms on the everyday life of the young person. Therefore, in addition to fulfilling (or not) diagnostic criteria, a supplementary approach is to ask about general symptomatology and to describe 'caseness'. This approach means that the person being assessed has enough symptoms to be defined as a clinical case if a certain threshold is reached, irrespective of what the diagnosis is on the classificatory system (Dogra *et al.*, 2003).

Table 8.1 gives a summary of the type of mental health disorders in children and young people that are frequently referred to CAMHS teams (Kurtz, 1992).

TABLE 8.1   *Mental disorders and illnesses*

Disorder	Symptoms
Emotional disorders	Phobias, anxiety states and depression. These may be made manifest in physical symptoms such as chronic headache or abdominal pain
Conduct disorders	Stealing, defiance, fire setting, aggression and antisocial behaviour
Hyperkinetic disorder	Disturbance of activity and attention and hyperkinetic conduct disorder
Developmental disorder	Delay in acquiring certain skills such as speech, social ability or bladder control. These may affect primarily one area of development or pervade a number of areas as in children with autism and those with pervasive developmental disorders
Eating disorders	Pre-school eating problems, anorexia nervosa, and bulimia nervosa
Habit disorders	Tics, sleeping problems and soiling
Post-traumatic syndromes	Post-traumatic stress disorder
Somatic disorders	Chronic fatigue syndrome
Psychotic disorders	Schizophrenia, manic depressive disorder, or drug-induced psychosis

Reproduced with permission from Kurtz (ed.) (1992) *With Health in Mind: mental health care for children and young people.* London: Action for Sick Children.

PREVALENCE OF MENTAL HEALTH PROBLEMS

Prevalence rates for the major disorders have been comprehensively studied by Meltzer *et al.* (2005) for the Office for National Statistics (Table 8.2).

Boys are more likely to have a mental disorder than girls, with 10 per cent of boys and 5 per cent of girls assessed as having a mental disorder between the ages of 5 and 10 years. The proportions change to 13 per cent of boys and 10 per cent of girls between the ages of 11 and 16 years. Meltzer *et al.* (2005) found that the number of young people in lone-parent families had double the rate of disorder compared with those in two-parent families. In reconstituted families, rates were 24 per cent compared with 9 per cent in families with no step children; 17 per cent of children with a parent who had no educational qualifications compared with 4 per cent of those with a parent of degree level qualification; and 20 per cent compared with 8 per cent where parents were not in full-time paid employment.

Economic disadvantage, disability benefit receipt, routine occupational groups, living in social housing and in deprived areas all correlated with higher statistics for mental health problems among young people.

POSSIBLE CAUSAL FACTORS

There is considerable debate about the causes of mental disorder and illness in children and young people (Hartley-Brewer, 2005). Recent analysis has shown

TABLE 8.2   *Percentage prevalence of mental disorders in 5- to16-year-olds by age and sex, as measured for 2004*

Type of disorder	Age (years)								
	5–10			11–16			All children		
	Boys	Girls	All	Boys	Girls	All	Boys	Girls	All
Emotional	2.2	2.5	2.4	4.0	6.1	5.0	3.1	4.3	3.7
Conduct	6.9	2.8	4.9	8.1	5.1	6.6	7.5	3.9	5.8
Hyperkinetic	2.7	0.4	1.6	2.4	0.4	1.4	2.6	0.4	1.5
Less common disorders	2.2	0.4	1.3	1.6	1.1	1.4	1.9	0.8	1.3
Any disorder	10.2	5.1	7.7	12.6	10.3	11.5	11.4	7.8	9.6

From Meltzer *et al.* (2005) *The Mental Health of Children and Young People in Great Britain 2004.* London: Office for National Statistics. Crown Copyright material is reproduced with the permission of the Controller of HMSO and the Queen's Printer for Scotland.

a rise in certain types of disorder across the developed countries, although there is now some evidence of a decline in the USA (Hagel, 2004).

Factors such as changing demography and family patterns in developed countries, pressures of examinations, commercialization of childhood, worsening diet, and even the increase in Caesarean section births have all been cited as plausible reasons for this rise in incidence. However, it is probably more relevant to talk about what biological and psychosocial factors *influence* rather than *cause* mental disorder and illness.

Risk

Broadly, the causes lie in three domains: in the child her/himself; in the family; and in the environment. The risk factors for mental health problems are set out in these categories in Box 8.1, and have been arrived at through a synthesis of research outcomes over a considerable time.

Each of these risk factors covers a considerable territory. For example, family breakdown and the subsequent separation of the parents has its own specific range of risks (Rutter, 1975). These are rooted in the fact that such changes may make problems worse in already troubled children. Younger children may be more affected as they are less able to understand what is happening. The secure relationship children need with their parents is likely to be disrupted as parents grapple with their own changes and loss, and children's need and wish for their parents' love and availability can become frustrated.

Poverty can affect fetal development as can substance misuse and alcohol misuse in the pregnant mother (Chasnoff *et al.*, 1980; Cleaver *et al.*, 1999; Harbin and Murphy, 2000). Children whose parents are in unskilled manual socioeconomic groups are more likely to experience serious childhood illness and disability (Meltzer *et al.*, 2005). Economic disadvantage has also been shown to affect cognitive function and some areas of mental health (Kuh *et al.*, 2004).

Box 8.1 Risk factors for mental health problems

Child

- Genetic influences
- Low IQ and learning disability
- Specific development delay
- Communication difficulty
- Difficult temperament
- Physical illness, especially if chronic and/or neurological
- Academic failure
- Low self-esteem

Family

- Overt parental conflict
- Family breakdown
- Inconsistent or unclear discipline
- Hostile and rejecting relationships
- Failure to adapt to child's changing developmental needs
- Abuse: physical, sexual and/or emotional
- Parental psychiatric illness
- Parental criminality, alcoholism and personality disorder
- Death and loss: including loss of friendships

Environmental

- Socio-economic disadvantage
- Homelessness
- Disaster
- Discrimination
- Other significant life events

From Health Advisory Service (1995) *Together we Stand: the commissioning role and management of child and adolescent mental health services*. London: HMSO, p.23. Crown Copyright material is reproduced with the permission of the Controller of HMSO and the Queen's Printer for Scotland.

The reference to early brain development in the first section of this chapter has significant messages for policy development. Policies that deal with adolescent behaviours need to pay attention to the nature of physiological change in the brain during the early developmental period and during adolescence. For example, it could be argued that a young person should not be punished for actions that might be outside her/his control and where treatment might be available but the clinical disorder has gone unrecognized. This is a difficult policy area in terms of balancing the needs of the individual with the needs of civil society.

Recent research also suggests some links between mental health and diet (Gesch *et al.*, 2002). Walker *et al.* (2006) reported a link between poor diet and reported psychosocial problems in Jamaican children in findings from a 2-year randomized controlled trial.

There is some evidence to show that diets lacking in certain fatty acids and vitamins can have a deleterious effect on mental health and also that certain food additives can adversely affect children's behaviour, particularly those with a precondition such as attention deficit hyperactivity disorder (ADHD) (Van de Weyer, 2005). This research is in its early days and needs further corroboration, as does research into the impact of substance misuse on mental health (Advisory Council on the Misuse of Drugs, 2005), but it suggests that these are areas we might need to be concerned about when assessing risk. A combination of these factors, particularly three or more (see Table 8.3) increases the likelihood of problems.

RESILIENCE

Studies suggest that there are factors which, when in combination, can provide a measure of protection against mental disorders. Factors that can build resilience within the individual child in different ways are shown in Table 7.1, p.155. The reasons why one child copes in adverse circumstances and another succumbs to mental ill-health are unclear. More research is needed, but the factors shown in Table 7.1 or combinations of factors do appear to help protect the child.

Many of these resilience factors are linked, and many depend on good early care-giving and continuing secure, confident parenting. This again underlines the importance of support when things are not going well.

Consistency of approach by professionals who may be involved with less-secure families is a recognized means of providing alternative positive attachment experiences when a child is at risk of mental health distress or illness. This is not an easy objective to achieve in the work environments that many practitioners experience, particularly in the context of the multiple new initiatives and service restructuring that continue to dominate the UK health and social care landscape. However child-centred planning and provision is central to England's *Every Child Matters: change for children* programme (HM Government, 2004). It is also a feature of policy planning in Wales, Scotland and Northern Ireland.

Throughout the literature on child mental health in developed countries we find references to building self-esteem. The repetition of reference to concepts of self-esteem has attracted many proponents in the field of children's mental health, and it needs some explanation. Self-esteem develops through the complex interrelationship between a sense of self, the place of the self in the world, and the relationships and experiences that enhance a strong sense of self. Positive self-esteem is inextricably linked with the development of a concept of the self in these analyses. A positive sense of self is believed to play an important part in confident approaches to new situations, confidence in personal ability and in the likelihood that the world is a safe, not an anxiety-provoking place. It seems self-evident that a child's self-esteem should be developed, *but high self-esteem is not essential to good mental health and achievement. In fact, it can be a limiting factor when the level of self-esteem is inappropriate.*

The most difficult problem in using the term self-esteem is that it is generally over-used and poorly conceptualized. Considerable conceptual work is needed before the term can be applied in a helpful way to public health practice in child and adolescent mental health.

TABLE 8.3   *Prevalence of specific child and adolescent mental health risk factors and impact on rate of mental disorder*

Risk factors	Impact on rate of disorder
In the child	
Physical illness	
Chronic health problems	3 times increase in rate overall
Brain damage	4 to 8 times increase in rate of disorder in youngsters with cerebral palsy, epilepsy or other disorder above the brainstem
Sensory impairments	
Hearing impairment (4 per 1000)	2.5 to 3 times more disorder
Visual impairment (0.6 per 1000)	No figures but rate of disorder thought to be raised
Learning difficulties	2 to 3 times increase in rate, higher in severe than moderate learning difficulties.
Language and related problems (2%, but better methods of identifying required)	4 times rate of disorder
In the family	
Family breakdown (divorce affects 1 in 4 children under 16 years of age); severe marital discord	Associated with a significant increase in disorders (e.g. depression and anxiety)
Family size	Large family size associated with increased rate of conduct disorder and delinquency in boys
Parental mental illness	
Schizophrenia	8 to 10 times increase in the rate of schizophrenia
Maternal psychiatric disorder	1.2 to 4 times increase in the rate of disorder
Parental criminality	2 to 3 times increase in the rate of delinquency
Physical and emotional abuse (of those on child protection registers, 1 in 4 suffer physical abuse and 1 in 8 neglect)	2 times the rate of mental disorder if physically abused and 3 times the rate if neglected
Sexual abuse (6.62% in girls and 3.31% in boys)	2 times the rate of disorder
Environmental risk factors	
Socio-economic circumstances	Gap in applicable evidence base
Unemployment	Gap in applicable evidence base
Housing and homelessness	Gap in applicable evidence base
School environment	9% in grades 1–9 are victims of bullying; 7–8% of children have self-reported bullying other children themselves
Life events	
Traumatic events	3 to 5 times rate of disorder. Rises with recurrent adversities

Reproduced from Wallace *et al.* (1997) *Child and Adolescent Mental Health*, with permission from Radcliffe Medical Press, Abingdon.

TREATMENT OPTIONS

It is impossible here to provide the public health practitioner with a thorough guide to the various treatment modalities that might be available in any specific locality for children and young people with mental disorders. Services are in continuous change and development. However, the main areas of treatment are specified in the substantive texts on treatments. The following section describes the main areas of treatment, but the substantive texts on treatments should be read in more detail.

Working from a sound evidence base is relatively new to many CAMHS practitioners. In some treatment areas there is still very little solid research on which to make choices about best outcomes. However the position is improving with the publication of randomized controlled trials (RCTs) as well as advice and guidance from the National Institute of Health and Clinical Excellence (NICE), the Care Services Improvement Partnership (CSIP), the Royal College of Psychiatrists and the Faculty for Children and Young People in the British Psychological Society (for websites see end of chapter). As with physical illness, the type and persistence of the problem dictates the level of response and the most appropriate intervention.

In addition the CAMHS Outcome Research Consortium (CORC):

> *is a collaboration between child and adolescent mental health services (CAMHS) across the UK. The consortium seeks to develop and implement an agreed model of routine outcome evaluation that can be used in meaningful and constructive ways to improve the provision of child and adolescent mental health services to children, young people and families'.*
> **(CAMHS Outcome Research Consortium, 2005)**

Mental health problems are, as we have seen above, low-level worries such as anxiety, low mood and mild phobias. These may have their roots in family or peer group events, but as long as the young person is able to talk to friends, a family member or another adult such as a teacher, most of these problems will reduce in a matter of weeks. The experience and sadness of loss and bereavement is not going to go away in that period, but with family and community supports the young person is helped to come to terms with loss and to move forward. In this process the emotional growth of the young person is enhanced.

If the young person is not able to confide in anyone and does not have opportunities to feel cared for and secure, or if there is some other factor at play, the problem(s) may escalate and require some professional intervention. Schools, friends, youth workers, family members may notice that there is a problem and, in particular, schools will use their own internal systems to support a vulnerable young person. These include the special education needs co-ordinator (SENCO), the school nurse, an educational psychologist or the behaviour support team. A GP might be the next port of call and he/she will want to watch and wait, seeing the young person regularly, before possibly referring the child to mental health specialists.

Where counsellors are available, often in schools, a referral may be made in order to offer a service to the young person in the least stigmatizing setting possible. Some counsellors are not trained to work with children and young people specifically and/or are not regularly professionally supervised. This situation should be challenged and appropriate safeguards put in place through local protocols, regular training and clinical supervision. Damage can be done if these essential safeguards are not in place. Other school- or community-based supports may also be accessible, depending on the young person's history and local service availability.

The school or primary healthcare system may refer the young person to a voluntary organization or to a primary mental health worker before a referral to a specialist CAMHS team is made.

Clinical child mental health specialists are frequently involved when there is evidence of a *mental disorder*, (e.g. moderate depression and anxiety, phobias, obsessive, abnormal, aggressive and hyperactive behaviours and eating disorders) as well as communication disorders such as autism, and *mental illnesses* such as bipolar disorders and psychoses. These specialists may be based at a local CAMHS clinic or may be available, for example, in GP surgeries, schools and family centres. Access differs in different localities and depends also on whether or not a multidisciplinary approach is needed (tier 3, see p.195) or whether treatment from a single CAMHS specialist (tier 2) is felt to be appropriate.

However, professional opinions vary about the types of treatments that are effective (Fonagy *et al.*, 2002). Evidence suggests that behaviour therapies are effective across a range of disorders, and the current trend is for solution-focused therapies that do not dwell on the past experiences of the young person but help to develop positive strategies for the future. Some of these approaches are likely to be more effective if combined with other supports such as parenting programmes or family therapy. Parenting programmes can work well, notably with the problems of behaviour that are experienced by younger families, if manualized programmes are followed carefully. They are also seen to be helpful for all families, hence the reasoning behind the government's Parenting Orders in the youth justice arena (www.yjb.gov.uk/en-gb/yjs/SentencesOrdersand Agreements/ParentingOrder/).

Many young people with conduct disorders, particularly those with childhood onset, are likely to need access to a CAMHS team on and off throughout their adolescence after an initial treatment, much as anyone with a chronic illness needs continued services. Access to appropriate levels of service has often been frustrated by long waiting lists and, to a certain degree, by service requirements to meet specific government targets. There is considerable debate and variable evidence about the efficacy of CAMHS treatment for conduct disorder. However, a recent health technology assessment by NICE shows effectiveness of parenting programmes for under 12s with conduct disorder (National Institute for Health and Clinical Excellence, 2006).

Psychodynamic psychotherapies have a less robust evidence base, but case studies bear witness to their effectiveness with entrenched problems. These treatments tend to be expensive because they can sometimes take many years to complete. However short-term treatments using these methods are being developed (Baruch, 2001).

Pharmacological interventions are an important component of treatment. Antidepressants, although not the treatment of choice, can be useful in stabilizing older adolescents prior to talking therapy. Their use with children has been reviewed by the Medicines and Health Care Products Regulatory Agency (MHPRA) and contraindications have been identified. The recent NICE (2005) guidelines describe the optimal treatment regime. Drug treatment for ADHD is effective in 70 per cent of cases, but should be combined with behaviour therapy for optimum outcome.

In cases of schizophrenia, the evidence is clear that the earlier drug treatment can begin after diagnosis, the less destructive the illness is in terms of the patient's ability to lead a normal life (Birchwood *et al.*, 1997). Patients have traditionally disliked drug treatments because of the unpleasant side-effects, but the newer drugs are better in this respect, making the outcomes for those with this illness much more hopeful than even a decade ago.

WHAT SORT OF SERVICES DO WE NEED FOR A PUBLIC HEALTH APPROACH TO CHILD AND ADOLESCENT MENTAL HEALTH?

From 1948 to 1997 in the UK, it is fair to say that child guidance clinics led by child psychiatrists and supported by psychotherapists, social workers and educational psychologists were mainly responsible for child mental health services. Over that period clinics grew in number, demand increased and waiting times lengthened with concomitant delays in treatment and pressures to prioritize the most severe and longstanding problems.

Little changed in this picture until evidence published in the 1990s suggested a need for policy and practice that could ensure services were able to improve child and adolescent mental health provision (Kurtz, 1992; Health Advisory Service, 1995; Audit Commission, 1999; Mental Health Foundation, 1999). Assembling findings of three influential pieces of research (Kurtz, 1992, 1996; Health Advisory Service, 1995), and combining their findings with new government policy after 1997 enabled the Audit Commission to design a set of guidelines for CAMHS providers (Audit Commission, 1999).

The Health Advisory Service report (1995) showed that CAMH services, i.e. the whole of the resources available for a particular population, which support children's mental health in any way, were being managed and delivered in many formal and informal contexts but without systematic co-ordination. From this came the tiered concept of CAMHS provision (tiers 1–4).

USING THE TIERED APPROACH TO BUILD A COHERENT SYSTEM

The current policy context for child and adolescent mental health services in the UK now emphasizes the need to build CAMH services through a partnership approach involving a range of agencies and including children, young people and their carers in the planning. *The National Service Framework for Children, Young People and Maternity Services* (Department of Health and DfES, 2004) has set out specifications in Standard 9:

> *All children and young people from birth to their eighteenth birthday who have mental health problems and disorders have access to timely, integrated, high quality, multi disciplinary mental health services to ensure effective assessment treatment and support for them and their families.*
>
> **(Department of Health and DfES, 2004, p. 4)**

This is commonly referred to as the model for *a comprehensive CAMH service.*

To achieve comprehensive care, specified services for children and young people need to be developed in a systematic way through interagency cooperation. This involves a number of key activities to ensure that services are built on known need and not merely on historical models of service provision. Key components of building a service continuum across agencies, and using the specialist skills within each, are predicated on a current needs assessment with an analysis of gaps in service provision. This is a formal public health approach. Furthermore, analysis needs to take into account the family, the environment and the factors personal to the child and his/her development.

In addition, it is necessary to audit the skills and competencies of the whole children's workforce in order to make best use of the staff already in the system and thus indicate where future recruitment needs should be targeted. The Department of Health for England requires that current needs assessment be undertaken by all primary care trusts (PCTs) in order to assess the level, degree and nature of local need for CAMHS.

Local CAMHS partnerships, which are designed to be fully representative of the range of services available, including voluntary organizations, are expected to consider the local public health needs assessment and gap analysis and to consider both in the context of staff skills. The national CAMHS mapping exercise in England (www.camhsmapping.org.uk) goes part way to helping with local authority and health workforce development planning for staff working with children. Such planning is also expected to take into account the number of professionals working with children and young people who share skills in addition to their profession specific skills.

To be truly comprehensive, all services need to be 'culturally competent', which means offering services in places and by staff who have been appropriately trained and who have the competency to understand the needs of children and young people from a wide variety of cultural, religious and ethnic backgrounds, including young asylum-seekers.

Most local CAMHS partnerships in England now use the tiered framework to help organize their thinking, plan operational services and develop workforce planning around a number of key themes, teams and areas of service development. (CAMHS partnerships are groups of key professionals, often managers, who meet to determine the priorities for CAMHS development within the tiered approach, including the local authority, health commissioners and CAMHS providers.)

The tiered approach

Tier 1 covers all those practitioners working with children in the universal services, most often based in primary care, schools and other local settings, provided by GPs, health visitors, teachers, youth workers, nursery nurses, Sure Start workers and other public services.

Tier 2 refers to practitioners with CAMH experience/qualifications who are working in a unidisciplinary way – usually in local settings. These include specialist social workers, community paediatricians, educational psychologists, community psychiatric nurses and primary mental health workers who work either in individually based GP practices or with other children's or other mental health services. Children's primary mental health workers (PMHWs) are a relatively recent addition to CAMHS. These posts have been helped into being by the CAMHS grant and are now frequently funded by CAMHS development funds through PCTs and local authorities. In some localities, actual or virtual 'teams' made up of CAMH specialists, but without a child psychiatrist, have developed. These 'tier 2 teams' offer early intervention services for families where problems are emerging and where easy access to other professionals for less specialist interventions such as parenting support and behavioural interventions can be helpful and can be provided locally.

Children's primary mental health workers (PMHWs) are a newly emerging category of CAMH worker. PMHWs are specialist CAMH professionals who offer a service in primary care settings, frequently non-clinic based. They offer multidisciplinary approaches, direct work, consultation, training and education to schools, children's services, non-statutory organizations and youth services. Primary mental health workers provide a 'bridge' between tiers 1 and 3, offering assessments, joint working, consultation and interventions in primary care. They often work alongside other key professionals. Some tier 2 work is conducted through primary mental health teams and others, such as singleton clinicians, are attached to tier 3 teams or work in PCTs with supervision from specialist CAMHS. Initially funded through a national CAMHS grant, their services are now more frequently commissioned through CAMHS development funds managed by PCTs and local authorities.

In *Tier 3*, the same specialist child and adolescent mental health practitioners, also including child psychiatrists, work together as a team. These teams provide a multiprofessional, multi-agency approach to diagnosis and treatment. They work from a clinic base, usually in the community, but sometimes in a local hospital. The teams offer the benefit of multidisciplinary approaches to assessment and treatment, specialist professional assessment and treatment, as well as many opportunities for joint working. The teams also offer liaison, consultation, supervision, education and training to a range of professionals within and outside their own service, in particular to children's social services, health visitors and school nurses, accident and emergency staff and teachers.

Targeted specialist CAMHS responses are also built into services for specific groups of vulnerable young people. These include specialist provision for looked after children, those with learning disability, services out of hours and youth offending services. Other targeted services are expected to include infant and perinatal mental health; services for young people on the autistic spectrum and those who have special educational needs, young people in local authority secure children's homes and the children of asylum seekers and refugees.

Other specialist services whose work includes a child mental health component include educational and clinical psychology; intensive support teams in schools for young people at risk of being excluded from school; youth inclusion support panels and teams; targeted youth support workers; voluntary and independent organizations; children's social services; children with disabilities teams; acute and community paediatrics; services for children with learning disabilities; behaviour education support teams; substance misuse teams; teenage pregnancy units and many others.

Tier 4 describes the very specialized inpatient services and outpatient/day care services for young people with mental illness; special units for sensory impairment or eating disorders; specialist neuropsychiatric services; secure forensic mental health and local authority services. Children and young people requiring these services are likely to be the most vulnerable.

Crucial to an understanding of the tiered approach is an appreciation of the need to manage the boundaries between each tier, and not use them as gate-keeping mechanisms to prevent access, but rather to facilitate a clear care pathway between services that support the young person. It is crucial that there are good working relationships and protocols for the safe and speedy movement of cases between the tiers and that consultation is available to staff at all levels of the structure. It is described as a structure but is actually a virtual structure whose prime purpose is to aid localities in the development of a comprehensive CAMHS, ensuring that staff at all tiers have the right and combined levels of competency, training and skill to provide a fully appropriate range of services for children and their families.

It is possible to describe children's needs in relation to the tiers (see Fig. 8.1), but the overriding imperative is to treat the child in the least stigmatizing setting where good consultation and liaison between practitioners at all levels can offer a child-centred service.

The National Service Framework for Children, Young People and Maternity Services (Department of Health and DfES, 2004) notes that a critical mass of staffing is required for services to be safe, timely, and effective and

> *able to respond to a wide range of demands which include the provision of specialist and multi disciplinary assessment and treatment services, research and audit; and support training, consultation and face to face work within primary care settings.*
>
> **(Department of Health and DfES, 2004,**
> **Standard 9 Section 9, Paragraph 1)**

This has called into question the level of staffing that is required to deliver such a comprehensive service. The National Service Framework (NSF) made its recommendation on the following basis:

> *. . . analysis of a number of attempts to estimate staffing need has suggested the following: a generic specialist multi disciplinary CAMHS at*

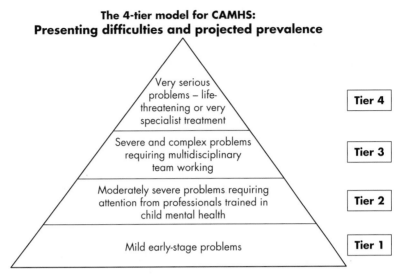

**The 4-tier model for CAMHS:
Presenting difficulties and projected prevalence**

Very serious problems – life-threatening or very specialist treatment — **Tier 4**

Severe and complex problems requiring multidisciplinary team working — **Tier 3**

Moderately severe problems requiring attention from professionals trained in child mental health — **Tier 2**

Mild early-stage problems — **Tier 1**

Figure 8.1 Child and Adolescent Mental Health Services (CAMHS): a tiered approach. (Adapted from Kurtz (1996) *Treating Children Well: a guide to using the evidence base in commissioning and managing mental health services for children and young people.* London: The Mental Health Foundation, p.25.)

> *Tier 3 with teaching responsibilities and providing evidence based interventions for 0–17 year olds would need a minimum of 20 whole time equivalents per 100 000 population, and a non teaching service, a minimum of 15 whole time equivalents.*
>
> **(Department of Health and DfES, 2004,
> Standard 9 Section 9, Paragraph 2)**

These figures have caused considerable discussion in the CAMHS community as the annual CAMHS mapping exercise demonstrates that most CAMH services are not adequately staffed, while the demands on them are increasing.

COMMISSIONING

This brings us to the role of CAMHS commissioners in the complex task of identifying need and commissioning the requisite number and type of services required to deliver to priority areas of need for children with mental health problems.

The CAMHS Grant guidance, the NSF, and more recently *Choosing Health* (Department of Health, 2004a) and *Commissioning a Patient Led NHS* (Department of Health, 2005) all emphasize the need to strengthen the commissioning function by means of structural changes in health and local authorities. Commissioning a 'patient-led' NHS and practice-based commissioning together imply commissioning structures that can provide a counterbalance to strong provider organizations. The policy intention is to encourage choice and contestability and to strengthen partnerships between health, education, local government and non-statutory organizations.

Following the Children Act 2004, social services departments merged with education services to become joint children's services departments under a children's services director, moving toward the provision of all children's services – including health – through children's trusts.

Future commissioning models will offer an inherent challenge to a health-dominated model of CAMHS, with greater emphasis on collaborative and joint commissioning structures. The 2003 Public Service Agreement emphasized that both health and children's services share the responsibility for commissioning CAMHS. This was further reinforced in 2005 when joint health and local authority performance targets were set for CAMHS to extend to young people aged 16 to 17 years; provision of 24/7 cover; services for children and young people with learning disability and services for those children with complex levels of health and social care need.

This is why it is important not only to have a CAMH needs assessment and a gap analysis, but for each local authority to have its own joint CAMH strategy with agreements about levels of investment in CAMHS across all local agencies. The intention is not only to be able to deliver a *comprehensive CAMHS,* as specified by the children's NSF, but also to ensure there are key linkages in terms of strategy and commissioning for services along the following lines:

• county-wide children and young people's plans – a legal responsibility for local authorities from April 2006
• youth offending service plans
• substance misuse plans
• joint area reviews
• local area agreements
• joint inspection services of health and local authorities.

The implicit message of *Every Child Matters: change for children* (HM Government, 2004) and the *National Service Framework for Children, Young People and Maternity Services* (Department of Health and DfES, 2004) is that practitioners and managers are expected to read both documents together; conduct planning together across disciplines and agencies; pool budgets where appropriate; jointly commission services, especially for children with complex care needs, and plan collaborative workforce development.

The English Department for Education and Skills published guidance on the joint planning and commissioning of children's services in 2006 and this should be read as a companion document to all health commissioning literature (DfES, 2006).

The policy aim of all commissioning processes is to improve the performance and management of all children's services; remain outcomes focused; establish clear and sensible care pathways that make sense to the child and their parents, and include children and young people in the planning of those services. This is a formidable and radical change of direction for child and adolescent mental

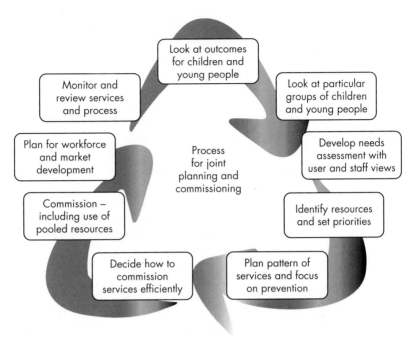

Figure 8.2 Process for joint planning and commissioning. (Reproduced from HM Government (2006) *The Common Assessment Framework for Children and Young People: practitioners' guide. Integrated working to improve outcomes for children and young people.* Nottingham: DfES Publications, p.1.) Crown Copyright material is reproduced with the permission of the Controller of HMSO and the Queen's Printer for Scotland.

health services, given that no significant policy change had occurred in the quarter century prior to the Health Advisory Service report in 1995.

The principle standard for commissioning CAMHS, as with all children's services in the UK, is to ensure that the right service should get to the right child at the right time, and in the most appropriate place. For this to happen effectively, agencies are expected to work together to build care pathways that reduce the historic duplication of effort and the need for families to 'tell their story' more than once.

The *Common Assessment Framework* (HM Government, 2006) and integrated children's information system is designed to assist with this process (see Fig. 8.2).

POLICY FRAMEWORK

The policy framework for CAMHS is influenced by a variety of sources and reflects the move in the UK to a multiprofessional, multi-agency, multisystem interpretation of child and adolescent mental health services based in the concept of the Health Advisory Service tier 1 to 4 system described earlier. Currently, the responsibility for much of the universal aspects of delivering a comprehensive CAMHS is now within the DfES. This shifts attention to work in schools where they can support mental health. The English Department of Health retains responsibility for the specialist services (tiers 2, 3, and 4) within its overall mental health remit.

Since devolution from Westminster Parliament in 1998, Wales, Scotland and Northern Ireland have acquired in-country responsibility for health and social care services. The direction of change varies in each but legislation such as the Children Act 2004, international agreements (UN Convention on the Rights of the Child 1989) and recommendations such as those arising from The Laming Inquiry (Department of Health and Home Office, 2003) apply across the UK.

Policy positions within health and social care, education, via the Healthy Schools programmes in each country, the youth justice system, the youth services, Sure Start and the early years services all impact on CAMHS. Broader housing, leisure and voluntary sector policies also play a part in constructing the framework within which the mental health of children and young people is supported or not.

The UK Parliament has set out its expectations in various planning documents. Most important are *The National Service Framework for Children, Young People and Maternity Services* (Department of Health and DfES, 2004) and *Every Child Matters: change for children* (HM Government, 2004) which are written as sister documents. Others of significant relevance are *Youth Matters* (DfES, 2005b), *Choosing Health* (Department of Health, 2005b), *Mental Health Needs and the Effectiveness of Provision for Young Offenders in Custody and in the Community* (Youth Justice Board, 2005), and the *National Service Framework for Mental Health (Adults)* (Department of Health, 1999).

Since 2000, the UK Government has invested specifically in CAMHS in England through the CAMHS Grant. The core CAMHS Grant is paid to councils with social services responsibilities (CSSRs) to enable them to carry forward their joint strategies with the NHS and other agencies to develop CAMHS. In 2004 and 2005 PCTs received specific funding for CAMHS, which is now within the PCT baseline budget allocation. The intention was that CAMHS partnerships should use the grant and the PCT monies to improve CAMHS in accordance with jointly agreed local needs and priorities as set out in local CAMHS development strategies.

When the CAMHS Grant was first introduced, and before the funds were released, localities were required to look at their commissioning patterns, which were largely historical, and to review the needs of their populations. In *Improvement, Expansion and Reform* (Department of Health, 2002) the Department of Health for England set targets for CAMHS. Comprehensive services were expected to be in development by 2006, including primary mental health worker (PMHW) posts, 24-hour cover, services for children and young people with learning disability and those aged 16 to 18 years, and a 10 per cent increase in resources year on year. This last requirement has been variously interpreted, but 2005 CAMHS mapping shows a 16 per cent increase in the number of CAMHS teams between 2003 and 2005 and an 11 per cent increase in the total number of staff by 2004–05 period ($n = 9876$). *National Standards,*

Local Action (Department of Health, 2004b) requires this specified level of service to be maintained, and the annual CAMHS mapping exercise supports commissioners by providing national statistics and comparators. It can be viewed at www.camhsmapping.org.uk.

In addition to government documentation, there have been a number of reports that have significantly influenced the development of child and adolescent mental health services in the UK in the 1990s. Key amongst these are *Together we Stand* (Health Advisory Service, 1995), *Bright Futures* (Mental Health Foundation, 1999) and *Children in Mind* (Audit Commission, 1999). They brought together child and adolescent mental health strategy and practice, as well as the experiences of users, and have established service standards.

The National Service Framework for Children, Young People and the Maternity Services (Department of Health and DfES, 2004)

Standard 9 of this NSF is specifically about mental health, although it can be argued that mental health has relevance to all the standards that, for example, cover chronic illness, children in hospital or children who suffer abuse. Standard 9 needs to be read alongside the other standards as they all cross-reference one to another and interface with the Green Paper *Every Child Matters* (Chief Secretary to the Treasury, 2003)

The NSF covers a 10-year period from 2003 and it is expected that the practice improvements set out in the standards will have been achieved within that time. It is not possible here to go into the detail, but broadly Standard 9 covers access, informed commissioning of CAMHS, ongoing multi-agency assessment and analysis of need; and workforce development. There is also a requirement to develop early intervention and prevention strategies; an expectation that user views will be sought; that the specific needs of black and multi-ethnic (BME) groups will be identified and met; that services will be local where possible, and that care pathways will be clear.

Particular groups such as those young people with learning difficulties who also have mental health problems are specifically highlighted for improved access to services. The age group for CAMHS is defined as up to the 18th birthday, formally adding an extra year to previous age guidelines and seeking to clarify existing age-range anomalies.

Emphasis on using the evidence base to underpin practice, and an expectation that practitioners will work across agency and professional boundaries is the premise on which services are expected to support the child and family. In this, the NSF fits neatly into the Change for Children programme.

Every Child Matters: change for children (HM Government, 2004)

This agenda – to raise the profile of the needs of children generally – stretches across the four countries of the UK and is underpinned by the Children Act

2004. The Act updates the 1989 Children Act and establishes the children's commissioner post in each country. Local authorities are required to appoint a director of children's services (bringing together social services and education) and to formalize the creation of a lead member for children. This has led to the development of real and virtual children's trusts, which, in some cases, include health. Changes are also made to child protection arrangements and to information sharing between agencies, and have been based on the recommendations of the Laming Report (Department of Health and Home Office, 2003), a government inquiry into the circumstances surrounding the death of Victoria Climbié.

There are five basic tenets within the Change for Children programme:

- being healthy
- staying safe
- enjoying and achieving
- making a positive contribution
- achieving economic well-being.

While mental health is integral to all these, it receives fairly minimal coverage in the Change for Children literature. CAMHS is cited as a partner in delivering services. Functional partnerships across agencies and the sharing of information underpin this agenda, which has at its root the intention to prevent the deaths of children through abuse. A common assessment framework, to be used by all agencies involved with the child, has been developed, and arrangements for information sharing are in progress. In addition, this programme provides opportunities to further integrate and co-ordinate services for children and their families, in places where access is easy and where co-location of teams and/or provision of services is possible. It also gives ample opportunity for CAMHS to be involved through primary mental health workers as well as specialist CAMHS team members, to link closely with the healthy schools agenda and to be part of the thinking behind children's trusts. These have been contentious issues for many practitioners and will, no doubt, continue to be complicated by the duty of confidentiality and how this is interpreted locally.

THINKING ABOUT THE CHALLENGES OF CHILD AND ADOLESCENT MENTAL HEALTH

There can be no doubt that well-resourced nurturing and support for the mental health of children and young people is essential for a stable society. It *is* everybody's business. Over the last two decades there has been increasing interest in, and understanding of, its importance within a burgeoning evidence base that links mental health problems and disorders in young people to increasing levels of problem behaviours.

From the mid-1990s, government funds have been targeted in order to improve traditional CAMHS. More recently, there has been government recognition of the part played by all children's services in delivering the CAMHS agenda. The stigma of mental illness remains, and for many children and young people this is still a potent factor in making much-needed services inaccessible. The challenge for CAMHS in the coming period is to engage effectively with all those in need, by providing services in the least stigmatizing settings and ensuring that interventions are timely, appropriate and evidence based in the true traditions of using public health theory to inform the design of strong and effective public services based on reliable evidence of need.

CONCLUSION

The mental health and well-being of our children and young people is dependent upon an understanding of the fundamentals of infant and child development and the management of the transitional stages of childhood. Health and local authority economies must build on the assessed needs of the under-18 population, taking a fundamental public health approach to maintaining the best of existing levels of service and reconfiguring others to ensure smooth transition through critical stages of development. Joint CAMH strategies are a key tool with agreed levels of investment against agreed priorities. However, there needs to be much greater emphasis on joint policy and service development and how to make the best use of well-trained and experienced staff in order to ensure that there are clear pathways of care for all those requiring a service on the spectrum of services that embrace the concept of child and adolescent mental health.

KEY POINTS

- The mental health of children and young people is everybody's business.
- Support to early parenting helps protect and nurture mental health.
- Attending to the mental well-being of parents is crucial to parents supporting emotionally healthy children.
- CAMH services must be accessible and acceptable and culturally appropriate, bearing in mind the potential stigma that can attach to these services.
- Commissioning of services must be based on known need and agreed joint priorities between agencies and not on historical patterns of provision.
- The consequences of failing to support vulnerable children, young people and families are highly significant for 'antisocial behaviours' and other negative outcomes for individuals, families and society as a whole.

REFERENCES

Advisory Council for the Misuse of Drugs (2005) *Further Consideration of the Classification of Cannabis under the Misuse of Drugs Act 1971*. London: Home Office.

Ainsworth M, Blehar M, Waters E, Wall S (1978) *Patterns of Attachment: a psychological study of the strange situation*. Hillsdale NJ: Lawrence Erlbaum Associates Inc.

American Psychiatric Association (1994) *Diagnostic and Statistical Manual of Mental Disorders (DSM IV)*. Washington DC: American Psychiatric Publishing Inc.

Astington J, Harris P, Olson D (1988) *Developing Theories of Mind*. New York: Cambridge University Press.

Audit Commission (1999) *Children in Mind: child and adolescent mental health*. London: Audit Commission.

Balbernie R (2001) Circuits and circumstances: the neurobiological consequences of early relationship experiences and how they shape later behaviour. *Journal of Child Psychotherapy* 27:237–55.

Baruch G (ed.) (2001) *Community-based Psychotherapy with Young People*. London: Brunner Routledge.

Birchwood M, McGorry P, Jackson H (1997) Early intervention in schizophrenia (Editorial). *British Journal of Psychiatry* 170:2–5.

Blair C (2001) The early identification of risk for grade retention among African American children at risk for school difficulty. *Applied Developmental Science* 5:37–50.

Blakemore SJ, Frith U (2005) *The Learning Brain: lessons for education*. Oxford: Blackwell Publishing.

Chasnoff IJ, Hatcher R, Burns W (1980) Early growth patterns of methadone addicted infants. *American Journal of the Disabled Child* 134:1049–51.

Chief Secretary to the Treasury (2003) *Every Child Matters* (Cm 5860). London: Stationery Office. www.everychildmatters.gov.uk/_content/documents/EveryChildMatters.pdf (accessed 17 January 2007).

Cicchetti D, Barnett D (1991) Attachment organisation in pre school-aged maltreated children. *Development and Psychopathology* 3:397–411.

Cleaver H, Unell I, Aldgate J (1999) *Children's Needs, Parenting Capacity*. London: HMSO.

CAMHS Outcome Research Consortium (2005) www.corc.uk.net (accessed 29 January 2007).

Department for Education and Skills (2005a) *Birth to Three Matters*. Nottingham: DfES Publications.

Department for Education and Skills (2005b) *Youth Matters*. Nottingham: DfES Publications.

Department for Education and Skills (2006) *Joint Planning and Commissioning Framework*. Nottingham: DfES Publications. www.everychildmatters.gov.uk/_files/312A353A9CB391262BAF14CC7C1592F8.pdf (accessed 29 January 2006)

Department of Health (1999) *National Service Framework for Mental Health (Adults)*. London: Department of Health.

Department of Health (2002) *Improvement Expansion and Reform – the Next 3 Years: priorities and planning framework 2003–2006*. London: Department of Health.

Department of Health (2004a) *Choosing Health*. London: Department of Health.

Department of Health (2004b) *National Standards, Local Action: health and social care standards and planning framework 2005/06–2007/08*. London: Department of Health.

Department of Health (2005) *Commissioning a Patient Led NHS*. London: Department of Health.

Department of Health and Department for Education and Skills (2004) *The National Service Framework for Children, Young People and Maternity Services*. London: Department of Health. www.dh.gov.uk/PolicyAnd Guidance/HealthAndSocialCareTopics/ChildrenServices/ChildrenServices Information/ChildrenServicesInformationArticle/fs/en?CONTENT_ ID=4089111&chk=U8Ecln (accessed 5 February 2007).

Department of Health and Home Office (2003) *The Victoria Climbié Inquiry. Report of an Inquiry by Lord Laming*. London: HMSO.

Dogra N, Parkin A, Gale F, Frake C (2003) *A Multi Disciplinary Handbook of CAMHS for Front Line Professionals*. London: Jessica Kingsley Publishers Ltd.

Elliot L (1999) *Early Intelligence: how the brain and mind develops in the first five years of life*. London: Penguin.

Fonagy P, Steele M, Steele H, Moran G, Higgins A (1991) The capacity for understanding mental states: the reflective self in parent and child and its significance for security of attachment. *Infant Mental Health Journal* 13:200–17.

Fonagy P, Target M, Cottrell D, Phillips J, Kurtz Z (2002) *A Critical Review of Treatments for Children and Adolescents*. New York: Guilford Publications.

Gesch CB, Hammond SM, Hampson SE *et al.* (2002) Influence of supplementary vitamins, minerals and essential fatty acids on the antisocial behaviour of young adult prisoners. *British Journal of Psychiatry* 181:22–8.

Graham H, Power C (2004) *Childhood Disadvantage and Adult Health: a lifecourse framework*. Lancaster: Institute for Health Research, University of Lancaster.

Hagel A (2004) *Time Trends in Adolescent Well-being*. London: Nuffield Foundation.

Harbin F, Murphy M (2000) *Substance Misuse and Child Care: how to understand, assist and intervene when drugs affect parenting*. Lyme Regis: Russell House Publishing.

Hartley-Brewer E (2005) *Perspectives on the Causes of Mental Health Problems in Children and Adolescents*. Report and discussion paper from a YoungMinds Symposium held in association with the Institute for Public Policy Research, March 2005, London. London: YoungMinds.

Health Advisory Service (1995) *Together we Stand: the commissioning role and management of child and adolescent mental health services*. London: HMSO.

HM Government (2004) *Every Child Matters: change for children*. Nottingham: DfES Publications. www.everychildmatters.gov.uk/_content/documents/ Every%20Child%20Matinserts.pdf (accessed 29 January 2007).

HM Government (2006) *The Common Assessment Framework for Children and Young People: practitioners' guide. Integrated working to improve outcomes for children and young people*. Nottingham: DfES Publications.

Kuh D, Power C, Blane D, Bartley M (2004) Socioeconomic pathways between childhood and adult health. In: Kuh DL, Ben-Schlomo YAA (ed.)

Life Course Approach to Chronic Disease Epidemiology, Tracing the Origins of Ill Health from Early to Adult Life (2e). Oxford: Oxford University Press, pp.371–98.

Kurtz Z (ed.) (1992) *With Health in Mind: mental health care for children and young people.* London: Action for Sick Children.

Kurtz Z (1996) *Treating Children Well: a guide to using the evidence base in commissioning and managing mental health services for children and young people.* London: The Mental Health Foundation.

Lyons-Ruth K (1996) Attachment relationships among children with aggressive behaviour problems – the role of disorganised early attachment patterns. *Journal of Consulting and Clinical Psychology* 64:64–73.

McLoyd AS (2001) The impact of economic hardship on black families and children: psychological distress, parenting and socioeconomic development. *Child Development* 61:311–46.

Meltzer H, Corbin T, Gatward R, Goodman R, Ford T. (2003) *The Mental Health of Young People looked after by Local Authorities in England.* London: HMSO.

Meltzer H, Green H, McGinnity A, Ford T, Goodman R (2005) *The Mental Health of Children and Young People in Great Britain 2004.* London: Office for National Statistics.

Mental Health Foundation (1999) *Bright Futures: promoting children and young people's mental health.* London: The Mental Health Foundation.

Murray L (1992) The impact of postnatal depression on infant development. *Journal of Child Psychology* 33:543–61.

National Institute for Health and Clinical Excellence (2005) *CG28 Depression in Children and Young People: NICE guideline.* www.nice.org.uk/page.aspx?o=cg028niceguideline (accessed 11 January 2007).

National Institute for Health and Clinical Excellence (2006) *TA102 Conduct Disorder in Children–parent-training/Education Programmes: quick reference guide.* www.nice.org.uk/page.aspx?o=345133 (accessed 11 January 2007).

Potts Y, Gillies ML, Wood SF (2001) Lack of mental well-being in 15-year-olds: an undisclosed iceberg? *Family Practice* 18:95–100.

Reder P, Duncan S, Gray M (1993) *Beyond Blame, Child Abuse Tragedies Revisited.* London: Routledge.

Rutter M (1971) Parent–child separation: psychological effects on the children. *Journal of Child Psychology and Psychiatry* 12:233–60.

Rutter M (1975) *Helping Troubled Children.* London and New York: Penguin.

Rutter M (2001) *Psychosocial Adversity and Child Psychopathology. Research and innovation on the road to modern child psychiatry.* London: Gaskell (Royal College of Psychiatrists).

Schaffer HR (1996) *Social Development.* Oxford: Blackwell.

Tagore R (1933) *My School.* (Lecture delivered in America). www.learningnet-india.org/lni/data/publications/revive/vol4/v4-2-m.php (accessed 29 January 2007)

Van de Weyer C (2005) *Changing Diets, Changing Minds.* London: Sustain.

Vygotskyi L (1978) *Mind in Society: the development of higher psychological processes*. Cambridge MA: Harvard University Press.

Walker SP, Chang SM, Powell CA, Simonoff E, Grantham-McGregor SM (2006) Effects of psychosocial stimulation and dietary supplementation in early childhood on psychosocial functioning in late adolescence: follow-up of randomised controlled trial. *British Medical Journal* 333:472–6.

Wallace SA, Crown JM, Cox AD, Berger M (1997) *Child and Adolescent Mental Health*. Abingdon: Radcliffe Medical Press.

World Health Organization (1992) *The ICD-10 Classification of Mental and Behavioural Disorders Clinical Descriptions and Diagnostic Guidelines*. Geneva: World Health Organization.

Youth Justice Board (2005) *Mental Health Needs and Effectiveness of Provision for Young Offenders in Custody and in the Community*. London: Youth Justice Board.

YoungMinds (2006) London. www.youngminds.org.uk/problems/ (accessed 29 January 2007).

Websites

Annual CAMH mapping exercise: www.camhsmapping.org.uk

CAMHS Outcome Research Consortium: www.corc.uk.net

Care Services Improvement Partnership: www.csip.org.uk

Department for Education and Skills: www.dfes.gov.uk/

Department of Health: www.doh.gov.uk

Every Child Matters: www.everychildmatters.gov.uk/

Faculty for Children and Young People in the British Psychological Society www.bps.org.uk/dcp-cyp/dcp-cyp_home.cfm

National CAMHS Support Service: www.camhs.org.uk

National Institute for Health and Clinical Excellence: www.nice.org.uk

National Service Framework for Children, Young People and their Families: www.dh.gov.uk/PolicyAndGuidance/HealthAndSocialCareTopics/Children Services/ChildrenServicesInformation/fs/en

Royal College of Psychiatrists www.rcpsych.ac.uk

Sure Start: www.surestart.gov.uk

The Standards Site: www.standards.dfes.gov.uk

Youth Justice Board: www.yjb.gov.uk

Act of Parliament

This Act is published by HMSO in London, and can be accessed from the UK Parliament website (www.publications.parliament.uk).

Children Act 2004

Susan Kirk

INTRODUCTION

The disabled child population is increasing and changing in character. Medical advances have improved the life expectancy for preterm infants and those with impairments and long-term conditions such as cystic fibrosis. In addition, increasing numbers of children are being diagnosed with autistic-spectrum conditions, attention deficit hyperactivity disorder and mental health problems. Consequently there are more children who have complex needs.

Defining disability is problematic and contested. Firstly there are debates in relation to social and medical models of disability, with the former seeing the barriers that disabled people face arising from a disabling environment, while the latter sees them emanating from impairment. Second, health, education and social care sectors may use different definitions based on different legislative frameworks, and third some people (for example, those with a long-term condition) may not define themselves as 'disabled'. In the UK, children with 'complex healthcare needs' is a term that is being used increasingly in practice, policy and research. Although there is no accepted definition of 'complex healthcare needs', it is generally considered to relate to children with high levels of health and social care needs, who require the support of a range of professionals and agencies and who have additional care needs specifically related to the use of medical technology (Glendinning *et al.*, 2001; Abbott *et al.*, 2005). Sometimes this term is used interchangeably with 'complex needs', which has recently been defined by the UK Government.

> Children with complex needs have a number of discrete needs – relating to their health, education, welfare, development, home environment and so on – that require additional support from more than one agency. Their needs are often chronic and may be life-long. Different needs tend to interact, exacerbating their impact on the child's development and well-being.
> **(Department for Education and Skills, 2006, p.37)**

However, the use of the term 'healthcare' is usually taken to suggest the presence of ongoing medical/nursing needs, often as a result of an unpredictable underlying long-term condition. Defining 'complex needs' has also been subject to analysis (Rankin and Regan, 2004) and it has been noted that it is not people's needs that are complex, but rather it is the systems and services they have to negotiate in order to meet their needs that are complex (Morris, 1999).

Children with complex healthcare needs form part of other 'groups' identified in the literature – disabled children, children with chronic illness/long-term conditions, technology-dependent children and children with life-limiting/-threatening conditions. Differentiating between these groups is problematic as, for example, some long-term conditions may be disabling and some disabled children may have a serious illness. Both can be progressive, episodic and medically unstable. Furthermore a child with complex healthcare needs may 'belong' to many or all of these different groups. Trying to categorize children risks pathologizing and marginalizing them and overlooking their individuality and the societal barriers they face. Consequently this chapter will provide a non-categorical, non-impairment-specific overview of research and debates in the area of children and young people with complex healthcare needs and long-term conditions, by drawing on the literature on disabled children, children with a chronic illness and children who need the support of medical technology (who may be associated with the terms 'technology-dependent', 'technology-assisted' or 'medically fragile' children). A social model perspective will be taken but one that incorporates the importance of understanding the individual experience of impairment in terms of identity and agency.

PREVALENCE AND CHARACTERISTICS

Knowledge of the prevalence, trends and socio-demographic characteristics of disabled children and their families is important to guide service development. Although data about disabled children are collected by a number of different organizations, how they are collected and the lack of standardization of definitions and categories mean that there is no straightforward way of aggregating data from different sources to produce a reliable overall estimate at either a national or local level (Blackburn et al., 2006). Moreover how disability is defined and conceptualized determines both the nature of the data being sought and the process of data collection; and the debate over whether disability can be measured remains unresolved (Blackburn et al., 2006). The most comprehensive and robust prevalence data date back to the national disability surveys of the 1980s (Bone and Meltzer, 1989). This survey identified over 320 000 disabled children in England and Wales but does not reflect more recent changes in prevalence or patterns of disability. Government departments are currently using the Family Resources Survey and have calculated that there are 770 000 disabled children under 16 years in the UK (7 per cent of all children aged 0–16 years) using the Disability Discrimination Act 1995 definition of disability (Department of Health/Department for Education and Skills (DfES), 2004).

Using the General Household Survey and data from the Family Fund Trust, the Office for National Statistics (2004) has provided further information on trends in childhood disability for those aged 0–19 years living in the UK. They report that the most frequent cause of mild disability (which includes long-standing illness) is asthma, and the most frequent cause of severe disability is autistic-spectrum and behavioural disorders. Severe disability was found to be more prevalent in boys, in the 0–4 years age group, and in those living in Wales and Northern Ireland. Prevalence rates for mild and severe disability were higher for those from lower socio-economic groups, and there appeared to be an increasing prevalence rate amongst minority ethnic groups, although they acknowledge that this might reflect an increasing uptake of services and benefits. In terms of children with complex healthcare needs, it has been estimated that there are 6000 technology-dependent children in the UK, the majority of whom are under 2 years old (Glendinning *et al.*, 2001). Other research has found that most disabled children have more than one impairment (Gordon *et al.*, 2000) and that a significant number of families have more than one disabled child (Lawton, 1998). It has also been identified that disabled children are more likely to experience abuse and neglect than non-disabled children (Sullivan and Knutson, 2000), that they are overrepresented in the 'looked after' children population and more likely to be placed in long-term residential settings (Pinney, 2005). The educational attainment of disabled children has been reported to be lower than that of non-disabled children (Prime Minister Strategy Unit, 2005). In recent years there has been more recognition of the disadvantage that disabled children and their families face in government policy and an increased emphasis placed on enabling disabled children to achieve their full potential and for families to live ordinary lives.

While parental experiences and needs have been the focus of most research, there is a developing body of research about disabled children themselves.

PARENTS' EXPERIENCES OF CARING

It is well documented how parents experience caring for disabled children and those with long-term conditions and the impact this has on their lives. Studies conducted over the past 30 years have provided a consistent picture of parents' experiences in spite of using different methodological approaches and focusing on different conditions and impairments. However, changes have occurred in how disabled children and their families are conceptualized. Sloper (1999) notes that the ideas that inform research, policy and practice in relation to disabled children have undergone change as a result of the growth of the disability and human rights movements, the increasing focus on the rights of children, the development of theoretical models of stress, coping and family systems approaches and the development of a carers' movement. This is in addition to wider policy changes such as the emphasis on obtaining the views of service users.

The reconceptualization of caring

Much of the early research has been criticized for pathologizing parents' experiences (Baldwin and Carlisle, 1994; Beresford 1994; McConachie, 1994;

McKeever and Miller, 2004). This pathological model saw parental stress and family burden as inevitable consequences of having a disabled child. Concepts such as grief, rejection, denial and overprotection were often central, reflecting a view of disability as an insurmountable tragedy. This approach pathologized individuals into homogenous problem groups and conceptualized them as passive recipients rather than active agents, responding to, and resolving, events affecting their lives (Beresford, 1994). The pathological approach is regarded as reflecting both society's devaluation of disabled people and the negative associations deeply embedded within it. Early studies on parents' experiences of caring for a child with a chronic illness have similarly been criticized for focusing on the dysfunctional and negative aspects of family functioning related to caring for a child with a chronic illness, rather than parental coping (Eiser, 1990; Coyne, 1997). To a large extent this perspective has informed professional practice (Kearney and Griffin, 2001).

The 1990s saw a change in the conceptualization and theorizing of disability research in relation to parents. This new approach is underpinned by theories of coping and focuses on parents' coping resources and strategies (Beresford, 1994; McConachie, 1994; Judge, 1998). This conceptualization redefines caring as not necessarily having a negative effect on parents, emphasizing that parents adapt and cope and actively manage their situation rather than responding passively (Beresford, 1994). In addition, the positive aspects of caring were revealed. However, the coping resources and strategies model has been criticized for neglecting the social and environmental factors that affect parents, for focusing on the individual and for overlooking the real stress parents experience (Dale, 1996).

Social consequences

A large number of studies over the past 30 years have identified the social isolation and the barriers to social participation that parents and families experience (Burton, 1975; Glendinning, 1983; Young et al., 1988; Aday et al., 1989; Diehl et al., 1991; Teague et al., 1993; Patterson et al., 1994; Bradley et al., 1995; Baumgardener and Burtea, 1998; Tozer, 1999; Townsley and Robinson, 2000; Dobson et al., 2001; Nelson, 2002; Heaton et al., 2003; Rehm and Bradley, 2005). This exclusion may be a result of transport and access problems and by having to contend with public reactions to their child (Tozer, 1999; Case, 2000; Dobson et al., 2001). In relation to children with complex healthcare needs, it may also be a consequence of fears over leaving their child, exhaustion from caring, the withdrawal of friends and the unwieldy nature of the equipment that needs to accompany the child. It may be compounded by the difficulty of finding baby-sitters who are both willing and able to care for a child with specialized needs. Family life may revolve around the child's needs, with no time for parents to meet their own individual needs (Stewart et al., 1994; Hatton et al., 1995; Heaton et al., 2003). Parents' daily life becomes dominated and routinized by the procedures relating to the technology (Wilson et al., 1998; Kirk et al., 2005). As a result, families can become physically and socially excluded from wider society.

Caring itself places a strain on parental relationships which can lead to relationship difficulties (Eiser, 1993; Teague *et al.*, 1993; Petr *et al.*, 1995). A number of studies have found that the risk of a breakdown in parental relationships is higher if there is a disabled child, and rises with the severity of the disability (Baldwin and Carlisle, 1994).

A consistent theme in the literature is parents' reports of sleep deprivation from their child's sleeping problems, parental anxiety about their child's condition, false monitor alarms, the need to provide care for their child or remain vigilant over them during the night (Andrews and Nielson, 1988; Aday *et al.*, 1989; Scharer and Dixon, 1989; Teague *et al.*, 1993; Clarke, 1995; Williams *et al.*, 1999; Townsley and Robinson, 2000; Heaton *et al.*, 2003). There is some evidence that suggests that behavioural interventions may be helpful in treating disabled children's sleeping problems (Lucas *et al.*, 2002). As will be discussed later, providing a break from caring (e.g. night-sitters) is an important way of supporting families.

Studies have also identified the housing problems that families may face, with as many as 50 per cent of families with a disabled child living in unsuitable housing (Beresford, 1995; Oldman and Beresford, 1998; Chamba *et al.*, 1999). This has a significant impact on caring and on children's independence. Major modifications of the home may be required to enable disabled children to be cared for at home. In the case of children with complex healthcare needs, the impact on the home milieu can be dramatic as it may be transformed by medical equipment and personnel into an environment associated more with a hospital intensive care unit (Smith, 1991; Kirk *et al.*, 2005). In addition this group of families often require a considerable amount of service support on a daily basis, with some families receiving home support services for up to 24 hours a day (Quint *et al.*, 1990; Leonard *et al.*, 1993; Kirk, 1999). Inevitably, this leads to a loss of privacy for families, as family life occurs under the gaze of the various support workers and professionals who visit or spend long periods of time in the home (Aday *et al.*, 1989; Scharer and Dixon, 1989; Leonard *et al.*, 1993; Clarke, 1995; Wilson *et al.*, 1998; Cohen, 1999; Kirk *et al.*, 2005). Hence the home may lose its association with comfort, security and privacy.

Financial consequences

It is well documented that childhood disability creates the need for additional expenditure, while at the same time, reducing income by restricting labour force participation (Baldwin and Carlisle, 1994; Dobson *et al.*, 2001).

Financial hardship

In the UK it has been estimated that 55 per cent of families with a disabled child live in poverty (Gordon *et al.*, 2000). The presence of financial difficulties and hardship has been reported in a large number of studies (Diehl *et al.*, 1991; Baldwin and Carlisle, 1994; Youngblut *et al.*, 1994; Beresford, 1995; Dobson and Middleton, 1998; Chamba *et al.*, 1999; Thyen *et al.*, 1999; Tozer, 1999; Emerson and Hatton, 2005). This is due to the additional financial costs of caring for a disabled child exceeding both family income and the financial support families receive. Mothers often have to leave employment, reducing family income at a time when the financial costs of caring rise (for example, increased electricity and water bills or long-distance travel to specialist centres) (Wheeler and Lewis, 1993; Thyen *et al.*, 1999; Glendinning *et al.*, 2001). In the UK it has been estimated that the costs of bringing up a disabled child are three times as much as for a non-disabled child (Dobson and Middleton, 1998). Not surprisingly, their financial situation has been identified by families as source of anxiety and stress (Teague *et al.*, 1993; Patterson *et al.*, 1994; Youngblut *et al.*, 1994).

Benefits have been found to inadequately compensate for the loss of earnings and the additional costs associated with disability such as laundry, transport and extra heating expenses (Dobson and Middleton, 1998; Kagan *et al.*, 1998). In addition to the direct costs to parents, there are also indirect costs from a loss of earnings. Families with a disabled child have significantly lower incomes than the general population (Beresford, 1995) and for those on very low incomes, any extra disability benefits they receive tend to be absorbed into the general household purse. In addition, there is reported to be confusion amongst families about eligibility for disability benefits (Beresford, 1994; Dobson and Middleton, 1998), with significant numbers not applying for benefits to which they are entitled (Roberts and Lawton, 1998). Minority ethnic families have been found to be less likely than white families to receive benefits, due in part to the lack of adequate and accessible information (Chamba *et al.*, 1999).

Labour market participation

Studies dating back to the 1970s have found that the parents of disabled children are less likely to be in paid employment (Burton, 1975; Bradshaw, 1980; Baldwin, 1985; Beresford, 1995; Gordon *et al.*, 2000; Emerson and Hatton, 2005). Parents perceive that caring for a disabled child affects their employment opportunities as they face considerable difficulties finding flexible work that will fit around their child's needs and appointments and appropriate childcare (Kagan *et al.*, 1998; Sloper *et al.*, 1991). In addition to the economic losses, there are occupational losses for parents, as caring may create barriers to both job promotion and mobility (Cohen, 1999; Thyen *et al.*, 1999).

Parents have reported the economic and psychological benefits that employment has for them and their children (Sloper *et al.*, 1991; Kagan *et al.*, 1998). Moreover a number of studies have found that the mothers of disabled children, who wished to work outside the home but were unable to, experienced higher levels of stress (Burton, 1975; Bradshaw, 1980; Glendinning, 1983; Gravelle, 1997).

Emotional consequences

The literature documents a range of emotions experienced by parents, including stress, guilt, anger, helplessness, frustration, depression, loneliness, anxiety, isolation, optimism and hope. Their feelings and attitudes also appear to change with time (Beresford, 1994). The main emotion investigated in the literature is parental stress. Studies have measured parents' mental health status, investigated the sources of the stress that they experience, and attempted to identify the predictive or causal factors that explain variation in parents' mental health status and stress levels. Other studies have investigated the coping resources and strategies that parents use to manage the stresses they encounter, and examined how parents and families adapt to their situation.

Parental stress

Baldwin and Carlisle (1994) conclude from their literature review that the evidence that parents of disabled children experience significant levels of stress is irrefutable. High levels of stress in parents have been identified in a number of studies (Bradshaw and Lawton, 1978; Sloper and Turner, 1992; Wallander and Varni, 1998; Pedersen *et al.*, 2004). It has been similarly reported that parents of children with long-term conditions report higher levels of stress and depression than parents of healthy children (Goldberg *et al.*, 1990; Patterson *et al.*, 1994; Labbe, 1996; Baumgardener and Burtea, 1998).

Sources of stress

The sources of stress are wide ranging. Initially the intense emotional impact of diagnosis engenders feelings such as shock, fear, anger, despair and many of the emotional reactions associated with bereavement (Burton, 1975; Gath, 1985; Eiser, 1990; Gibson, 1995; Nelson, 2002). The diagnosis of a genetic condition, in particular, may give rise to feelings of guilt (Chapple *et al.*, 1995; Ahmad *et al.*, 2000). The distress that parents experience may be further compounded by the insensitive manner in which the diagnosis is disclosed to parents. Parents may have to live with uncertainty, in relation to not only their child's long-term prognosis, but also their health on a day-to-day basis (Andrews and Nielson, 1988; Patterson *et al.*, 1994; Atkin and Ahmad, 2000; O'Brien, 2001). Other sources of stress identified in the literature include parents' concerns about the effect on siblings and parental relationships, sleepless nights, social isolation, parents' unfulfilled aspirations and interactions with services (Baldwin and Carlisle, 1994; McConachie, 1994).

Another major source of anxiety may relate to the nature of the care parents provide, such as suctioning airways, giving injections, physiotherapy. The type of procedures they perform are not only potentially dangerous, but they may also involve parents inflicting pain on their child, something which is in direct conflict with a parent's natural desire to protect and show affection to their child (Hatton *et al.*, 1995; Wilson *et al.*, 1998; Atkin and Ahmad, 2000; Kirk *et al.*, 2005).

The unrelenting and sometimes overwhelming practical work involved in caring (the 'daily grind') as a source of stress is well documented: washing, feeding, carrying, managing incontinence, managing sleep and behaviour problems (Wilkin, 1979; Glendinning, 1983, 1986; Sloper and Turner, 1992; Brinchmann, 1999). In addition there is the time-consuming and unrelenting regime of treatments and the management of symptoms; the physiotherapy, medications and special diets (Burton, 1975; Jerrett, 1994; Stewart *et al.*, 1994; Hatton *et al.*, 1995; Gravelle, 1997). Parents with children with complex healthcare needs can feel overburdened with the continuing care demands placed upon them, as well as the need to be constantly on alert for a crisis (Andrews and Nielson, 1988; Aday *et al.*, 1989; Quint *et al.*, 1990; Ostwald *et al.*, 1999; Judson, 2004; Rehm and Bradley, 2005). Meeting a disabled child's needs is physically and emotionally demanding, and it is therefore not surprising that having a break from caring is one of most frequently reported needs and is a key support service enabling parents to continue to care at home. However, the stress parents experience may not all be a direct consequence of having a disabled child, as there may be other sources of stress within the family (Beresford, 1994).

Studies have attempted to identify the predictors of parental stress, for example, lone parenthood, the nature of the functional impairment, low family income and caregiver burden. However, there is a lack of consensus regarding the predictors of caregiver stress owing, in part, to methodological problems: for example, sample differences, omission of important predictors, different measurement tools or disregard of socio-economic status (Baldwin and Carlisle, 1994; Canning *et al.*, 1996). Baldwin and Carlisle (1994) argue that instead of attempting to identify the predictors of parental stress, it is more productive to focus on how parents cope with their situation.

Parental coping

In recent years, both quantitative and qualitative studies have examined how parents cope with caring in terms of coping resources and coping strategies. This work is based upon a number of different theoretical models of coping (see for example, Lazarus and Folkman, 1984). The strength of this approach is that the diversity between families is emphasized. Parents vary widely in terms of their coping resources and strategies, which suggests the need for flexible, individualized service provision.

Coping resources

Coping resources are a range of personal and social factors that may protect the individual from stress (for example, physical and mental health, beliefs about locus of control, social support, money, housing). Individuals with few coping resources are regarded as being vulnerable to experiencing greater stress. The importance of emotional, practical and financial support in mediating stress has been highlighted (Sloper and Turner, 1992; McConachie, 1994; Hentinen and Kyngas, 1998). A number of studies have identified social support as an important factor in promoting coping and mediating stress, and there is evidence to suggest that a perceived lack of social support negatively affects parents' psychological status (Florian and Krulik, 1991; Stewart *et al.*, 1994). Beresford (1994) found that the strength and quality of the parent–child relationship contributed to how well parents managed stress.

Coping strategies

Coping strategies are the conscious cognitive or behavioural efforts made by individuals to alleviate stress, i.e. the actions people take in the face of illness or impairment (Affleck and Tennen, 1993). Research has identified an enormous range of coping strategies that parents use to deal with the stresses they encounter. Examples include problem solving, information seeking, taking control, self-maintenance such as parents developing other interests outside the family, approaches to life such as reframing, and building and using support systems (Burton, 1975; Baldwin and Carlisle, 1994; Beresford, 1994; Hatton *et al.*, 1995; Atkin and Ahmad, 2000). It has been suggested that behavioural interventions in relation to specific issues and coping skills training might be helpful (Beresford *et al.*, 2003).

Positive aspects of caring

The negative aspects of caring are balanced by the child themselves and the parent–child relationship. Research has often overlooked the rewards that the children themselves bring to family life and has instead focused on their impairment or condition. Studies have documented how parents are rewarded by their child's personality and their achievements and that they feel a deep sense of love and commitment towards their child (Burton, 1975; Beresford, 1994; McKeever and Miller, 2004). Parents may also enjoy their caring role, obtaining personal satisfaction and enrichment from it (Beresford, 1994; Jerrett, 1994; Gravelle, 1997; Baumgardener and Burtea, 1998; Cohen, 1999; Landesman, 1999; Kearney and Griffin, 2001; McKeever and Miller 2004). Other studies have noted that the experience of caring is paradoxical, as children are both a source of joy, fulfilment and rewards and a source of sorrow (Larson, 1998; Landesman, 1999; Scorgie and Sobsey, 2000; Kearney and Griffin, 2001; Nelson, 2002).

PARENTS' EXPERIENCES OF SERVICES AND PROFESSIONALS

There are consistent messages from research in terms of parents' support needs and their experiences of services.

Parents' expressed needs

Parents perceived needs have been consistently identified (Sloper and Turner, 1992; Baine *et al.*, 1995; Beresford, 1995; Bamford *et al.*, 1997; Case, 2000; Mitchell and Sloper, 2001; Audit Commission, 2003). They express needs for accessible information; counselling; assistance with helping their disabled child maximize their potential such as Portage and physiotherapy; help in managing behavioural problems; practical help such as housing adaptations, equipment, financial support and domestic assistance; a break from caring; help during school holidays; social support, for example, from parent support groups or the extended family; and parental involvement in decision making about their child's care.

Parents value professionals who are approachable, open and honest; who provide information; listen to their concerns; respect their ideas and expertise; are empathetic of their needs and situation, and who see their child as an individual (Sloper and Turner, 1992; Baldwin and Carlisle, 1994; Mitchell and

Sloper, 2001). Continuity of relationships with professionals is important, particularly for one professional to have a key worker role (Glendinning, 1983, 1986; Sloper and Turner, 1992; Baldwin and Carlisle, 1994; Stewart et al., 1994; Baine et al., 1995; Gravelle, 1997; Mitchell and Sloper, 2001; Kirk and Glendinning, 2004).

There is evidence in the literature of substantial levels of unmet need (Pelletier et al., 1993; Baldwin and Carlisle, 1994; Beresford, 1995; Middleton, 1998; Sloper, 1999), even for those families who have frequent contact with the service system (Harris and McHale, 1989; Sloper and Turner, 1992). Particularly high levels of unmet needs have been identified in families with profoundly impaired children (Beresford, 1995), who have older disabled or chronically ill children (Pelletier et al., 1993; Beresford, 1995), minority ethnic families (Anderson, 1990; Chamba et al., 1999; Atkin et al., 2000) and those with more than one disabled child (Lawton, 1998).

Obtaining appropriate services

A number of studies document how parents themselves have to be advocates for their child and 'fight' for support from services. Families often face a lottery of service provision, which means that the support they receive relates more to the area in which they live rather than their support needs (Audit Commission, 2003). In addition, families can experience long waits for services, adaptations and equipment.

The type and amount of home-based support parents receive in relation to their child's healthcare needs is variable (Kirk, 1999). Studies highlight parents' concerns over the competency of the nursing staff who are available to support them in caring at home for a child with specialized healthcare needs (Young et al., 1988; Aday et al., 1989; Wheeler and Lewis, 1993; Townsley and Robinson, 2000).

Obtaining medical equipment can be problematic sometimes, as a result of funding disputes between agencies (Aday et al., 1989; Quint et al., 1990; Kirk, 1999; Townsley and Robinson, 2000). Parents can also experience problems in maintaining equipment, in dealing with equipment breakdowns, and with the collection and delivery of supplies. Beresford (2003) has also identified unmet equipment needs in relation to areas such as lifting, communication, mobility support and bathing.

In relation to education services, there are reports of parents experiencing problems in getting their child's needs assessed, with transportation to school and with the educational provision for children with specialized healthcare needs (Diehl et al., 1991; Wheeler and Lewis, 1993; Clatterbuck et al., 1998). It has recently been reported that parents feel that mainstream teaching staff have a low level of awareness about children's medical conditions, and that there is insufficient support to help children catch up with missed schoolwork (Asprey and Nash, 2006). Children in mainstream schools also appear to be at a greater risk of not receiving appropriate therapy (Clarke et al., 2001; Parkes et al., 2004).

Experiences of service delivery

There is considerable evidence to suggest that families are dissatisfied with how services are delivered. Recurring problems are poor information giving, difficulties in obtaining a break from caring, a lack of service co-ordination, and problematic relationships with professionals.

Information

A large number of studies over a long period of time have found that parents feel they receive inadequate information about their child's condition and care; support services and entitlement to benefits (for example, Glendinning, 1983; Sloper and Turner, 1992; Stallard and Lenton, 1992; Beresford, 1994, 1995; Jerrett, 1994; Coyne, 1997; Cavet, 1998; Oldman and Beresford, 1998; Kagan *et al.*, 1998; Case, 2000; Noyes, 2000; Townsley and Robinson, 2000; Kirk and Glendinning, 2004). Access to information has been identified as being particularly difficult for minority ethnic families, due to language barriers and poor interpreting support (Chamba *et al.*, 1999; Atkin and Ahmad, 2000). Parents of children with complex healthcare needs can feel inadequately prepared for caring for them at home (Andrews and Nielson, 1988; Diehl *et al.*, 1991). Mitchell and Sloper (2002) have identified the elements of good practice in relation to information giving.

A break from caring

A break from caring is one of the most frequently reported needs of parents. It is important in relieving stress and is seen as enabling parents to continue to care for their child at home. Baldwin and Carlisle (1994) note that until the mid-1980s 'respite care' (as it was then known) was seen as a service to relieve parents of the burdens of caring and was often provided in long-stay hospitals. Oswin's (1985) study uncovered the unsuitability of this type of accommodation for children, and parents' dissatisfaction with it. This, coupled with Glendinning's (1983) research that had revealed parents' unhappiness over the way in which their child was viewed as a burden to them and their unwillingness to use poor services, led to the recognition that a break from caring for parents had to offer something positive for the child as well. While family-based schemes are associated with a higher level of parental satisfaction and have been found to be advantageous for parents and children in a number of ways (for example, continuity of care, development of wider social networks), some parents have described feelings of ambivalence about their child being cared for by another family, and prefer residential provision or support within the family home (Baldwin and Carlisle, 1994). Obtaining a break from caring has been repeatedly reported to be problematic, as has the quality of the services available (Hubert, 1991; Beresford, 1995; Hall, 1996; Chamba *et al.*, 1999; Robinson *et al.*, 2001).

A consistent theme in this literature is that of particular problems parents with a child with complex healthcare needs face in obtaining a break from caring because of their childrens' specialized nursing needs (Diehl *et al.*, 1991;

Wheeler and Lewis, 1993; Youngblut *et al.*, 1994; Petr *et al.*, 1995; Kirk, 1999; Heaton *et al.*, 2003; Kirk and Glendinning, 2004). Usual services provided for disabled children and social support networks are often inappropriate, as support workers, relatives and friends need the appropriate clinical skills. Even when services are specifically developed for this group of children, they may lack the flexibility to respond to children's and families' changing needs (Olsen and Maslin-Prothero, 2001). Initiatives in the UK such as Direct Payments or Individualised Budgets, where parents/young people are given the funding to develop their own packages, may enable them to purchase more individualized support.

Service co-ordination and key working

Different agencies are involved in providing services to support families, and it has been reported that over the course of a year families have contact with at least 10 different professionals and attend at least 20 appointments (Abbott *et al.*, 2005). Hence, co-ordination is important in ensuring families receive seamless services. A key worker to co-ordinate services has been recommended in numerous studies and reports over the past 30 years. However, many studies and reports have reported that services are fragmented, duplicated and poorly co-ordinated, with only a minority of families having a key worker who can provide a first point of contact and co-ordinate a complex range of services for families (Glendinning, 1983; Young *et al.*, 1988; Diehl *et al.*, 1991; Hubert, 1991; Sloper and Turner, 1992; Haylock *et al.*, 1993; Wheeler and Lewis, 1993; Beresford, 1995; Hall, 1996; Gravelle, 1997; Chamba *et al.*, 1999; Kirk, 1999; McConachie *et al.*, 1999; Tozer, 1999; Townsley and Robinson, 2000; Audit Commission, 2003; Kirk and Glendinning, 2004). As long ago as 1986, there was evidence of the positive benefits of keyworking for families, in terms of higher morale, more practical help and less isolation (Glendinning, 1986). Sloper and Turner (1992) found that parents without a keyworker had significantly more unmet needs. In a recent evaluation, Greco *et al.* (2005) found that keyworkers had positive impact on families' lives and that their collaborative working facilitated families' access to services. However, their effectiveness was found to be dependent upon how the service was managed, how clearly the keyworker role was defined, and the provision of training and supervision for keyworkers.

In the UK the lack of clarity in relation to funding responsibilities for care packages for children with complex healthcare needs has been found to be a barrier to discharge and to contribute to service fragmentation (Kirk, 1999; Noyes, 2000; Kirk and Glendinning, 2004). Such difficulties in obtaining services lead to parents having to play an active role in service planning and organization in addition to their caring responsibilities (Clatterbuck *et al.*, 1998; Kirk, 1999).

Multi-agency working and collaboration as a means to improve co-ordination, communication and integration is a key policy priority in the UK (Audit Commission, 2003; HM Government, 2004; Department of Health/DfES, 2004; Welsh Assembly, 2005). Currently however, there is little evidence on the effectiveness of multi-agency working or of different models of multi-agency working in terms of producing improved outcomes for children and families, although there are consistent findings on the facilitators and barriers to multi-agency working (Sloper, 2004).

As will be discussed later, poor multi-agency working at transition from school to further/higher education or employment/unemployment; from the family home to independent living or residential settings; from child health and social care services to adult health and social care services pose enormous problems for disabled young people and their families (Ward, 1999). Young people with complex healthcare needs can face particular problems during this time (Morris, 1999).

Services and professionals as a source of stress

Relationships with professionals may not be supportive but constitute an additional source of stress for parents (Pelletier *et al.*, 1993; Beresford, 1994, 1995; Stewart *et al.*, 1994; Hall, 1996; Coyne, 1997; Atkin and Ahmad, 2000). Problems identified by parents in their relationships with professionals include a lack of emotional support, a lack of empathy, and an apparent failure to acknowledge parents' knowledge and expertise. The quality of parent–professional relationships appears particularly important, as even parents who have high levels of contact with professionals can report extensive unmet needs and dissatisfaction with services (Sloper and Turner, 1992). Baldwin and Carlisle (1994) in their review note that numerous studies have found that professionals do not develop appropriate ways of working with parents.

Parents can experience conflict and confrontation in their relationships with professionals (Beresford, 1994; Jerrett, 1994; McKeever and Miller, 2004). One reason for this appears to be professionals' failure to acknowledge parents' expertise in caregiving (Stewart *et al.*, 1994; Gibson, 1995; Kirk and Glendinning, 2002; Judson, 2004). Another reason derives from the finding that parents feel that they need to fight to receive support, which may lead to the development of adversarial relationships with professionals (Glendinning, 1986; Hubert, 1991; Beresford, 1994, 1995; Gravelle, 1997; Larson, 1998; Chamba *et al.*, 1999; Atkin and Ahmad, 2000). Professionals may be perceived as being unaware of parents' emotional needs (Bradford, 1991; Pelletier *et al.*, 1993; Ray and Ritchie, 1993; Stewart *et al.*, 1994). They may lack an understanding of what life with a disabled child is like in reality, and allow their own beliefs and values to pervade their interactions with parents (Beresford, 1995; Larson, 1998; Atkin and Ahmad, 2000). Problematic issues highlighted in relation to children with complex healthcare needs are control over caregiving and decision making, and parental trust in professionals' expertise and competence (Young *et al.*, 1988; Aday *et al.*, 1989; Scharer and Dixon, 1989; Diehl *et al.*, 1991; Wilson *et al.*, 1998; Kirk and Glendinning, 2004).

Hospitalization can be a major stressor for parents as they have to contend with both the stress of their child being sick and the impact of long periods of hospitalization on their other children and their jobs. In addition, their expertise in caring may be unrecognized by professionals, with whom they may have to battle for control over caregiving, resulting in confrontational relationships with professionals (Hayes and Knox, 1984; Robinson, 1985; Burke *et al.*, 1991).

Consequently there are reports of a lack of congruence between parents and professionals' conceptions of parenting roles in hospital (Hayes and Knox, 1984).

It appears to be important to parents that professionals work in partnership with them, recognize their expertise and knowledge, listen to them and respect their ideas, and recognize the individuality of the family (Patterson *et al.*, 1994; Clatterbuck *et al.*, 1998; Mitchell and Sloper, 2001; Audit Commission, 2003; Beresford *et al.*, 2003).

THE EXPERIENCES OF CHILDREN AND YOUNG PEOPLE

While there is now a well-established body of knowledge about how parents experience life with a disabled child and the support they require, children's own experiences and views have been under-researched (Baldwin and Carlisle, 1994; Robinson and Stalker, 1998).

The reconceptualization of childhood disability

As with research focusing on parents' experiences, some of the research about children's lives has been underpinned by a medical model definition of disability that has taken a pathological approach, focusing on how children have adapted psychologically and emotionally to the 'personal tragedy' of disability (Connors and Stalker, 2003). This work has put impairment-related concerns at the centre, constructing issues in terms of 'biological vulnerability' and 'developmental delay', and has conceptualized disabled children as dependent rather than active social agents (Clarke, 2006). However, there has been other research that has examined children's experience of disability and long-term illness and their social lives and aspirations (e.g. Watson *et al.*, 2000; Atkin and Ahmed, 2001; Connors and Stalker, 2003).

In the past, parents' and professionals' reports have been relied upon as proxies but there is now an increasing awareness of how children and parents have different perspectives (Mitchell and Sloper, 2001; Havermans *et al.*, 2006). There has also been an increasing recognition of children's and disabled people's rights. Increasingly the social model of disability is underpinning research (and policy) emphasizing the environmental, social and attitudinal barriers that disable and exclude disabled children and their families. In addition within the social sciences there has been a reconceptualization of children as competent social actors who actively respond to and shape their social worlds. Consequently in recent years there has been a growth of interest in directly seeking children's views, and consideration of the arising methodological and ethical issues (Beresford, 1997; Morris, 1998a; Ward, 1998).

Children's understandings of disability

Few studies have explored children's understanding of disability. Connors and Stalker (2003) examined how far and in what ways children perceive and try to make sense of their difference. The children in their study seemed happy with themselves, and displayed a practical, pragmatic approach to life. They were not looking for a 'cure' and did not view their impairment as a tragedy, with none describing feelings of loss. Although they saw their impairment in medical and functional terms, generally they saw themselves as much the same as other children until situations arose that illustrated their difference from their non-disabled peers. Largely they understood disability through concrete experience that made them feel different, such as physical restrictions, institutional barriers and the reactions of others. Closs (1998) also found that young people may be made to feel 'different' through the words and actions of others. While some may experience this difference positively, other young people may conceal their impairment or present themselves as 'normal' in order to protect their self-identity (Cavet, 1998; Prout *et al.*, 1999; Sartain *et al.*, 2000; Atkin and Ahmad 2001; Gjengedal *et al.*, 2003).

Social lives and relationships

Social contacts and social interaction with peers are as important to young disabled people as they are to non-disabled young people. Friendships are important, they enjoy participating in clubs and other leisure activities and have similar interests and aspirations to their non-disabled peer group (Flynn and Hirst, 1992; Mitchell and Sloper, 2001; Murray, 2002; Connors and Stalker 2003; Herrman, 2006). While they want to participate in mainstream leisure activities, they also want to have opportunities to meet other young disabled people (Bignall *et al.*, 2002; Murray, 2002). The considerable barriers to living the ordinary life that they desire are well documented. These difficulties mainly relate to social barriers to their participation in mainstream society: poor physical access to buildings, open spaces and transport; the negative reactions and attitudes of other people, and lack of personal assistance (Cavet, 1998; Watson *et al.*, 2000; Murray, 2002; Connors and Stalker, 2003). Attending a segregated school outside their community can also mean that social contacts are limited to other disabled young people who may live some distance away and there may be less contact with local children (Watson *et al.*, 2000; Connors and Stalker, 2003). Consequently disabled young people can experience loneliness and exclusion. Disabled young people have been reported to be less likely to go to discos or the cinema, or to take part in or watch sports (Flynn and Hirst, 1992; Hirst and Baldwin, 1994). Activities such as staying at friends or going on school trips may be difficult (Cavet, 1998). Many are dependent on parents for assistance in getting out, though an adult presence at social events becomes less acceptable as they grow older (Cavet, 1998; Connors and Stalker, 2003). For young people with long-term conditions, their condition and the associated regimens can interrupt and restrict their social lives (Kyngas *et al.*, 2000; Gabe *et al.*, 2002; Herrman 2006).

Young people describe having close relationships with their parents, who are seen as sources of both practical and emotional support (Closs, 1998; Hendey and Pascall 2002; Connors and Stalker, 2003). However, at the same time, young people can find them overprotective, and struggle in developing independence

(Atkin and Ahmad 2001; Connors and Stalker, 2003; Hussain *et al.*, 2002). In relation to young people with long-term conditions, parents may be reluctant to relinquish responsibility for decision making (Buford, 2004). Siblings are also seen as being important in disabled children's lives, but their relationship with them has been described as complex and diverse, with evidence of both conflict and support (Connors and Stalker, 2003). As noted earlier, friends are important to young disabled people, and peer support can be an important coping resource (Skinner *et al.*, 2000; Bignall *et al.*, 2002; Herrman, 2006). It has been reported that it is important to young people that services value and protect friendships (Mitchell and Sloper, 2001). Friendships are also affected by parent's willingness to give disabled children the freedom to have friends. However, being bullied and feeling excluded are also commonly reported, as will be discussed later.

School life

Over the past 20 years the importance of the inclusion of disabled children in mainstream education has been emphasized in policy, and there has been an increasing body of research documenting its benefits in terms of educational and social opportunities (Mukherjee *et al.*, 1999; DfES, 2004; O'Connell, 2005). The Disability movement has made the distinction between *integration* where children are taught separately in units on mainstream educational sites, and *inclusion* where they are taught alongside their non-disabled peers. In mainstream schools, disabled children usually have access to additional support such as aids, equipment, adaptations, assistants and individual learning programmes (Shaw, 1998). Shaw (1998) found that disabled pupils had a matter-of-fact attitude to this additional support and felt that it fitted unproblematically into their everyday school life. However, young people can still face considerable barriers accessing mainstream education, and it has been reported that only one in ten mainstream schools are fully accessible (O'Connell, 2005).

It has been noted that disabled children can spend most of their time in school in the company of adults, with their day being dominated by inter-actions with adults and adult surveillance (Watson *et al.*, 2000; Rehm and Bradley 2006). Indeed Rehm and Bradley (2006) found that interaction with non-disabled peers was limited and not encouraged by staff. Young people can have a complex and ambivalent relationship with care assistants in school. Their presence can be seen as having an adverse effect on inclusion, creating a barrier to making friends (Connors and Stalker, 2003; Shaw, 1998), although young people also recognized that their support can also enable their participation in activities. Children's views on the help they need in school may clash with adult views on appropriate level of support in school and can undermine independence (Shaw, 1998).

In general, disabled children appear to enjoy school and are positive about the friendships and social opportunities provided (Connors and Stalker, 2003; O'Connell, 2005). However, bullying at school has been reported in a number of studies (Shaw, 1998; Connors and Stalker, 2003; Watson *et al.*, 2000). Disabled children in mainstream schools have been reported to have less access to augmentative and alternative communication systems (Clarke *et al.*, 2001) and to talk less openly about impairment.

Research that has investigated disabled young people's experiences of residential schools has found that while young people can have positive experiences in terms of making friends and independence, they can also experience distress at being separated from their family, lack of privacy and respect and lack of consultation, particularly if they do not communicate verbally (Morris, 1998b; Abbott *et al.*, 2001).

Young people with long-term conditions may not always be recognized as having 'special educational needs' or receive additional support (Closs, 1998). Education staff may lack both knowledge of their condition and empathy (Closs, 1998). Frequent school absences can disrupt social relationships and impede academic progress (Mukherjee *et al.*, 1999; Sartain *et al.*, 2000; Atkin and Ahmad, 2001).

Information

Information is an important coping resource, and young people have a range of information needs that relate not just to medical information about their condition and treatment but also about how to manage everyday living and deal with various situations and emotions (Beresford and Sloper, 2000). Information needs are individualized, and different information needs may be met from different sources such as the internet (Nettleton *et al.*, 2004), multimedia programs (McPherson *et al.*, 2006), or condition-/impairment-specific groups (Closs, 1998; Beresford and Sloper, 2000), as well as parents.

There is evidence to suggest that young people are dissatisfied with information giving from professionals (Cavet, 1998; Beresford and Sloper, 2000). Problems reported include professionals withholding information, excluding young people in information-giving situations, using complex language and giving conflicting information.

CHILDREN AND YOUNG PEOPLE'S EXPERIENCES OF PROFESSIONALS AND SERVICES

This group of young people are experienced users of services, particularly health and education. Staff social skills and empathetic approach are important to young people. They have been reported to value professionals who have knowledge about their condition; who have a caring, sensitive approach; who include them in discussions and listen to their views, answer questions and provide explanations; and who take notice of their opinions and enable them to make choices (Atkin and Ahmad 2001; Mitchell and Sloper, 2001; Dixon-Woods *et al.*, 2002).

Some studies have found that professionals can be seen as having negative assumptions about disabled young people and to be overly focused on their impairments (Stone, 2001). Professional's communication styles can also exclude and intimidate young people, and lack of time, continuity and privacy may create additional barriers (Closs, 1998; Dixon-Woods *et al.*, 2002). There is some evidence that communication training for professionals working with children can have positive effects on information giving, inclusion of children and children's satisfaction (Clark *et al.*, 1998; Lewis *et al.*, 1991). However, professionals may need training to meet the particular communication needs of disabled children.

In relation to short-term care, Connors and Stalker (2003) found that children were rarely satisfied with their arrangements. Other studies suggest that young people appear to enjoy family-based short-term care and holiday schemes (McGill, 1996; Prewett, 1999), but that they can be unhappy with residential short breaks (Minkes *et al.*, 1994; Marchant *et al.*, 1999).

Participation

There has been increasing recognition of all children's rights and competence to be involved in decision making about health and welfare issues, and the need to involve disabled children in particular in decisions concerning them is supported in law, policy and professional practice (Cavet and Sloper, 2004) However, it has been noted that the growth of participation has been slower in relation to disabled children than it has been in relation to non-disabled children (Franklin and Sloper, 2005).

While the reasons why all children should be enabled to participate apply equally to disabled children, there are additional reasons as to why it is particularly important for disabled children. Dickins (2004) has identified these as being: they are subject to a much higher degree of adult intervention but their opportunities for making decisions and choices relating to this are often severely limited; they are significantly more vulnerable to abuse; they are more likely to be subject to medical interventions, treatments and various assessment processes; they are more likely to be excluded from consultation and decision-making processes as these are often reliant on written and verbal communication methods; and parents and staff are more likely to see themselves as advocates than listeners.

Research suggests that disabled children can express views about a range of issues such as the care/services they receive, leisure activities, information needs, psychosocial issues (Cavet and Sloper, 2004). Moreover they value being involved, and report that involvement increases their self-esteem and confidence and that they enjoy the social opportunities it can offer (Lightfoot and Sloper, 2002, 2003). However, there is a lack of evidence on the effects of participation on changes to services and on outcomes for children.

There is some evidence to suggest that disabled children are excluded from decision making and are less actively involved than non-disabled children (Noyes, 1999, 2000; Cavet and Sloper, 2004). A national survey looking at involvement within the health service found few initiatives and even fewer that went beyond consultation to actual involvement in decision making (Lightfoot and Sloper, 2002; Sloper and Lightfoot, 2003). Children under 12 years old were less likely to be consulted and only half of the schemes provided feedback on the outcomes of consultation to young people. A recent survey of social service departments by Franklin and Sloper (2005) found that the majority were involving disabled young people in both service development (mostly in relation to play/leisure services) and in decision making regarding their own care. There was some indication that children with communication impairments were being increasingly involved. However, participation was not embedded in all departments. Studies have usefully identified the barriers and enablers to the participation of disabled children (Lightfoot and Sloper, 2002; Cavet and Sloper, 2004; Franklin and Sloper, 2005).

Transition

The literature presents a consistent picture of difficulties for young disabled people during transition to adult health, social care and education services and employment. These include a lack of effective multi-agency communication, assessment, planning and co-ordination between children's and adults' services, and the lack of key/transition workers to co-ordinate transition (Rosen, 1995; Forbes et al., 2001; O'Sullivan, 2001; Morris, 2002; Beresford, 2004; Townsley et al., 2004; Hudson, 2006). Young disabled people without a statement of special educational need may miss out on specialized transition support (Fiorentino et al., 1998; O'Sullivan, 1998). In addition, adult and children's services tend to be organized differently and to have different cultures (Viner, 1999; Tuffrey and Pearce, 2003; McDonagh and Viner, 2006).

It appears that young people are inadequately prepared and involved in transition planning, as well as having a lack of information about the choices and options open to them (Fiorentino et al., 1998; Morris, 2002; Tarleton, 2004). There is a tendency for services and support (e.g. therapy services and specialized health care) to fall away at transition as young people move into adult services where there may be no equivalent service (Fiorentino et al., 1998; Morris, 1999). Transition is also a time when young people lose contact with people who are familiar with their individual needs and ways of communication (Morris, 1999). Currently there is little evidence about what is effective, and few studies take a holistic view of transition, focusing only on one aspect or the process within a single agency.

The difficulties surrounding organizational transitions are compounded by concurrent social status and family life transitions as young people move towards adulthood and independence (Forbes et al., 2001; Beresford, 2004). Status transitions, which include paid employment, financial independence, independent living, adult social relationships and parenthood may be difficult to attain (Riddell, 1998). Young disabled people have aspirations for independent adulthood, but combining both work and independent living can be difficult (Hendey and Pascall, 2002). They face multiple barriers to independence, such as lack of personal support; inaccessible transport; lack of provision of communication technology; negative attitudes of non-disabled people and a high degree of adult surveillance (Morris, 1999, 2002). Some markers of adult status, however, are culturally specific. Hussain et al. (2002) found that gaining independence and leaving home may not have same significance for disabled young people from minority ethnic groups, as they wanted control over their lives but they also wanted to continue to play an active role within the family.

Transition to adult services has received increasing attention in recent policy guidance, with a common theme of co-ordinated, holistic, person-centred transition planning based on informed choice (Department of Health, 2001; DfES, 2004; Department of Health/DfES, 2004, 2006).

Siblings of disabled children and young people

The siblings of disabled children have received relatively little attention from either research or services (Connors and Stalker, 2003). Some studies have suggested that they can experience behavioural and emotional problems (Beresford *et al.*, 2003). However, there is limited evidence that having a disabled sibling has a negative psychosocial impact, and it appears there is variability in how siblings respond, suggesting that this is more likely to be linked to family functioning and relationships (Connors and Stalker, 2003; Beresford *et al.*, 2003; Barlow and Ellard, 2006). It appears that growing up with disabled sibling brings both rewards and difficulties, and the experience may relate more to family coping styles and circumstances than the nature of the impairment (Connors and Stalker, 2003). Positive aspects include parents' perceptions that non-disabled siblings are more caring, responsible and independent (Connors and Stalker, 2003; Barlow and Ellard, 2006). Research has found that siblings contribute to caregiving, not only helping with domestic chores but they can also be involved in providing care for their disabled sibling (Heaton *et al.*, 2003). Connor and Stalker's (2003) research about siblings' experiences found that accounts of their lives were mainly positive and that their relationships were little different from those between non-disabled siblings – rarely conflict free but underpinned by mutual affection and support. They reported a strong sense of siblings having an ordinary life, although some siblings reported experiencing bullying at school, having less attention from parents and restricted social activities.

Siblings have their own particular needs. They may have concerns over their disabled sibling and need information and explanations about their condition, how to help them and how to deal with others' responses. They may need support in accessing social activities and may value attending sibling support groups (Clarke, 2006).

CONCLUSION

There are consistent messages from research about how parents would like to be supported in caring for their disabled child; however, there remain gaps in our knowledge. We know comparatively little about what support works, for whom and in what circumstances. Assessing the effectiveness of interventions is fraught by methodological problems such as defining and measuring outcomes and disentangling the effects of multiple interventions. More also needs to be known about the lives and aspirations of disabled young people themselves, and their siblings, and reliable data on the prevalence and pattern of childhood disability are needed for planning at a local and national level.

In the UK there have been significant policy developments in recent years in relation to disabled children (Department of Health, 2001; Department of

Health/DfES, 2003, 2004; Prime Minister's Strategy Unit, 2005). Much of this focuses on multi-agency working as a way of integrating assessment, planning and a co-ordinated service delivery. This is, however, difficult to achieve in practice, and often requires changes that challenge professional cultures. There is also increasing awareness of the social barriers to participation that families and children face, and a social model now underpins much policy formulation (Department of Health, 2001, 2004; Prime Minister's Strategy Unit, 2005). However, transforming families and young people's experiences and enabling them to achieve social inclusion and live ordinary lives requires fundamental changes, not only in how support is provided but also in societal attitudes towards disability.

KEY POINTS

- The disabled child population is increasing and changing in character, and there are more children who have complex needs.
- Recent calculations have suggested that there are 770 000 disabled children under 16 years in the UK. However, lack of standardization of definitions and categories and how data are collected means that producing a reliable estimate of the prevalence of childhood disability at either a national or local level is problematic.
- Studies conducted over the past 30 years have provided a consistent picture of parents' experiences of caring for disabled children and those with long-term conditions, and the impact this has on their lives. There are also consistent messages from research about parents' support needs and their experiences of services. However, relatively little is known about what support works, for whom and in what circumstances.
- Recently, research has started to explore young peoples' experiences of disability and long-term illness. These studies suggest that social contacts and social interaction with peers is as important to young disabled people as it is to non-disabled young people, and that they have similar aspirations.
- Young people face considerable barriers to living the ordinary life they desire. These difficulties mainly relate to social barriers to their participation in mainstream society.
- The literature presents a consistent picture of difficulties for young disabled people during transition to adult health, social care and education services, and employment.

REFERENCES

Abbott D, Morris J, Ward L (2001) *The Best Place to be? Policy, practice and the experience of residential school placements for disabled children.* York: Joseph Rowntree Foundation.

Abbott D, Townsley R, Watson D (2005). Multi-agency working in services for disabled children: what impact does it have on professionals? *Health and Social Care in the Community* 13:155–63.

Aday LA, Wegener DH, Anderson R, Aitkin M (1989) Home care for ventilator assisted children. *Health Affairs* 8:137–47.

Affleck G, Tennen H (1993) Cognitive adaptation to adversity. Insights from parents of medically fragile children In: Turnbull A (ed). *Cognitive Coping, Families and Disability.* Baltimore, MD: Brookes, pp.135–50.

Ahmad WIU, Atkin K, Chamba R (2000) Causing havoc among their children: parental and professional perspectives on consanguinity and childhood disability. In: Ahmad WIU (ed.) *Ethnicity, Disability and Chronic Illness.* Buckingham: Open University Press, pp.28–44.

Anderson J (1990) Home care management in chronic illness and the self-care movement: an analysis of ideologies and economic processes influencing policy decisions. *Advances in Nursing Science* 12:71–83.

Andrews MM, Nielson DW (1988) Technology-dependent children in the home. *Pediatric Nursing,* 14 (2), 111–114, 151.

Asprey A, Nash T (2006) The importance of awareness and communication for the inclusion of young people with life limiting and life threatening conditions in mainstream schools and colleges. *British Journal of Special Education* 33:10–18.

Atkin K, Ahmad WIU (2000) Family care-giving and chronic illness: how parents cope with a child with a sickle cell disorder or thalassaemia. *Health and Social Care in the Community* 8:57–69.

Atkin K, Ahmad W (2001) Living a 'normal' life: young people coping with thalassaemia major or sickle cell disorder. *Social Science and Medicine* 53:615–26.

Audit Commission (2003) *Services for Disabled Children: a review of services for disabled children and their families.* London: Audit Commission.

Baine S, Rosenbaum P, King S (1995) Chronic childhood illnesses: what aspects of care-giving do parents value? *Child: Care, Health and Development* 21:291–304.

Baldwin S (1985) *The Costs of Caring: families with disabled children.* London: Routledge and Kegan Paul.

Baldwin S and Carlisle J (1994) *Social Support for Disabled Children and their Families: a review of the literature.* London: HMSO.

Bamford D, Griffiths H, Long S, Kernohan G (1997) Analysis of consumer satisfaction in cerebral palsy care. *Journal of Interprofessional Care* 11:187–93.

Barlow J, Ellard D (2006). The psycho-social wellbeing of children with chronic disease, their parents and siblings: an overview of the research evidence base. *Child: Care, Health and Development* 32:19–31.

Baumgardener DJ, Burtea ED (1998) Quality of life in technology-dependent children receiving home care, and their families: a qualitative study. *Wisconsin Medical Journal* 97:51–5.

Beresford B (1994) *Positively Parents: caring for a severely disabled child.* York: Social Policy Research Unit, University of York.

Beresford B (1995) *Expert Opinions: a national survey of parents caring for a severely disabled child.* Bristol: Policy Press.

Beresford B (1997) *Personal Accounts: involving disabled children in research.* York: Social Policy Research Unit, University of York.

Beresford B (2003) *The Community Equipment Needs of Disabled Children and their Families*. York: Social Policy research Unit, University of York.

Beresford B (2004) On the road to nowhere? Young disabled people and transition. *Child: Care, Health and Development* 30:581–9.

Beresford B, Sloper B (2000) *The Information Needs of Disabled Young People*. York: Social Policy Research Unit, University of York.

Beresford B, Sloper B, Baldwin S, Newman T (2003) *What works for Children? Meeting the needs of families with disabled children: what works and what looks promising* (2e). London: Barnados.

Bignall T, Butt T, Agarani D (2002) *Peer Support Groups and Young Black and Minority Ethnic Disabled and Deaf People*. York: Joseph Rowntree Foundation.

Blackburn C, Read J, Spencer N (2006) Can we count them? Scoping data sources on disabled children and their households in the UK. *Child: Care, Health and Development (Online Early Articles)* www.blackwell-synergy.com/doi/abs/10.1111/j.1365-2214.2006.00646.x (accessed 22 January 2007).

Bone M, Meltzer H (1989) *The Prevalence of Disability amongst Children*. OPCS Surveys of Disability in Great Britain, Report 3. London: HMSO.

Bradford R (1991) Staff accuracy in predicting the concerns of parents of chronically-ill children. *Child: Care, Health and Development* 17:39–47.

Bradley RH, Parette HP, Van Bierliet A (1995) Families of young technology-dependent children and the social worker. *Social Work in Pediatrics* 21:23–37.

Bradshaw J (1980) *The Family Fund: an initiative in social policy*. London: Routledge and Kegan Paul.

Bradshaw J, Lawton D (1978) Tracing the causes of stress in families with handicapped children. *British Journal of Social Work* 8:181–92.

Brinchmann BS (1999) When the home becomes a prison: living with a severely disabled child. *Nursing Ethics* 6:137–43.

Burke SO, Kaufmann E, Costello E, Dillon M (1991) Hazardous secrets and reluctantly taking charge: parenting a child with repeated hospitalisations. *Image: Journal of Nursing Scholarship* 23:39–45.

Buford T (2004) Transfer of asthma management responsibility from parents to their school-age children. *Journal of Pediatric Nursing* 19:3–12.

Burton L (1975) *The Family Life of Sick Children*. London: Routledge and Kegan Paul.

Canning RD, Harris ES, Kelleher KJ (1996). Factors predicting distress among caregivers to children with chronic medical conditions. *Journal of Pediatric Psychology* 21:735–49.

Case S (2000) Refocusing on the parent: what are the social issues of concern for parents of disabled children? *Disability and Society* 15:271–92.

Cavet J (1998) *Children, Young People and Their Families Living with a Hidden Disability*. Findings (228). York: Joseph Rowntree Foundation.

Cavet J, Sloper P (2004) The participation of children and young people in decisions about UK service development. *Child: Care, Health and Development* 30:613–21.

Chamba R, Ahmad W, Hirst M, Lawton D, Beresford B (1999) *On the Edge: minority ethnic families caring for a severely disabled child.* Bristol: The Policy Press.

Chapple A, May C, Campion P (1995) Parental guilt: the part played by the clinical geneticist. *Journal of Genetic Counselling* 4:179–91.

Clark NM, Gong M, Schork M *et al.* (1998) Impact of education for physicians on patient outcomes. *Pediatrics* 101:831–6.

Clarke JE (1995) Rural home care of a technology-dependent infant. *Canadian Family Physician* 41:1051–6.

Clarke H (2006) *Preventing Social Exclusion of Disabled Children and their Families.* London: Department for Education and Skills.

Clarke M, McConachie H, Proce T, Wood P (2001) Speech and language therapy provision for children using augmentative and alternative communication. *European Journal of Special Needs Education* 16:41–54.

Clatterbuck CC, Jones D, Turnbull HR, Moberly RL (1998) Planning educational services for children who are ventilator assisted. *Children's Health Care* 27:185–204.

Closs A (1998) Quality of life of children with serious medical conditions. In: Robinson C, Stalker K (eds). *Growing up with Disability.* London: Jessica Kingsley, pp. 111–27.

Cohen M (1999) The technology-dependent child and the socially marginalised family: a provisional framework. *Qualitative Health Research* 9:654–68.

Connors C, Stalker K (2003) *The Views and Experiences of Disabled Children and their Siblings.* London: Jessica Kingsley.

Coyne I (1997) Chronic illness: the importance of support for families caring for a child with cystic fibrosis. *Journal of Clinical Nursing* 6:121–9.

Dale N (1996) *Working with Families of Children with Special Needs: partnership and practice.* London: Routledge

Department for Education and Skills (2004) *Meeting Special Educational Needs: a programme of action.* Nottingham: DfES Publications.

Department for Education and Skills (2006) *Multiagency Working Glossary.* London: Department for Education and Skills.

Department of Health (2001) *Valuing People: a new strategy for learning disability in the 21st century.* London: Department of Health.

Department of Health and Department for Education and Skills (2004) *The National Service Framework for Children, Young People and Maternity Services: disabled child.* London: Department of Health.

Department of Health and Department for Education and Skills (2006) *Transition: getting it right for young people.* London: Department of Health.

Dickins M (2004) *Listening as a Way of Life: listening to young disabled children.* London: National Children's Bureau.

Diehl S, Moffitt K, Wade SM (1991) Focus group interviews with parents of children with medically complex needs: an intimate look at their perceptions and feelings. *Children's Health Care* 20:170–8.

Dixon-Woods M, Anwar Z, Young B, Brooke A (2002) Lay evaluation of services for childhood asthma. *Health and Social Care in the Community* 10:503–11.

Dobson B, Middleton S (1998) *Paying to Care: the cost of childhood disability.* York: York Publishing Services.

Dobson B, Middleton S, Beardsworth A (2001) *The Impact of Childhood Disability on Family Life.* Findings (631). York: Joseph Rowntree Foundation.

Eiser C (1990) *Chronic Childhood Disease: an introduction to psychological theory and research.* Cambridge: Cambridge University Press.

Eiser C (1993) *Growing Up with a Chronic Disease: the impact on children and their families.* London: Jessica Kingsley.

Emerson E, Hatton C (2005) *The Socio-economic Circumstances of Families Supporting a Child at Risk of Disability in Britain in 2002.* Lancaster: Institute for Health Research, Lancaster University.

Fiorentino L, Datta D, Gentle S *et al.* (1998) Transition from school to adult life for physically disabled young people. *Archives of Disease in Childhood* 79:306–11.

Florian V, Krulik T (1991) Loneliness and social support of mothers with chronically ill children. *Social Science and Medicine* 32:1291–6.

Flynn R, Hirst M (1992) *This Year, Next year, Sometime . . . Learning Disability and Adulthood.* London: National Development Team.

Forbes A, While A, Ullman R *et al.* (2001) *A Multi-method Review to Identify Components of Practice which may Promote Continuity in Transition from Child to Adult Care for Young People with Chronic Illness or Disability.* Report for the National Co-ordinating Centre for NHS service Delivery and Organisation R and D. London: London School of Hygiene and Tropical Medicine.

Franklin A, Sloper P (2005) Participation of disabled children and young people in decision-making within social services departments: a survey of current and recent activities in England. *British Journal of Social Work* 36:723–42.

Gabe J, Bury M, Ramsay R (2002) Living with asthma: the experiences of young people at home and at school. *Social Science and Medicine* 55:1619–33.

Gath A (1985) Parental reactions to loss and disappointment: the diagnosis of Down's syndrome. *Developmental Medicine and Child Neurology* 27:392–400.

Gibson CH (1995) The process of empowerment in mothers of chronically ill children. *Journal of Advanced Nursing* 21:1201–10.

Gjengedal E, Rustoen T, Wahl A, Hanestad B (2003) Growing up and living with cystic fibrosis: everyday life and encounters with health care and social services – a qualitative study. *Advances in Nursing Science* 26:149–59.

Glendinning C (1983) *Unshared Care: parents and their disabled children.* London: Routledge and Kegan Paul.

Glendinning C (1986) *A Single Door: social work with the families of disabled children.* London: Allen and Unwin.

Glendinning C, Kirk S, Guiffrida A, Lawton D (2001) Technology-dependent children in the community: definitions, numbers and costs. *Child: Health, Care and Development* 27: 321–34.

Goldberg S, Morris P, Simmons RJ, Fowler RS, Levison H (1990) Chronic illness in childhood and parenting stress. *Journal of Pediatric Psychology* 15:347–58.

Gordon D, Parker R, Loughran F, Heslop P (2000) *Disabled Children in Britain: a reanalysis of the OPCS disability surveys*. London: The Stationery Office.

Gravelle AM (1997) Caring for a child with a progressive illness during the complex chronic phase: parents' experience of facing adversity. *Journal of Advanced Nursing* 25:738–45.

Greco V, Sloper P, Webb R, Beecham J (2005) *An Exploration of Different Models of Multi-agency Partnerships in Key Worker Services for Disabled Children: effectiveness and costs*. London: Department for Education and Skills.

Hall S (1996) An exploration of parental perception of the nature and level of support needed to care for their child with special needs. *Journal of Advanced Nursing* 24:512–21.

Harris VS, McHale SM (1989) Family life problems, daily care-giving activities and the psychological well-being of mothers of mentally retarded children. *American Journal on Mental Retardation* 94:23–9.

Hatton DL, Canam C, Thorne S, Hughes S (1995) Parents' perceptions of caring for an infant or toddler with diabetes. *Journal of Advanced Nursing* 22:569–77.

Havermans T (2006) Assessment of agreement between parents and children on health related quality of life in children with cystic fibrosis. *Child: Care, Health and Development* 32:1–7.

Hayes V, Knox J (1984) The experience of stress in parents of children hospitalised with long-term disabilities. *Journal of Advanced Nursing* 9:333–41.

Haylock CL, Johnson MA, Harpin VA (1993). Parents' views of community care for children with motor disabilities. *Child: Care, Health and Development* 19:209–20.

Heaton J, Noyes J, Sloper P, Shah R (2003) *Technology-dependent Children and Family Life*. Research Works 2003–02. York: Social Policy research Unit.

Hendey N, Pascall G (2002) *Becoming Adult: young disabled people speak*. York: Joseph Rowntree Foundation.

Hentinen M, Kyngas H (1998) Factors associated with the adaptation of parents with a chronically ill child. *Journal of Clinical Nursing* 7:316–24.

Herrman J (2006) Childrens and young adolescents voices: perceptions of the costs and rewards of diabetes and its treatment. *Journal of Pediatric Nursing* 21:211–21.

Hirst M, Baldwin S (1994) *Unequal Opportunities: growing up disabled*. London: HMSO.

HM Government (2004) *Every Child Matters: change for children*. Nottingham: DfES Publications. www.everychildmatters.gov.uk/_content/documents/Every%20Child%20Matinserts.pdf (accessed 17 January 2007).

Hubert J (1991) *Home-Bound: crisis in the care of young people with severe learning difficulties: a story of twenty families*. London: King's Fund Centre.

Hudson B (2006) Making and missing connections: learning disability services and the transition from adolescence to adulthood. *Disability and Society* 21:47–60.

Hussain Y, Atkin K, Ahmad W (2002) *South Asian Disabled Young People and Their Families*. Bristol: The Policy Press.

Jerrett MD (1994) Parents' experience of coming to know the care of a chronically ill child. *Journal of Advanced Nursing* 19:1050–6.

Judge SL (1998) Parental coping strategies and strengths in families of young children with disabilities. *Family Relations* 47:263–8.

Judson L (2004) Protective care: mothering a child dependent on parenteral nutrition. *Journal of Family Nursing* 10:93–120.

Kagan C, Lewis S Heaton P (1998) *Caring to Work: accounts of working parents of disabled children.* London: Family Policy Studies Centre.

Kearney PM, Griffin T (2001) Between joy and sorrow: being a parent of a child with developmental disability. *Journal of Advanced Nursing* 34:582–92.

Kirk S (1999) Caring for children with specialised health care needs in the community: the challenges for primary care. *Health and Social Care in the Community* 7:350–7.

Kirk S, Glendinning C (2002) Supporting 'expert' parents – professional support and families caring for a child with complex health care needs in the community. *International Journal of Nursing Studies* 39:325–35.

Kirk S, Glendinning C (2004) Developing services to support parents caring for a technology-dependent child at home. *Child: Health, Care and Development* 30:209–18.

Kirk S, Glendinning C, Callery P (2005) Parent or nurse? The experience of being the parent of a technology dependent child. *Journal of Advanced Nursing* 51:456–64.

Kyngas H, Kroll T, Duffy M (2000) Compliance in adolescents with chronic diseases: a review. *Journal of Adolescent Health* 26:379–88.

Labbe E (1996) Emotional states and perceived family functioning of caregivers of chronically ill children. *Psychological Reports* 79:1233–4.

Landesman G (1999) Does God give special kids to special parents: personhood and the child with disabilities as gift and as giver. In: Layne LL (ed.) *Transformative Motherhood: on giving and getting in a consumer culture.* New York: New York University Press.

Larson E (1998) Reframing the meaning of disability to families: the embrace of paradox. *Social Science and Medicine* 47:865–75.

Lawton D (1998) *Complex Numbers: families with more than one disabled child.* Social Policy Reports 8. York: Social Policy Research Unit, University of York.

Lazarus RS, Folkman S (1984) Coping and adaptation. In: Gentry WD (ed.). *Handbook of Behavioural Medicine.* New York: The Guilford Press, pp.282–325.

Leonard B, Brust JD, Nelson R (1993) Parental distress: caring for medically fragile children. *Journal of Pediatric Nursing* 8:22–30.

Lewis CC, Pantell RH, Sharp L (1991) Increasing patient knowledge, satisfaction and involvement: randomised trial of a communication intervention. *Pediatrics* 88:351–8

Lightfoot J, Sloper P (2002) *Involving Young People in Health Service Development.* York: Social Policy Research Unit, University of York.

Lightfoot J, Sloper P (2003) Having a say in health: involving young people with a chronic illness or disability in local health services development. *Children and Society* 17:277–90.

Lucas P, Liabo K, Roberts H (2002) Do behavioural treatments for sleep disorders in children with Down's syndrome work? *Archives of Disease in Childhood* 87:413–14.

McConachie H (1994) Implications of a model of stress and coping for services to families of young disabled children. *Child: Health, Care and Development* 19:37–46.

McConachie H, Salt A, Chaidry Y, McLachlan A, Logan S (1999) How do health development teams work? Findings from a UK national survey. *Child: Care, Health and Development* 26:429–44.

McDonagh R, Viner R (2006) Lost in transition: between paediatric and adult services. *British Medical Journal* 332:669.

McGill P (1996) Summer holiday respite provision for the families of children and young people with learning disabilities. *Child: Care, Health and Development* 22:203–12.

McKeever P, Miller K (2004) Mothering children who have disabilities: a Bourdieusian interpretation of maternal practices. *Social Science and Medicine* 59:1177–91.

McPherson A, Glazebrook C, Forster D, James C, Smyth A (2006) A randomised controlled trial of an interactive educational computer package for children with asthma. *Pediatrics* 117:1046–9.

Marchant R, Jones M, Martyn M (1999) *Tomorrow I will go: what you told us about Dorset Road.* Brighton: Triangle.

Middleton L (1998) Consumer satisfaction with services for disabled children. *Journal of Interprofessional Care* 12:223–31.

Mitchell W, Sloper P (2001) Quality in services for disabled children and their families: what can theory, policy and research on children's and parents' views tell us? *Children and Society* 15:237–52.

Mitchell W, Sloper P (2002) Information that informs rather than alienates families with disabled children: developing a model of good practice. *Health and Social Care in the Community* 10:74–81.

Minkes J, Robinson C, Weston C (1994) Consulting the children: interviews with children using residential respite care services. *Disability and Society* 9:47–57.

Morris J (1998a) *Don't Leave us Out: involving disabled children and young people with communication impairments.* York: Joseph Rowntree Foundation.

Morris J (1998b) *Still Missing? Vol 1 The experiences of young disabled children living away from home.* London: The Who Cares? Trust.

Morris J (1999) *Hurting into the Void: transition to adulthood for young disabled people with complex health and support needs*. Brighton: Pavilion Publishing Ltd.

Morris J (2002) *Moving into Adulthood*. York: Joseph Rowntree Foundation.

Mukherjee S, Lightfoot J, Sloper P (1999) Supporting pupils in mainstream school with an illness or disability: young people's views. *Child: Care, Health and Development* 25:267–84.

Murray P (2002) *Disabled Teenagers' Experiences of Access to Inclusive Leisure*. York: Joseph Rowntree Foundation.

Nelson AM (2002) A metasynthesis: mothering other-than-normal children. *Qualitative Health Research* 12:515–30.

Nettleton S, Burrows R, Watt I (2004) *Children, Parents and the Management of Chronic Illness in the Information Age*. Economic and Social Research Council (ESRC) Final Report (Innovative Health Technologies Programme). York: Department of Sociology, University of York.

Noyes J (1999) *Voices and Choices: young people who use assisted ventilation: their health, social care and education*. London: The Stationery Office.

Noyes J (2000) Enabling young 'ventilator-dependent' people to express their views and experiences of their care in hospital. *Journal of Advanced Nursing* 31:1206–15.

O'Brien ME (2001) Living in a house of cards: family experiences with long-term childhood technology-dependence. *Journal of Pediatric Nursing* 16:13–22.

O'Connell P (2005) *A better future? Young adults with complex physical and communication needs in mainstream education*. Paper presented at the British Educational Research Association Conference, 17 September 2005, University of Glamorgan, Wales. www.leeds.ac.uk/disability-studies/archiveuk/o%27connell/oconnellp%20a%20better%20future%20bera%202005.pdf (accessed 22 January 2007).

Office for National Statistics (2004) Disability. *The Health of People and Young People*. London: Office for National Statistics.

O'Sullivan T (1998) *The Transition of Young Adults with Disability: a study of the effectiveness of inter-agency transitional planning*. Executive Summary. www.info.doh.gov.uk/doh/refr_web.nsf/0570b366e8e90a0a802567e7004f3bb0/cbabbc30f3b4d72300256951004b0d86?OpenDocument&Highlight=0, transition (accessed 22 January 2007).

O'Sullivan T (2001) *Young Adults Transition Project: draft summary*. London: Optimum Health Services NHS Trust (now Community Health South London NHS Trust).

Oldman C, Beresford B (1998) *Housing, Disabled Children and Their Families*. Findings (018). York: Joseph Rowntree Foundation.

Olsen R, Maslin-Prothero P (2001) Dilemmas in the provision of own-home respite support for parents of young children with complex health care needs: evidence from an evaluation. *Journal of Advanced Nursing* 34:603–10.

Ostwald SK, Leonard B, Choi T *et al.* (1999) Caregivers of frail elderly and medically fragile children: perceptions of ability to continue to provide home health care. *Home Health Care Services Quarterly* 14:55–80.

Oswin M (1985) *They Keep Going Away: a critical study of short term residential care services for children who are mentally handicapped.* London: King Edward's Hospital Fund.

Parkes J, Donnelley M, Dolk H, Hill N (2004) Use of physiotherapy and alternatives by children with cerebral palsy: a population survey. *Child: Care, Health and Development* 276:469–77.

Patterson J, Jernell J, Leonard B, Titus JC (1994) Caring for medically fragile children at home: the parent professional relationship. *Journal of Pediatric Nursing* 9:98–106.

Pedersen S, Parsons H, Dewey, D (2004) Stress levels experienced by the parents of enterally fed children. *Child: Care, Health Development* 30:507–13.

Pelletier L, Godin G, LePage L, Dussault G (1993) Social support received by mothers of chronically ill children. *Child: Care, Health and Development* 20:115–31.

Petr CG, Murdock B, Chapin R (1995) Home care for children dependent on medical technology: the family perspective. *Social Work in Health Care* 21:5–22.

Pinney P (2005) *Disabled Children in residential placements.* London: Department for Education and Skills.

Prewett B (1999) *Short-break, Long-term Benefit: family-based short-term care for disabled children and adults.* York: Joseph Rowntree Foundation.

Prime Minister's Strategy Unit (2005) *Improving the Life Chances of Disabled People.* London: Prime Minister's Strategy Unit.

Prout A, Hayes L, Gelder L (1999) Medicines and the maintenance of ordinariness in the household management of childhood asthma. *Sociology of Health and Illness* 21:137–62.

Quint RD, Chesterman E, Crain L, Winkleby M, Boyce T (1990) Home care for ventilator dependent children. *American Journal of Diseases in Children* 144:1238–41.

Rankin J, Regan S (2004) *Meeting Complex Needs: the future of social care.* London: Institute for Public Policy Research.

Ray LD, Ritchie JA (1993) Caring for chronically ill children at home: factors that influence parents' coping. *Journal of Pediatric Nursing* 8:217–25.

Rehm R, Bradley J (2005) The search for social safety and comfort in families raising children with complex chronic conditions. *Journal of Family Nursing* 11:59–78.

Rehm R, Bradley J (2006) Social interactions at school of children who are medically fragile and developmentally delayed. *Journal of Pediatric Nursing* 21:299–307.

Riddell S (1998) The dynamic of transition to adulthood. In: Robinson C, Stalker K (eds) *Growing up with Disability.* London, Jessica Kingsley, pp.189–201.

Roberts K, Lawton D (1998) *Reaching its Target? Disability Living Allowance for children.* York: Social Policy research Unit, University of York.

Robinson CE (1985) Parents of hospitalised chronically-ill children: competency in question. *Nursing Papers* 17:59–68.

Robinson C, Jackson P, Townsley R (2001) Short breaks for families caring for a disabled child with complex health needs. *Child and Family Social Work* 6:67–75.

Robinson C, Stalker K (1998) Introduction. In: Robinson, C, Stalker K (eds) *Growing up with Disability.* London: Jessica Kingsley, pp.7–11.

Rosen D (1995) Between two worlds: bridging the cultures of child health and adult medicine. *Journal of Adolescent Health* 17:10–16.

Sartain S, Clarke C, Heyman R (2000) Hearing the voices of children with chronic illness. *Journal of Advanced Nursing* 32:913–21.

Scharer K, Dixon D (1989) Managing chronic illness: parents with a ventilator dependent child. *Journal of Pediatric Nursing* 4:236–47.

Scorgie K, Sobsey D (2000) Transformational outcomes associated with parenting children who have disabilities. *Mental Retardation* 38:195–206.

Shaw L (1998) Children's Experiences of School. In: Robinson C, Stalker K (eds) *Growing up with Disability.* London: Jessica Kingsley, pp.73–84.

Skinner TC, John M, Hampson SE (2000). Social support and personal models of diabetes as predictors of self-care and well-being: a longitudinal study of adolescents with diabetes. *Journal of Pediatric Psychology* 25:257–68.

Sloper P (1999) Models of service support for parents of disabled children. What Do We know? What do we need to know? *Child: Care, Health and Development* 25:85–99.

Sloper P (2004) Facilitators and barriers for coordinated multi-agency services. *Child: Care, Health and Development* 30:571–80.

Sloper P, Lightfoot J (2003). Involving disabled and chronically ill children and young people in health service development. *Child: Care, Health and Development* 29:15–20.

Sloper P, Turner S (1992) Service needs of families of children with severe disability. *Child: Care, Health and Development* 18:250–82.

Sloper P, Knussen C, Turner S, Cunningham C (1991) Factors relating to stress and satisfaction with life in families of children with Down's syndrome. *Journal of Child Psychology and Psychiatry* 32:655–76.

Smith SJ (1991) Promoting family adaptation to the home care of the technology-dependent child. *Issues in Comprehensive Paediatric Nursing* 14:249–58.

Stallard P, Lenton S (1992) How satisfied are parents of pre-school children who have special needs with the services they have received? A consumer survey. *Child: Care, Health and Development* 18:197–205.

Stewart M, Ritchie J, McGrath P, Thompson D, Bruce B (1994) Mothers of children with chronic conditions: supportive and stressful interactions with partners and professionals regarding caregiving burdens. *Canadian Journal of Nursing Research* 26:61–82.

Stone E (2001) *Consulting with Disabled Children and Young People.* York: Joseph Rowntree Foundation.

Sullivan PM, Knutson JF (2000) Maltreatment and disabilities: a population-based epidemiological study. *Child Abuse and Neglect* 24:1257–73.

Tarleton B (2004) *The Road Ahead? Information for young people with learning difficulties, their families and supporters at transition. A review of the evidence for the Social Care Institute for Excellence.* Bristol: Norah Fry Research Centre.

Teague BR, Fleming J, Castle A *et al.* (1993) High tech home care for children with chronic health conditions: a pilot study. *Journal of Pediatric Nursing* 8:226–32.

Thyen U, Kuhlthau K, Perrin JM (1999) Employment, child care and mental health of mothers caring for children assisted by technology. *Pediatrics* 103:1235–42.

Townsley R, Robinson C (2000) *Food For Thought: effective support for families caring for a child who is tube fed.* Bristol: Doveton Press, Norah Fry Research Centre, University of Bristol.

Townsley R, Abbott D, Watson D (2004) *Making a difference? Exploring the impact of multi-agency working on disabled children with complex health care needs, their families and the professionals who support them.* Bristol: Policy Press.

Tozer R (1999) *At The Double: supporting families with two or more severely disabled children.* London: National Children's Bureau.

Tuffrey C, Pearce A (2003) Transition from paediatric to adult medical services for young people with neurological problems. *Journal of Neurology, Neurosurgery and Psychiatry* 74:1011–13.

Viner R (1999) Transition from paediatric to adult care: bridging the gaps or passing the bucks? *Archives of Disease in Childhood* 81:271–5.

Wallander JL, Varni JW (1998) Effects of pediatric chronic physical disorders on child and family adjustment. *Journal of Child Psychology and Psychiatry* 39:29–46.

Ward L (1998) *Seen and Heard: involving disabled children and young people in research and development projects.* York: Joseph Rowntree Foundation.

Ward L (1999) Supporting disabled children and their families. *Children and Society* 13:394–400.

Watson N, Shakespeare T, Cunningham-Birley S *et al.* (2000) *Life as a Disabled Child: a qualitative study of young people's experiences and perspectives.* Edinburgh: University of Edinburgh.

Welsh Assembly (2005) *National Service Framework for Children, Young People and Maternity Services in Wales.* Carfiff: Welsh Assembly.

Wheeler T, Lewis CC (1993) Home care for medically fragile children: urban versus rural settings. *Issues in Comprehensive Paediatric Nursing* 16:13–30.

Wilkin D (1979) *Caring for the Mentally Handicapped Child.* London: Croom Helm.

Williams PD, Press A, Williams AR *et al.* (1999) Fatigue in mothers of infants discharged home on apnea monitors. *Applied Nursing Research* 12:69–77.

Wilson S, Morse J, Penrod J (1998) Absolute involvement: the experience of mothers of ventilator-dependent children. *Health and Social Care in the Community* 6:224–33.

Young L, Creighton D, Sauve R (1988) The needs of families of infants discharged home with continuous oxygen therapy. *Journal of Obstetric, Gynaecological and Neonatal Nursing* 17:187–93.

Youngblut J, Brennan P, Swegart L (1994) Families with medically fragile children: an exploratory study. *Pediatric Nursing* 20:463–8.

Act of Parliament

This Act is published by HMSO in London, and can be accessed from the UK Parliament website (www.publications.parliament.uk).

Disability Discrimination Act 1995

10 LIFESTYLE

Emma Croghan

INTRODUCTION

Supporting a healthy lifestyle for children and young people is an essential function of contemporary public health activities. Most governments in developed countries recognize the importance of child-centred public health in their strategic policies, and most base their statements on the United Nations Convention on the Rights of the Child (UNCRC) 1989, Article 24. This requires participating countries to:

> recognise the right of the child to the enjoyment of the highest attainable standard of health and to facilities for the treatment of illness and rehabilitation of health [and] to strive to ensure that no child is deprived of the right of access to such health care services.

The UNCRC thus commits nation states to delivery of services that respond to acute health needs in a reactive manner, but also to be proactive in helping children and young people to develop healthy habits and lifestyles.

This chapter places in context the importance of lifestyle choices for children and young people, and examines the impact that health-related behaviour choices have on health and well-being as children progress through childhood and grow up. It traces the challenges for public health practice in achieving health-enhancing behaviour choices during the school-age years.

CONTROL OF LIFESTYLE CHOICE AND SOCIALIZATION TO HEALTHY NORMS

For adults, individual lifestyle health behaviours are dependent on other health determinants such as employment, education, income, social and community networks, and cultural factors. Healthy lifestyles, in other words, do not emerge in a vacuum of individual choice, but are influenced by a multitude of interconnected, and often external, factors.

For children and young people, who may have little control over the immediate environment in which they live and develop, 'healthy' lifestyle choices are a matter of less personal decision making. It is unusual to find 5-year-olds who control exactly what food is bought and cooked for their personal consumption, although they may influence this choice through what is commonly known as 'pester power'– a major marketing strategy for some food and drink companies.

Most lifestyle choices are based on normative values and imply a level of socialization to immediate community norms. Socialization is the process by which individuals learn to partake of the attitudes, values and behaviours of a society or community. Primary socialization, which occurs in early childhood, is usually based on family and societal norms within the familial and cultural community environment. Secondary socialization is the process of learning appropriate behaviour from a smaller, often peer- and friendship-led group. This next stage is particularly noticeable in adolescence and is part of a growing individualization. There is also a recognized process of anticipatory socialization, the ways in which a child or young person 'rehearses' for the future (i.e. visualization of a desirable adult identity that includes future work and social relationships).

Primary socialization theories lead us to suggestions that changing behaviours in childhood can lead to healthier behaviours throughout life. These periods of socialization are important in helping to explain lifestyle choices, both

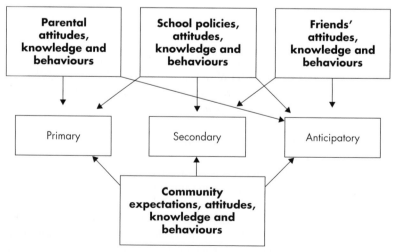

Figure 10.1 Lifestyle choice: gaining attitudes, knowledge and behaviour.

in early and later childhood. They also partially explain why it is important to intervene early in order to imbue children with the knowledge, attitudes and behaviours that can underpin a healthy lifestyle, and to reinforce these throughout the school years. For example, young children at school can be particularly open to messages about dental hygiene, nutrition, exercise, bicycle and road safety, and other forms of self-care.

In theory, early intervention to promote healthy decisions about lifestyle behaviours can reduce the impact of poor influences on health for a young child. In this thinking, both the primary and secondary socialization that occur through reinforcement of healthy lifestyle choices can lead to children taking increasingly responsible decisions about their own health behaviours.

It is critical, however, to understand the complexity of factors that interact throughout the socialization period from early childhood and through transition into adult independence. Figure 10.1 indicates a framework for those interactions.

SOCIAL HEALTH AND LIFESTYLE

Choosing to be part of a community and associating with that community is a positive lifestyle choice. For example, children acquire capacity to 'choose' friends and community as a consequence of growing up and acquiring access to adult independence.

But children who are isolated, or who isolate themselves from communities, have restricted choices. It has been often stated that varying degrees of isolation are 'socially unhealthy', and multiple forms of disadvantage can be a result (Acheson, 1998). In this thinking, a socially healthy child is able to make informed decisions and choices, the consequences of which impact on themselves and potentially on those around them. The UNCRC 1989 in Article 12 states that all children and young people have the right to express their views freely on all matters affecting them. Therefore, a healthy lifestyle choice in respect of social health and well-being would imply the right to participate in a local school or cultural community and to participate in decisions about their own health care. Of course, children are not citizens within civil society, in that they are disenfranchised. Formal choices, therefore, about personal health and social care generally remain in the hands of adults as proxies (see Chapters 2 and 11).

Yet, for children, it can be argued that participation skills can be enhanced in decision making about their own health and social care via participation in school councils, school elections and other democratic and influential processes within their personal environments. For example, it has been suggested that school friendships are the forerunners of subsequent relationships in later life. But Hartup (1992) argues that only 27 per cent of the youth population attain this.

> *Peer relations contribute substantially to both social and cognitive development and to the effectiveness with which we function as adults. Indeed, the single best childhood predictor of adult adaptation is not school grades, and not classroom behaviour, but, rather, the adequacy with which the child gets along with other children.*
>
> *(Hartup, 1992, p.1)*

This suggests that isolated children need to be encouraged to make and maintain friendships, and that community networks, and school health should support and facilitate this process. Peer pressure or bullying, for example, can impact negatively upon personal choice. In an American study of the influence of peer pressure and bullying on risk-taking behaviour, 'dares' were reported most frequently by 8th grade students (age 13 to 14 years). About 50 per cent of the 'dares' encouraged problem behaviours that placed the children (or others) at risk of personal injury, or the potential development of habits hazardous to their health (Lewis and Lewis, 1984).[1] Peer association, or being part of a group of similar-minded people, is important to young people. But it is the choice about which group the person joins that is significant.

BRAND LOYALTY AND THE BUSINESS MODEL

Socialization theories have suggested to big business that it is important to establish brand loyalty at the earliest possible age and then reinforce it continually over time. Market research undertaken in Ireland designed to help marketing departments understand this sector of the consumer market suggested five major groupings, or clusters, of young people:

1 *the cheerleader*: the active, healthy, fulfilled and happy, 27 per cent of the youth population (identifier: Lois and Clark, Superman)

2 *the passivist*: the inert, content, non-mover, 17 per cent of the youth population (identifier: Homer, the Simpsons)

3 *the man behaving badly*: lad culture, 17 per cent of the youth population (identifier: Gary, Men Behaving Badly)

4 *the image-led, style-conscious female*: 22 per cent of the youth population (identifier: Britney Spears)

5 *the self-assured, well-travelled, techno-aware and judgmental*: 16 per cent of the youth population – male and female (identifier: Frasier and Lilith, Frasier).

Understanding the typology of children and young people is as important for health and social care services as for big business. Public health practitioners need to understand and appreciate the diverse ideologies of lifestyle in order to promote healthy behaviours appropriately and from an early age. In this thinking, it is feasible to establish patterns of health promotion and thus health behaviours that can have resonance as the child gradually acquires the capacity for freer personal choice. Because there is more than one type of sensibility amongst young people, public health practitioners need to market their messages appropriately both for age and for typology of sensibility.

---

[1] Lewis and Lewis (1984) described this as 'lad' culture and argued that it affected 17 per cent of the youth population in the US (pp.580–4).

RISK TAKING

Risk taking is the willingness to make mistakes, to advocate unconventional or unpopular positions, or to tackle extremely challenging problems without obvious solutions, such that one's personal growth, integrity, or accomplishments are enhanced. The very nature of learning requires risk taking. A child would never learn to walk, talk, or socially interact without taking risks, experiencing successes and failures, and then monitoring and adjusting behaviours accordingly.

Risk taking can be understood as 'going against the norm' as much as a reference to problematic or health-decreasing risk. In fact, when talking about 'risk taking' in relation to young people, we are often talking about health-detracting behaviours such as truancy, smoking, or participating in extreme sports. The usual definition of risk taking, when applied to children and young people, tends to trigger an impression of taking a chance that something bad will happen as a result of the decision that is made. It is useful to look at some examples:

- *reasonable (healthy) risk-taking thoughts and decision-making processes*: 'I could probably gain something positive or I will probably lose little or nothing of value and probably cause little or no harm to myself or others'
- *unreasonable (unhealthy) risk-taking thoughts and decision-making processes*: 'I will probably gain nothing positive or I could probably lose something of value and probably cause harm to myself or others'.

To go through the process of deciding to take a risk, however, it is likely that a young person will follow two lines of thought:

- first, he/she must consider whether to take the risk or not
- second, he/she must weigh up personal perceptions of loss and gain if taking the risk.

To influence the likelihood of the risk being taken or not, public health practitioners must try to influence the weighting that happens during the second part of the decision-making process (see Fig. 10.2).

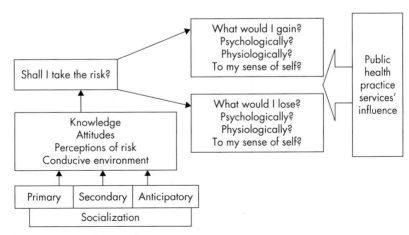

Figure 10.2 Decision-making process.

Most risk taking that is potentially damaging to health is integral to lifestyle choices in the following areas:

• poor dietary choices and sedentary lifestyles
• sexual health
• smoking
• drinking
• illegal drug use
• actions leading to accidents and injury.

PHYSICAL HEALTH AND LIFESTYLE

Obesity

Children who are overweight are more likely to grow up into adults who are overweight. They therefore have a higher risk of developing serious health problems in later life, including heart attack and stroke, type 2 diabetes, bowel cancer, and high blood pressure. The risk of health problems increases the more overweight a person becomes. Being overweight as a child can also cause psychological distress. Teasing about their appearance affects children's confidence and self-esteem and can lead to isolation and depression (Young-Hyman *et al.*, 2003).

Obesity in childhood differs from obesity in adults. Children need nutritious food in order to grow and develop. Growth in childhood is only possible if energy intake exceeds energy output. During puberty, a child will, on average, double in weight and height will increase by 20 per cent. Simple measures used in adulthood to diagnose obesity are more problematic when used in childhood, and therefore multiple measures should be used, for example, body mass index (BMI) percentile that is age- and sex-matched (Association for the Study of Obesity, 2006).

There is international and national concern about the increasing prevalence of obesity in children in developed countries. The number of overweight and obese children in the UK has risen steadily over the past 20 years. Since 1990, obesity among UK children has increased rapidly. In 1990, 5 per cent of all children were noted as above the 95th percentile for BMI, and 2 per cent were above the 98th percentile; 11 per cent of 6-year-olds and 17 per cent of 15-year-olds were overweight or obese (above the 95th percentile) in 1996 (Department of Health, 1996), while in 2002 30 per cent of all children aged 2 to15 were above the 95th percentile, and 16 per cent were classed as obese, which means above the 98th percentile (Department of Health, 2002). There is also a great deal of media concern about the issue. Yet, foods high in fats and sugars continue to be overtly and covertly advertised to children through product placement and through direct advertising in comics, on the television, and in the cinema.

Data on children's height and weight were collected in the National Study of Health and Growth (NSHG, published every year 1975–94), and since 1995 by the Health Survey for England (HSE, published every year since 1995). The prevalence of obesity doubled between 1984 and 1994 among 4 to12-year-olds in England, rising from 0.6 per cent to 1.7 per cent in boys and from 1.3 per cent to 2.6 per cent in girls. The most recent HSE estimates suggest that by 2001,

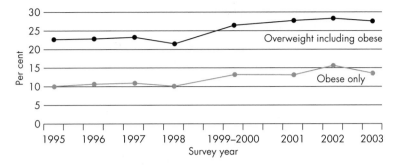

Figure 10.3 Overweight and obesity prevalence among children aged 2–10 years 1995–2003. From Department of Health (2005c) *Obesity among Children under 11 in England.* London: Department of Health, Figure 1. Crown Copyright material is reproduced with the permission of the Controller of HMSO and the Queen's Printer for Scotland.

some 8.5 per cent of 6-year-olds and 15 per cent of 15-year-olds were obese. But the different studies (NHSG and HSE) used different definitions of obesity and overweight and are thus not strictly comparable.

A similar rise in the prevalence of obesity has also been reported in children in Scotland (British Medical Association, 2005). This increase in childhood obesity also reflects a wider trend among the adult population in the UK and in other developed countries. The prevalence of obesity among adults in England has almost trebled in the last 20 years (see Fig. 10.3, Department of Health, 2005c), but by 2020 the predicted prevalence of childhood obesity will be in excess of 50 per cent.

The main factors that raise the child's risk are:

- an income-poor family background
- parents or carers with a high BMI (BMI is a measure based on height/weight ratio, which determines weight category)
- home in a deprived area
- home in an inner-city area
- age 6 to10 years (Wardle 2005).

There are occasionally physical causes for obesity such as Prader–Willi syndrome, Cushing's disease and others, but these are unusual. The most common cause is taking in more calories than are used by the body, either in growth and daily activities or in physical activity.

Only around one in eight children in the UK eats the recommended five portions daily of fruit and vegetables (Wardle, 2005). Most children do not choose water as their primary drink of choice. However, drinking plenty of water regularly throughout the day can protect health and contribute to well-being and can help prevent a range of short- and long-term health problems, from headaches, bladder, kidney and bowel problems to cancer. For schools, increasing the water intake of children matters because with dehydration, mental performance can deteriorate by up to 10 per cent. Children also experience increased thirst, tiredness and irritability. Most other drinks contain sugar, which causes sharp energy and mood swings and decreases concentration. Excess sugar has been associated with panic attacks, nightmares, hyperactivity and chronic tiredness. It is also associated with increased risk of overweight and obesity in children and develops a palate in children for lifelong use of sweetened drinks with little or no nutritional value.

Exercise

It has been estimated that excess weight and physical inactivity together could account for about one-third of all premature deaths. According to the Chief Medical Officer (CMO) for England's report on physical activity and health, regular physical activity helps control weight and can reduce the risk of becoming obese (Donaldson, 2004). It also brings important reductions in risk of mortality and morbidity for those who are already overweight. Physical activity has a range of benefits during childhood, including healthy growth and development, maintenance of energy balance, and psychological well-being. It also has a direct link in preventing the development of cardiovascular disease risk factors (e.g. obesity, raised blood pressure, adverse lipid profiles). Furthermore, sufficient physical exercise can prevent excess weight gain during childhood and can promote weight loss in overweight children (Donaldson, 2004).

The English CMO recommends that:

> . . . *children and young people (aged 5–18 yrs) should achieve a total of at least 60 minutes of at least moderate intensity physical activity each day. At least twice a week this should include activities to improve bone health, muscle strength and flexibility. This can be gained in one session, or through several shorter bouts of activity of 10 minutes or more.*
> **(Donaldson, 2004, p.2)**

At present 70 per cent of English boys and 61 per cent of girls between the ages of 2 and 15 years (Department of Health, 2003) are achieving the recommended amount of activity per week.

Management of obesity and inactivity

Management strategies for preventing and reducing obesity in children and adolescents should involve holistic, therapeutic interventions that ideally include the whole family. Often a child will have limited control over exercise and activity choices. This means that the efficacy of any intervention can be reduced if the controllers of these choices are not involved.

Management of obesity in growing children should not aim for the child to lose weight but for the child to maintain weight while height increases, or for weight to increase at a reduced rate compared to height growth rate, unless the child is under the care of a specialist team. For older children, care must be taken to ensure that slow weight loss is achieved in line with nutrient requirements, and that activity is increased wherever possible while healthier choices are made about food intake.

Management strategies need to focus on new tastes, healthy tastes and increased activity, while activity is designed such that it is perceived to be fun. In good public health practice, the child could be asked to consider how activity makes them feel before and after each type of activity.

SEXUAL HEALTH

Rates of teenage conceptions and rates of sexually transmitted infections (STIs) among young people continue to be a source of concern to policy makers and healthcare providers (Department of Health, 2004). The main source of controlled and credible information for all young people is through the delivery of sex and relationships education (SRE) in schools and colleges (Department of Health, 2004). SRE in England is mainly offered on an *ad hoc* basis. There is also no specialist youth sexual health service for all young people. The use of generalist family planning nurses to provide sexual health services for young people can be stressful for some of these nurses.

A survey of general nurses providing such a service found that, although 65 per cent of these nurses had worked on a gynaecology unit for more than 5 years, there was poor knowledge, an inconsistent pattern of nursing interventions and negative perceptions of the service offered. A majority of the nurses (87 per cent) had not received any specific training in how to nurse teenagers with sexual health issues, and 65 per cent reported that the quality of sexual health services offered to teenagers was poor. Unexpected findings included poor general knowledge of local teenage sexual health services, the emotional effect on some nurses caring for young teenagers undergoing medical terminations of pregnancy, and a complete lack of training and protocols for taking a sexual history (Jolley, 2001).

Both the school health service and the youth services currently offer a disparate and geographically diverse service of advice and support around sexual health matters. Empirically, the youth services have suggested that they do not offer such services routinely, owing to lack of protocols, training and clear guidance. A specialist outreach sexual health service runs in some areas only of the UK. These services are often managed separately from either standard sexual health or standard school health services. The disparate nature of these services, their divided management, and their low profile has resulted in great variation in quality and access for young people, depending on which part of the UK they live in.

There is a paucity of robust evidence about providing sexual health services to young people. Recent surveys of youth-orientated sexual health service users found that young people often think about and take steps to obtain adequate protection only after having sexual intercourse for the first time. Of the 747 respondents, 29 per cent had used a sexual health service before ever having sex, most commonly 'to be prepared'. In contrast, 61 per cent of respondents had used a service after sexual debut. The authors conclude that

> *Young people need to be realistic about the possibility of having sex. Service use could be increased by providing more youth-specific services and by improving publicity and links between the youth, education and health sectors to dispel fears and myths about services.*
> **(Social Exclusion Unit, 1999, p.130)**

The main governmental outcome measure for adolescent sexual health services is a reduction in unplanned teenage pregnancy and a reduction in sexually transmitted diseases amongst this age group (Ermisch, 2003). Social, emotional and educational outcome measures may also offer good measures of the success of disease-prevention and health-promotion programmes for young people. In England, the target is to halve the numbers of conceptions in those aged under 18 years by 2010, and to set a firm downward trend in conceptions amongst under-16-year-olds (Ermisch, 2003).

Just over 5 per cent of young women aged between 15 and 17 years become pregnant each year. In 66 per cent of cases this leads to a full pregnancy and birth for the young woman. The consequences of having a pregnancy and birth at this age show consistent associations through childhood and early adulthood that generally reflect poorer outcomes the younger the mother. Research suggests that having a teen-birth, particularly when under the age of 18 years, makes it more difficult to find and retain a partner. These young women are also more likely to partner with more unemployment-prone and lower-earning men. Teenage mothers are much less likely to be a homeowner later in life, and living standards, as measured by equivalent household income, is about 20 per cent lower than it is for non-teenage parents (Pevalin, 2003).

The effects on the child of being born to a young mother can be physical, emotional and social. Specifically, babies born to younger mothers are more likely to be born preterm or with low birth weight. They are likely to achieve less educationally in the long term, and are more likely to become teenage parents themselves (Department of Health, 2001). These findings add to social, economic and health inequalities for these young parents. It is currently not possible to identify statistically how many of these teenage pregnancies are unwanted or unintended pregnancies. This is an area that needs more research. We need to find out more about the numbers of young people who are choosing pregnancy as a life choice, indeed a career alternative, compared with how many are conceiving from lack of sexual health information and knowledge.

SMOKING, DRINKING AND DRUG USE

Smoked tobacco

Amongst young people, tobacco smoking is defined as at least one cigarette per week (Boreham and McManus, 2003). National rates of regular smoking vary by age and over time (see Fig. 10.4), peaking in 1996 with an overall average of 13 per cent, and falling thereafter to an overall average of 9 per cent in 1999. This rose to 10 per cent in 2000 and remained at 10 per cent in 2001 (Boreham and McManus, 2003; Department of Health, 2004), dropping to 9 per cent in 2003 (Boreham and McManus, 2003; Department of Health, 2004, 2005a).

Girls are more likely to be regular smokers than boys (11 per cent compared with 9 per cent), and regular smoking increases sharply with age. One per cent of all 11-year-olds were regular smokers in 2002, compared with 22 per cent of 15-year-olds. The proportion of young people who have ever smoked reached

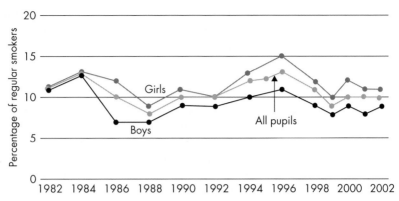

Figure 10.4 Regular cigarette smoking by sex 1982–2002. From Boreham and McManus (2003) *Smoking, Drinking and Drug Use among Young People in England in 2002*. London: Office for National Statistics, p.24. Crown Copyright material is reproduced with the permission of the Controller of HMSO and the Queen's Printer for Scotland.

a peak in 1984 at 55 per cent, and has followed a downward trend since with 44 per cent of girls and 39 per cent of boys in 2002 described this way (Boreham and McManus, 2003). Most adult smokers in the UK commenced their smoking habit before the age of 16 (82 per cent) and nearly two-thirds (63 per cent) of 16-year-olds have tried smoking or still are smokers (Jarvis, 1997).

Adolescent smoking poses a concern because of the numbers and proportions of young people who begin smoking in adolescence and then go on to become long-term adult smokers (around 50 per cent), thus affecting their life chances. There are correlations between smoking prevalence and community deprivation indices for adult smokers, but there is no social class difference among adolescents who experiment with smoking (Croghan *et al.*, 2003). There is, however, a large social class differentiation between those who go on to become adult smokers. Those in lower socio-economic groups have an increased risk of becoming a long-term smoker (Health Development Agency, 2004). This group is also more likely to go on to suffer increased rates of morbidity and lower mortality rates from their smoking than do their counterparts in other socio-economic groups. It can be argued that this increases inequalities not just around health but also around wealth, with smokers in the lowest socio-economic groups spending a higher proportion of their household income on cigarettes than other groups.

Smoking in adolescence is potentially less entrenched as a habit than it is for adults, although this has not been proven. The reasoning is that young people have been smoking for a shorter period of time and often do so in response to social and other peer pressures. On the other hand, a smoking habit may be calculated as more entrenched if, for example, an adolescent smoking habit were assessed as a percentage of a lifetime. For example, a 16-year-old who has smoked for 4 years has done so for 25 per cent of his or her life, whereas in an adult smoking for the same length of time it represents a smaller lifetime percentage.

Among young people, the short-term health effects of smoking include damage to the respiratory system, addiction to nicotine and, arguably, the associated risk of other drug use. Long-term health consequences of youth smoking are reinforced by the fact that, on past experience, most young people who smoke regularly continue to smoke throughout adulthood. Smoking hurts young people's physical fitness in terms of both performance and endurance – even among young people trained in competitive running.

Smoking among youth can hamper the rate of lung growth and the level of maximum lung function. The resting heart rates of young adult smokers are often two to three beats per minute faster than those of non-smoking young adults.

Among young people, regular smoking can lead to cough and increased frequency and severity of respiratory illnesses. The younger people start smoking cigarettes, the more likely they are to become strongly addicted to nicotine. Smoking is associated with a host of other risky behaviours such as fighting and engaging in unprotected sex, or multiple risk taking (Lindberg et al., 2000).

Smoking is associated with poor overall health and a variety of short-term adverse health effects in young people, and may also be a marker for underlying mental health problems such as depression among adolescents. In the US, high school students who are regular smokers and who began smoking by age 13 years have been found to be 2.4 times more likely than their non-smoking peers to report poorer overall health; 2.4 to 2.7 times more likely to report cough with phlegm or blood, shortness of breath when not exercising, and wheezing or gasping; and 3 times more likely to have seen a doctor or other health professional for an emotional or psychological complaint (Centers for Disease Control and Prevention [CDC], 1994).

All four countries of the UK report that around half of the teenagers who continue to smoke will eventually be killed by tobacco-related morbidities, and that half of these will die in middle age – between the ages of 35 and 69 years (Department for Education and Skills, 2005).

It could be argued that the single most important health behaviour that young people can adopt in order to improve personal health, wealth and social outcomes in life is to stop smoking or avoid starting in the first place.

Alcohol drinking

Alcohol is the most commonly used lifestyle drug for children and young people. In the US, one in five young people between the ages of 12 and 20 years regularly binge drink (five or more drinks on one occasion). In England, 22 per cent of young people between the ages of 11 and 15 years regularly (weekly) drink alcohol. This is double the number who smoke regularly in England (Department of Health, 2005a). More than 80 per cent of 11–16-year-olds in the UK have tried alcohol. Just under 5 per cent of 8-year-olds have consumed a whole alcoholic drink. Fourteen per cent of girls and 21 per cent of boys between the ages of 10 and 11 drink each week. By the age of 13, drinkers outnumber those young people who do not drink alcohol. Over half of 14 and

15-year-olds drink alcohol each week. In one research survey, by the age of 14 or 15 young people reported that they drink in order to:

- have fun and experience the buzz
- get drunk and experience losing control
- socialize with others – alcohol can break down boundaries
- enhance sex appeal (CDC, 1994).

In other words, according to young people themselves, most drink alcohol in order to get the effects of being drunk. More than 90 per cent of the alcohol consumed by 12–20-year-olds is drunk when they are binge drinking – often a conscious act or choice. Young people are more tolerant of drunkenness than are adults. They consciously plan to binge drink and think their friends approve of this (Wright, 1999). In fact, the drinks that young people choose are now more often stronger brands than they were in the past, chosen for the ability to speed drunkenness. Nearly one-third of young drinkers choose extra-strength brands of alcohol (Department of Health, 2006).

The UK has some of the highest levels of drunkenness among young people in Europe. Hibell *et al.* (2000) found that 76 per cent of 15–16-year-olds reported having been drunk at least once, and 29 per cent reported having been drunk 20 times or more. Fifty per cent of English 15–16-year-olds reported having been drunk during the last 30 days (Department of Health, 2005a). When drunk, young people are less inhibited and are more likely to make other risky decisions that can impact upon health. A survey into adolescent health found that regular heavy-drinking and binge-drinking behaviours are associated with a range of problems that include antisocial behaviour, violence, accidental injury, physical and mental health problems, and poor school performance (British Medical Association, 2005).

Sensible drinking, as part of a healthy social lifestyle is not the outcome for many young people. They are likely to drink with friends via informal networks (i.e. not in a public house or bar but when out with friends during casual socializing time [Department of Health, 2006]). Figure 10.5 shows mean alcohol consumption in one week in England by school-age pupils. Young people have reported that drunkenness is the preferred outcome of alcohol consumption, and this is the perception that needs to be challenged by public health practitioners.

Illegal drug use

The use of recreational drugs amongst young people is steadily increasing in England as it is in other countries (see Fig. 10.6 for England). The use of volatile substances (mainly sniffing glue and aerosols) is more commonly seen in younger age groups (children between the ages of 11 and 13 years), while the use of cannabis and class A drugs (cocaine, heroin, crack etc.) increases with age (Department of Health, 2006).

Young people who regularly partake in any one of these behaviours (smoking, drinking alcohol, using volatile substances or other drugs) are also more

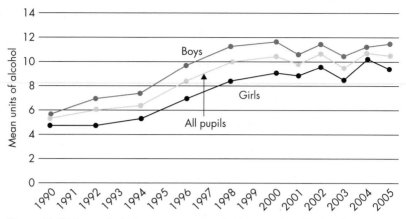

Figure 10.5 Mean alcohol consumption in the last week in England. (Reproduced with permission from Department of Health [2006] *Drug Use, Smoking and Drinking among Young People in England in 2005.* London: HMSO. Copyright © 2006 The Information Centre. All rights reserved. This work remains the sole and exclusive property of the Information Centre and may not be used or reproduced in any manner except with the express written permission of the Information Centre.)

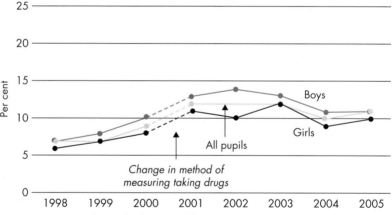

Figure 10.6 Drug use in the last month in England, by sex. (Reproduced with permission from Department of Health [2006] *Drug Use, Smoking and Drinking among Young People in England in 2005.* London: HMSO. Copyright © 2006 The Information Centre. All rights reserved. This work remains the sole and exclusive property of the Information Centre and may not be used or reproduced in any manner except with the express written permission of the Information Centre.)

likely to engage in other risk behaviours, including sexual health risks, substance abuse and truancy. Particularly strong interrelationships are seen between cannabis use, tobacco smoking and alcohol use (Department of Health, 2006). The use of such substances is also related to social class, with the least advantaged in society most likely to use substances damaging to health. Educational attainment, personal aspirations and social norms are also correlated with the kinds and degrees of risk-taking lifestyle behaviours of young people. This returns us to theories of primary, secondary and aspirational socialization.

SICKNESS ABSENCE AND LEARNT HEALTH-ENHANCING BEHAVIOURS

Authorized absence rates from schools in England and Wales have remained fairly stable over the last decade at around 5 per cent in England, Wales, Scotland and Northern Ireland. This figure relates to all authorized absences. By this we mean absence that has been reported to the school by a parent or carer, and in which an explanation has been received that satisfies the school. Although it is not possible to define how much of this is due to pre-agreed family holidays and how much is due to sickness absence, it can be assumed that a high proportion of this is due to sickness absence. Estimates suggest around 1–2 per cent of authorized absences are for family holidays, thereby leaving around 3–4 per cent of all authorized absence from school due to sickness.

Individual schools keep an account of their own sickness absence rates among pupils, and this can be one way of evaluating the efficacy of any interventions with pupils and their families.

The main causes of sickness absence in the school-age population are:

• accidents, burns and accidental poisoning
• submersion/drowning in water (domestic baths and swimming pools)
• infectious diseases (World Health Organization [WHO], 2005).

The United States CDC estimated in 1998 (for 1995) that the average school-age child missed approximately 1 week annually due to illness-related absenteeism in 1995. The most common infections transmitted in school environments are respiratory and diarrhoeal illnesses.

Most infections occur at a constant and low level, but occasionally general outbreaks do occur resulting in increased absenteeism. Hand-to-hand contact is the primary mechanism for transmission of these illnesses. Proper hand-hygiene techniques have been endorsed as the first defence in reducing the risk of infection transmission. Most infectious diseases are spread through the close contact of children in schools.

Preventing the spread of infection is an important function for schools because of the impact on the school itself of an outbreak of an infectious disease. An outbreak of any infectious disease, though not usually serious, can have debilitating results. Teacher and ancillary staff absence; parental absence from work to care for the sick child (thus increasing financial pressures and income inequalities); and pupil absence (particularly damaging in formative environments such as the early years when initial socialization into the group dynamics are taking place) can all be consequences of an outbreak. Often these outbreaks can take a long time to dissipate because of continued re-infection or a long period of the disease organism infecting new people. Routine hand washing with soap and water has been cited by the World Health Organization (WHO, 2005) as being 'the most important hygiene measure in preventing the spread of infection' (p.3).

ACCIDENTS

Around half of all accidents involving bicycles and that led to hospitalization in England and Wales in 2004 were seen in those under the age of 11 years (Department of Health, 2005b). These range from falling from a bicycle to serious collisions with motorized vehicles including cars, motorcycles and buses. Accidents with fireworks, at the home and in the school, also account for high levels of hospitalization. Less serious accidents that do not result in hospitalization are a frequent occurrence in this age group, and there is a need for education to raise awareness and skills in order to avoid such injuries.

Providing information, education and increasing knowledge in both parents and children about the dangers of unsupervised bathing is an area where schools can work together with parents and carers to support healthy socialization.

CONCLUSIONS

Children and young people take risks as part of healthy development from childhood to adulthood. Young people make decisions about taking risks based on a number of external and internal influencing factors, some of which are more important than others. The importance of each variable is individual to the young person, although there are similarities between some groups. These similarities can be used to identify messages that will 'speak' to different groups of young people in order to 'sell' the idea of healthy lifestyles.

For young people to reach maturity and to develop into socially and physically productive adults, healthy habits need to be established at an early age and need to be reinforced throughout the lifetime – i.e. iterative and age specific. It is therefore important to support healthy lifestyles by use of 'brands' of health that are developed and marketed to children and young people. Ideas such as 'water is cool in school' and 'an apple a day keeps the doctor away' are simple but effective messages.

Providing children and young people with the opportunity to gain the knowledge and skills they need in order to influence their attitudes and behaviours takes a lifestyle-led approach. 'What could you do in your current situation to help yourself and why?' is more effective than a medical, paternalistic and negative model, 'This is what is good for you so do it or else you will be unwell'. This latter approach is the one that has been most prominent until recently, and it seems that this approach, failing as it does to take account of the rituals, meanings and questions of the transition period between childhood and adult independence, has failed. It is important for public health practitioners to take steps to support children and young people in reaching their full potential as healthy and well-developed members of society.

KEY POINTS

- Understanding the reasons why children and young people make lifestyle choices, as well as understanding the consequences of unhealthy lifestyle choices are areas of concern for policymakers and public health practitioners alike.
- Decisions about food, physical activity, sexual health, tobacco, alcohol and illicit drug use have consequences that can include time away from school, but can also include longer-term health outcomes such as reduced life chances.
- Supporting health education and the wider social marketing of healthy lifestyle choices is one function of public health practice, and these tasks must compete with current youth markets.
- Understanding the context in which children and young people make decisions about risk behaviours is integral to public health practice. What is the balance between healthy and unhealthy risk taking in child growth and development?
- Lifestyle choice is an area of intervention for public health practice that exists within the context of an ethical and legal framework that needs to have the capacity to enhance health and safety.

REFERENCES

Acheson D (1998) *Independent Inquiry into Inequalities in Health*. London: Department of Health.

Association for the Study of Obesity (ASO) (2006) www.aso.org.uk (accessed 26 January 2007).

Boreham R, McManus S (2003) *Smoking, Drinking and Drug Use among Young People in England in 2002*. London: Office for National Statistics.

British Medical Association (2005) *Adolescent Health*. London: BMA Board of Science and Education.

Centers for Disease Control and Prevention (1994) *Preventing Tobacco Use among Young People: a report of the Surgeon General*. Atlanta: US Center for Disease Control.

Croghan E, Aveyard P, Griffin C, Cheng KK (2003) The importance of social sources of cigarettes to school students. *Tobacco Control* 12:67–73.

Department for Education and Skills (2005) *National Drug Strategy for Young People*. London: HMSO.

Department of Health (1996) *Health Survey for England 1995*. London: HMSO.

Department of Health (2001) *Drinking, Smoking and Drug Use in Young People 2000*. London: HMSO.

Department of Health (2002) *Health Survey for England 2001*. London: HMSO.

Department of Health (2003) *Health survey for England 2002*. London: HMSO.

Department of Health (2004) *Drinking, Smoking and Drug Use in Young People in 2003*. London: HMSO.

Department of Health (2005a) *Drinking, Smoking and Drug Use in Young People 2004*. London: HMSO.

Department of Health (2005b) *Hospital Episode Statistics*. www.hesonline. org.uk/Ease/servlet/ContentServer?siteID=1937&category=192 (accessed 26 January 2007).

Department of Health (2005c) *Obesity among Children under 11 in England*. London: Department of Health.

Department of Health (2006) *Drug Use, Smoking and Drinking among Young People in England in 2005*. London: HMSO.

Donaldson L (2004) *At Least Five a Week: evidence on the impact of physical activity and its relationship to health: a report from the CMO*. London: The Stationery Office.

Ermisch JF (2003) *Does a 'Teen-Birth' Have Longer-Term Impacts on the Mother? Suggestive evidence from the British Household Panel Study*. Colchester: Institute for Economic and Social Research. http://ideas.repec.org/p/ese/iserwp/2003-32.html (accessed 17 March 2007).

Hartup W (1992) *Having Friends, Making Friends and Keeping Friends Relationships as Educational Contexts*. Univeristy of Illinois: Eric Digest.

Health Development Agency (2004) *The Smoking Epidemic in England*. London: Health Development Agency.

Hibell B, Andersson B, Ahlström S *et al* (2000) *The 1999 ESPAD Report. Alcohol and other drug use among students in 30 European countries*. Stockholm: CAN (Swedish Council for Information on Alcohol and Other Drugs).

Jarvis L (1997) Smoking among Secondary School Children in 1996: England. London: The Stationery Office.

Jolley S (2001) Promoting teenage sexual health: an investigation into the knowledge, activities and perceptions of gynaecology nurses. *Journal of Advanced Nursing* 36:246.

Lewis CE, Lewis MA (1984). Peer pressure and risk-taking behaviors in children. *American Journal of Public Health* 74:580–4.

Lindberg LD, Boggess S, Porter L, Williams S (2000) *Teen Risk Taking: a statistical portrait*. Washington, DC: Urban Institute.

Pevalin DJ (2003) *Outcomes in Childhood and Adulthood by Mother's Age of Birth: evidence from the 1970 British Cohort Study*. Working Paper of the Institute for Social and Economic Research, Paper 2003-31. Colchester: University of Essex.

Social Exclusion Unit (1999) *Teenage Pregnancy*. London: HMSO.

US Centers for Disease Control and Prevention and the National Center for Health Statistics (1998) *Current Estimates from the National Health Interview Survey 1995*. Atlanta: Centers for Disease Control and Prevention.

Wardle H (ed.) (2005) *Obesity in Children Under 11 National Statistics*. London: Department of Health.

World Health Organization (2005) *Hospital Infection Control Guidance*. www.who.int/csr/surveillance/infectioncontrol/en/print.html (accessed 17 January 2007).

Wright L (1999) *Young People and Alcohol: what 11 to 24 year olds know, think, and do?* London: Health Education Authority.

Young-Hyman D, Schlundt DG, Herman-Wenderoth L, Bozylinski K (2003) Obesity, appearance, and psychosocial adaptation in young African American children. *Journal of Pediatric Psychology* 28:463–72.

11 THE CHILD'S PERSPECTIVE AND SERVICE DELIVERY

Tina Moules and Niamh O'Brien

INTRODUCTION

Since the beginning of the 1990s there has been a drive towards involving children and young people in the development and delivery of public services in the UK. At no other time in our history has there been so much focus on enabling children and young people to participate in the lives of their communities. UK Government policies rhetorically stress that every opportunity must be taken to listen to the voices of the young and for their perspectives to be heard.

At the same time, children and young people are starting to take advantage of this change in thinking and are beginning to want to be part of the decision-making processes that govern their lives (Kirby and Bryson, 2002; Stafford *et al.*, 2003; Hill *et al.*, 2004). The children who took part in the Children's Summit on Corporal Punishment in Sweden in 2001[1] reflect what many others have said:

> *Politicians often refer to us children as being the future of Europe. But we are living right now . . . Our childhood is happening now and not in the future. We do not think it is enough for decision-makers (for example politicians and public officials) to speak a lot about children and how important they are . . . We want them to listen to us. We want to see action!*

> ***(Children's Summit, Sweden 2001)***

However, though there is a growing trend in developed economies towards listening to children's perspectives, a culture of non-participation in public life

[1] Children's Summit, Sweden. www.endcorporalpunishment.org/pages/frame.html

and in decision making about services is still the norm. What constitutes 'participation' by children is interpreted in many different ways. Often the degree to which they are encouraged or enabled to participate depends largely on the attitude of adults around them and the interpretation those adults place on the term 'participation'. As a result, the current focus in the UK on children's participation runs the risk of being implemented in a meaningless way or not implemented at all.

If children's 'participation' is to have substance, it will require those who work with children to seek to ensure children's perspectives are taken into account when developing health and social care services. As the importance of promoting health in childhood is foregrounded, we may become more interested in finding out what children have to say about their own health. This chapter examines the case for children's participation in service delivery and the policy drivers that underpin the current situation in the UK. Some of the barriers to participation are examined before moving on to a review of examples of children's views about services.

THE CASE FOR INCLUDING THE CHILD'S PERSPECTIVE IN SERVICE DELIVERY

Laws (1998) concluded in her study that it is important for services to recognize the capacity of children to evaluate service provision and give reasoned opinions. One clear reason for involving children in service delivery is the potential for services to improve because of children's involvement. Involving children in all levels of service planning, delivery and evaluation can lead to services that are more appropriately equipped to meet their needs. As Hart and Chesson (1998, p.1602) argue, 'unless children's perceptions . . . are known, services cannot respond to their needs and improvements to achieve high quality care cannot be instigated'.

Research has shown that the involvement of children leads to better decision making, which is more likely to be based on accurate information and therefore more likely to be implemented and subsequently to have beneficial outcomes (Thoburn, 1992; Hodgson, 1996). In the health arena, Lightfoot and Sloper (2001) noted that when children's perspectives about services were taken into consideration, compliance with treatment improved. In a series of studies aimed at developing effective ways of consulting with children who experience mental health problems, Laws (1998) found that children were capable of not only giving relevant, considered views on the services they encountered, but also of actively participating in the process of identifying problem areas and collecting information.

In a review of Scotland's children's hearings system in 2004, the Deputy Education Minister stated that 'it's vital that we listen to children and young people's views if we are to have a hearings system which addresses their needs' (Robson, 2004). The review specifically set out to hear children's views more directly, to ensure that they would be at the heart of any new system. Research on outcomes and children's views can tell us about the types of needs that services supporting children should address. Indeed Aubrey and Dahl (2006) propose that children's perspectives on the services that they receive can contribute to the development of new knowledge and to the development of more democratic communities. The children in their study held many valid views related to their relationships with service providers. In addition, Aubrey and Dahl found that the children would have welcomed more involvement in decisions about services that affected them.

Importantly, children themselves have indicated that they want to be involved and, more importantly, that they want to be listened to. Primarily they want to be part of decisions about matters that concern them closely, including the education system, public transport, health, education and advice (Borland *et al.*, 2001). Children give a variety of reasons why they believe they should participate in decision making about services, including the fact that it offers them new skills, builds their self-esteem and leads to better outcomes, and because they think children have different perceptions from adults (Lansdown, 2001; Kirby *et al.*, 2003). In a study by Lightfoot and Sloper (2003), children reported the benefits of their involvement as being:

> *the chance to make a difference; personal development, such as improved confidence and self-esteem and learning to take responsibility; feeling valued/respected; useful in a CV for potential employers and (for those who worked in groups) an opportunity to have fun and meet people.*
> **(Lightfoot and Sloper, 2003, p.283)**

A large national survey (RBA Research Ltd, 2002) found that more than half the respondents (aged 5–16 years) wanted to have a say on a range of personal and public issues such as how schools and local services could be improved, how police treat young people, how the government sets policies and how young people can take action on big issues like the environment. According to Lansdown (2001), the children surveyed by Euronet, a children's rights network, reported that they wanted to be given the chance to be heard and to be taken more seriously, and according to Nagel (1987, p.14), participation in decision making can lead to 'an enhanced sense of one's own individual worth and an intensified identification with one's community'.

So, social and political arguments for involving children in service delivery rest on the fact that they share the same world as adults, coping with similar factors that affect their lives. As Willow (1997) points out, failing to involve children or consult with them also fails to take into account their specific views and experiences. It fails to recognize them as future citizens and ignores their 'presentness' thereby leaving them without a voice. With no voice, it could be argued that they have no responsibility to contribute to society's norms and rules, which can be 'seen as a form of social exclusion' (Johnson and Ivan-Smith (1998, p.7). A society that does not value the contribution of all its members breeds inequality and divisiveness (Willow, 1997). Promoting children's participation increases their visibility, brings their needs to the attention of adults and can lead to better decision making. In a report on effective government structures for children, Hodgkin and Newell (1996, p.38) argue that if children and young people are given more opportunities to participate in the running of society, 'they will be more willing to engage in the processes of democracy'.

POLICY DRIVERS

A range of policies in the UK underpins the growing regard for the role of children as social actors. Recognition of the importance of acknowledging the participation rights of children and young people is evident in current government policy (Cavat and Sloper, 2004; Street and Herts, 2005). At the end of 1991 the British Government signed up to the United Nations Convention on the Rights of the Child (1989). This international treaty gives children a voice, and at the same time presupposes a more socially active role for them. By acknowledging that children still need protection and provision by adults, as well as the right to participate in decisions affecting their lives, it recognizes the role of children as social actors. The Department of Health and the former Department of Education and Enterprise (DfEE) (now the Department for Education and Skills [DfES]) stated in 1996 that the views of children should be given 'due weight' in services delivered for them (Cavat and Sloper, 2004). Children's participation has also been fundamental to the development of *The Quality Protects Programme* (Department of Health, 1999[2]) through which, in order to hear the views and opinions of children, a number of events have been organized and run specifically to hear directly from those in the care system.

In November 2000, the English Government launched the Children and Young People's Unit (CYPU)[3]. In its guidance for involving children and young people, the CYPU states that:

> *Giving children and young people an active say in how services are developed, provided, evaluated and improved should ensure that services more genuinely meet their needs.*
>
> ***(CYPU, 2001, p.8)***

Furthermore, the CYPU has stated that all government departments should have an active policy on involving children and young people within each department (Street and Herts, 2005), claiming that involving children and young people in all levels of planning, delivery and evaluation of government services can lead to benefits for all involved. The unit specifies that 'the benefits of better policies and services provide the most immediate and powerful driver for action' (CYPU, 2001, p.6).

In 2003 the commitment to improving the lives of children, young people and their families was strengthened by the publication of the Green Paper

---

[2] www.dfes.gov.uk/qualityprotects. *The Quality Protects Programme* is a key part of the Government's wider strategy for tackling social exclusion. It focuses on working with some of the most disadvantaged and vulnerable children in our society – those children looked after by councils; in the child protection system; and other children in need.

[3] In 2003 the CYPU was taken over by the Children, Young People and Families Directorate, responsible to the Minister of State for Children, Young People and Families.

Every Child Matters (Chief Secretary to the Treasury, 2003), which proposed changes in policy and legislation in England to intensify the focus of services around the needs of children, young people and their families. Support for the proposals was clearly evident in its intention to base services on outcomes identified by children themselves rather than via prescribed organizational change alone. At the beginning of March 2004, the Children Bill was published alongside *Every Child Matters: the next steps* (DfES, 2004) and the Bill received Royal Assent in November 2004. The Children Act (2004) provides the legal framework for the programme of reform outlined in the Green Paper *Every Child Matters* (Chief Secretary to the Treasury, 2003). The Act is an attempt by Parliament to shift the focus from crisis-driven, hard-end-service delivery towards prevention and early detection by the formation of new children's services authorities managed by strategic partnerships that will integrate the planning, commissioning and delivery of services. The Act also made provision for the appointment of a Children's Commissioner for England. The devolved administration in Wales established a Children's Commissioner in 2001; a Children's Commissioner was appointed in Northern Ireland in June 2003, and Scotland's Parliament appointed their commissioner in February 2004. Their role is to ensure that the views of children are heard in the national public arena.

Children's wishes to participate in decision making in relation to the English appointment was evident in July 2002, when more than 150 children and young people went to the House of Commons to question the Minister of State for Children about the proposals for the Commissioner for England. The young people were clear in their message. They wanted the Children's Commissioner for England to be an independent champion for their rights, with equal powers to those already commissioned in Scotland, Wales and Northern Ireland. However, constraints on the post in England mean that the commissioner will have limited powers to carry out formal inquiries into individual children's cases.

The other main area of policy development has been the publication of the *National Service Framework* (NSF) *for Children, Young People and Maternity Services* in September 2004 (Department of Health and DfES, 2004). The NSF is part of the UK Government's wider *Every Child Matters: change for children* programme (HM Government, 2004) linking to the wider policies on children's services and the government's policy around tackling inequalities and poor access, and stressing the importance of involving children in the improvement of their services (Curtis *et al.*, 2004).

Central to all the recent UK national policies in relation to children, young people and their families has been a strong emphasis on listening to and consulting with them. For example, there is pressure for health and social services to consult with their service users about policy and planning (Poulton, 1999), and this applies to children as service users as well as adults. The policy is clear. Participation by children and young people as individuals in their own right, acknowledged for their 'presentness', has its benefits. However, the barriers that mitigate against children's rights to participate can lead to their voices being ignored.

BARRIERS TO PARTICIPATION IN SERVICE DELIVERY

The concept of participation does not refer only to the token involvement of children and young people. It is about finding ways of incorporating their views into decision-making processes within the context of what is possible both institutionally and culturally (Moules, 2005). Many instances of initiatives that attempt to make children's voices heard can be found in the literature (Chawla and Kjorholt, 1996; Edwards, 1996), but sometimes participation is reduced to a token gesture whereby children and young people are asked to give their views but have very little choice about the subject or topic for review. Or children's views are 'decoration', where children and young people are used to promote a cause without really understanding the issue, as described by Hart (1992). When participation is done badly it can act against the interests of the child and it can suggest that a low value is being placed on the child's views (Phillips, 2000). Expectations can be raised and then dashed, leading to disillusionment and further isolation (Johnson, 1996). Children and young people involved in any participatory project or initiative where they have no real power will quickly become disillusioned and will perceive their efforts to be useless, 'they smell manipulation and ... they will be resentful' (Woolcombe, 1996, p.45).

In 1998, Sinclair asked children about their experiences of participating in care planning and reviews, and found that they often felt unprepared for meetings and, more importantly, felt that, though they were listened to, what they had to say had little effect on the outcome. When children and young people feel 'ignored, bored, put on the spot or talked about as if they were not there' (Department of Health, 2000, p.20), it is unlikely that any benefits will be accrued. By failing to hear young people's views, opinions and suggestions about service delivery, it is possible that they will become unwilling to participate further in the service on offer and thus in its improvement (Curtis *et al.*, 2004).

In particular, there tends to be a view that adults know best and that children in general do not have the knowledge required to bring about change or indeed make any difference to practice (Poulton, 1999). Indeed it would appear that children themselves recognize that they are not generally understood as having the relevant knowledge to contribute to changing their own and others' lives (Aubrey and Dahl, 2006). Linked to this is a belief by many, perhaps most, that children's views about services can safely be represented by parents or other adults as proxies. Relying solely on adults' perceptions of services provided for their children fails to recognize the diversity and complexity of children's views and opinions, in the same way as reporting by proxy measures the impact of an illness on the proxy rather than on the child (Hart and Chesson, 1998). This view stems from historical presumptions about the nature of childhood and the role that adults have as those who know more than children do, who are thereby responsible for decision making on their behalf, generally up to the age of maturity. There can be no doubt that children are comparatively more vulnerable than adults to exploitation and harm, and require special measures to protect them.

Because children need protection, adults are vested with powers to act on their behalf. Lansdown (1995) argues that this need for protection is used to justify continued resistance to giving children more control over decision making in their lives. This actual power that adults can hold over children can lead adults to believe that they know more than children do about all aspects of childhood, about children's own wishes and needs, and that they can understand the needs of children without having to ask them. Thus adults always know what is 'in the best interests of children', and therefore it does not matter if the children's voices are not heard. Even if the child's voice is heard, it can safely be ignored because it can always be replaced by the more reliable adult source. The adult who is in a position to speak on behalf of children is, at the same time, more able to disregard their voices. Lee (2001) describes this as the 'silencing of children', and goes on to suggest that this view of children and childhood also gives adults reason to doubt whether children are capable of speaking for themselves. Mayall (1996) supports this view and goes on to suggest that adults speak for children on the Piagetian basis that children are not able to 'think' like adults until they reach a certain age of development, though there is no clear definition of when this is. Even when adults affirm children's rights to be heard and taken seriously, they inevitably question children's competence to participate (Lee, 1999).

Competence is not, however, a fixed measurable truth, and the assumption that children and young people are not competent to participate in decision making is open to challenge, especially as children grow in developmental maturity and gain independence (Moules, 2005). Indeed, some studies have explored the competence of children and young people to participate in decisions, especially in relation to their own healthcare treatment. Weithorn and Campbell (1982) concluded that 14-year-olds did not differ from adults in their capacity to make competent decisions, and though 9-year-olds were less competent than adults, they were still able to participate meaningfully in decision making about personal treatment. While these authors acknowledge the limitations of their research, they concur with work carried out by Alderson (1993) who found that children who experience major surgery develop a capacity for understanding and decision making that far exceeds commonly held perceptions about children's capabilities and competencies.

Thus, rather than define children by what they cannot do, we should consider what they could do, and acknowledge that development is not just chronological but is also related to the way in which a child's knowledge of any given issue (and therefore ability to contribute to debates about service delivery) will be affected by their direct experience in that area. This may mean that we have to reconsider the way in which we view children in our society today.

In the late 1990s a new sociology of childhood emerged as a political challenge by sociologists to cultural views of childhood that positioned children in a passive role without agency. James and Prout (1997, p.10) refer to this view as a 'dominant perspective' of childhood in Western cultures, where the value of the child is seen mainly in relation to his or her position as a future adult. In the 'dominant perspective', according to Lee (2001), children are not viewed as social actors but as recipients of socialization, and any opinions and views they might have would not thereby be recognized. The dominant perspective, therefore, has the consequence of muting children's voices and rendering their contributions invisible. It reinforces the power and authority of adults and hides children behind the figure of the 'universal child' (Lee, 2001, p.44). Within this perspective, children are rarely engaged directly as subjects, rather they tend to be subsumed within the family in both statistical and empirical studies (Hill, 1997).

In contrast, in the new sociology of childhood:

> *Children are and must be seen as active in the construction and deter-*
> *mination of their own social lives, the lives of those around them and of*
> *the societies in which they live.*
>
> ***(James and Prout, 1997, p.8)***

This conceptual shift positions children as competent and formed human beings, not as 'human becomings', and recognizes them as individuals in their own right alongside adults. Within this new discourse on childhood, children are allocated a conceptual autonomy, and as a consequence they are recognized as individuals with perspectives of their own and with their own strategies for dealing with the social world around them. The new sociology of childhood takes account of the here and now of children's voices, hearing them as independent from the adults around them. Children are seen as causal and/or interpretive agents and do not necessarily therefore need adults to make them socially significant. The new sociology of childhood calls for children to be understood as social actors, and its key aim is to bring their marginal status to the foreground, thereby constituting childhood as a key feature of the social stratification system (Wyness, 2000). In this way the position of children is less likely to be neglected (Wyness, 2000) and the 'being child' can be understood in its own right (James *et al.*, 1998).

WHAT CHILDREN HAVE TOLD US ABOUT SERVICES: SOME EXAMPLES OF CHILDREN'S PERSPECTIVES

In line with current UK policy there is a significant increase in the level of participation by children in service development and delivery across a range of statutory and voluntary organizations, though only a few examples can be explored here. A range of organizations are engaging with children, building up a wealth of experience to inform good practice and showing that it is possible for children and adults to work together on some very complex issues. This is evidenced by the involvement of children in the inspection of children's services, the *National Service Framework* (Department of Health and DfES, 2004); *Every Child Matters* (HM Government, 2004) *Youth Matters* (DfES, 2005) and many more (Cavat and Sloper, 2004). This is also clear from the many children-led programmes and projects initiated in the last decade (e.g. Article 12, UNCRC) but in particular to the creation of Children's Commissioners for each country of the UK. A study by Kirby *et al.* (2003) set out to find agencies that were listening to children and where children's voices had influenced service planning, delivery or evaluation. A database of 146 agencies was identified, and whilst

Kirby and coworkers recognize that this is not representative, they suggest that it provides a useful summary of the range of current activity. The service areas with the greatest representation in the database are youth work and regeneration projects, but there is evidence of participation by children in other services such as sports and leisure, education, arts and culture, and health.

In the health arena, an increase in the extent to which children and young people were asked their views about hospital experiences was already evident from the mid-1990s. Recognition of the need to talk directly to children and to listen to what they had to say led to a flurry of activity in this field. The Department of Health consultation draft on child health in the community (Department of Health, 1995) stressed the importance of taking into account the provisions of the UNCRC (1989) when considering the principles on which to base services. A number of research studies and consultation exercises have since begun to bring the views of children to the fore, and have served to increase the attention paid to what they have to say about services.

In 1995 Doorbar involved more than 700 children and young people (mean age 13 years) in a qualitative study to find out what children thought about the healthcare services they received in a particular health authority. The children gave their views in 'abundance', and were keen to give valuable suggestions about how services could be improved. Several factors that made experiences positive were identified. Nurses were seen as being the major caregivers. Nurses who were friendly, who took time to listen and to give explanations that were honest and clear, who treated children and young people with respect and made them feel more comfortable were more likely to produce positive responses. A follow-up to the initial project (Doorbar, 1996) found that a number of changes in the presentation and practice of services had taken place as a direct result of the feedback given by children. The follow-up also gave an opportunity for children involved in the initial project to be given feedback about the impact the findings had had on practice.

Laws (1998) cites a series of projects aimed at developing effective ways of consulting with young people who are experiencing mental health problems. The results, following projects involving a total of 110 young people from the age of 13 years upwards, showed that the young people were not only capable of giving relevant, considered views on the services they encountered, but were also capable of actively participating in the process of identifying problem areas and collecting information. The programme concluded that it is important for services to recognize the capacity of young people to evaluate provision and give reasoned opinions. More recently, against a growing awareness of limited information from children themselves about Child and Adolescent Mental Health Services (CAMHS), a series of projects has been undertaken by YoungMinds over the last five years. In the most recent study by Street et al. (2005), which focused on the accessibility and acceptability of services for Black and ethnic minority young people, the barriers facing them included a patchy geographical spread of services, a lack of staff from Black and ethnic minority groups and a lack of staff able to speak languages other than English. In addition, other barriers (noted by children across a range of services) include long waiting times, lack of staff continuity, a lack of age-appropriate resources, and services only available to them at times that were difficult for them.

A report by Lightfoot and Sloper (2001) noted an apparent increased interest among NHS organizations in involving children and young people in service development. This national survey of health authorities and NHS trusts in England revealed a limited, but growing range of initiatives involving children and young people with chronic health problems in decisions about service development (Lightfoot and Sloper, 2001). Twenty-seven initiatives that concentrated on the involvement of children and young people were identified in the survey. The focus of these initiatives was mainly on practical aspects of service provision, and in 17 cases children's views were sought on hospital in-services. Limitations inherent in the survey method were acknowledged, thus giving rise to a possible 'understating' of the true volume of activity. Lightfoot and Sloper applied Treseder's (1997) 'wheel of participation' to evaluate the degree to which the children and young people had participated in the initiatives. They found that, though all the initiatives included consultation with children and young people, the majority of initiatives were characterized by limited involvement of the children, and in only 11 cases were the children actually involved in the process of decision making.

A study by Moules (2005) explored the role children can play in monitoring the quality of services in hospital, with a total of 138 children. The findings support the notion that children will freely give their views on the hospital care they receive if they are asked for them. Furthermore, the majority of children in this study were able to conceptualize that contribution. Because they were the ones who would be receiving care, they argued that they should be the ones, rather than their parents alone, to express a view about its quality. Though some acknowledged that their parents/carers might have opinions about the quality of care, most wanted to give their own views, believing that they have the right to do so because they are the ones who experience the care. The study also found that children tend to value qualities related to characteristics of the provider as being more important than those relating to the physical environment. Thus, they want staff to be technically skilled, friendly, caring and respectful, and able to assist them in making care choices, where possible, by giving them information. Furthermore, it was possible to present these five quality criteria in some order of priority. Omission of any of the first three – technical expertise, friendly staff and respect, during clinical interventions or during general care – is likely to lead to care being rated as poor. Though the latter two – choice and explanations – are important, their omission would not necessarily lead to the children rating care as poor. The findings of the research are a clear demonstration that children and young people are capable of making rational, competent evaluations of the quality of care they receive and would like to receive.

Connexions is a government support service established for all young people aged 13 to 19 years in England.[4] It provides advice and support for young

---

[4] www.connexions.gov.uk/partnerships/index.cfm?CategoryID=3

people in relation to education, training, jobs, money, health, volunteering and other needs by 'personal advisers' (PAs). During its planning and development stages, Connexions sought the views of 13–19-year-olds on how best to deliver this service, and it was young people who came up with the name 'personal advisers'. These PAs work across a range of settings including schools, colleges, one-stop shops and on an outreach basis. Connexions believe their success greatly depends on the involvement of young people. This is done through listening to and taking seriously their views and opinions in relation to how this service is continually designed and delivered.

In 2003 the first evaluation survey of Connexions was carried out, and in total over 52 000 young people responded to it (Deakin *et al.*, 2004). In 2004 a second wave of the survey was carried out and over 18 000 young people were consulted using a variety of measures such as face-to-face interviews, telephone interviews, postal and self-completion questionnaires. In relation to the use of Connexions and whether it has made an impact on young people and the decision-making process, 53 per cent reported that while they were in contact with the service they felt much more confident. Those who were receiving higher levels of support were more likely to report an even greater increase in confidence. In relation to how young people in general viewed the staff at Connexions, this was very positive. They reported that staff were '. . . friendly, knowledgeable and to a slightly lesser extent, easy to contact' (Deakin *et al.*, 2004).

In a study to evaluate the use of Children's Fund projects, Moules and Kirwan (2005) worked with a group of children as co-researchers. The children were instrumental in identifying a number of factors that would mitigate against their using existing services. An inability to get to a service was identified as being an important factor in the non-use of services. A variety of factors make access to services difficult – lack of transport in rural areas, the time of day a project runs, and the cost of services. It seems that a lack of awareness about the services that are available may be an issue for some children, young people and their families. All respondents reported a lack of knowledge about where services are located. Both children and their parents/carers want services to do more to advertise their activities and make them better known. For the children, being with friends, fitting in and/or being with friendly people in services is extremely important. This is especially so when children first begin attending a service and/or when they have to attend by themselves. For example, some children would only use a service if a friend were also attending.

A report edited by Kirwan *et al.* (2005) shows how children and young people in one English county can work effectively with adults in relation to the decision-making process. It shows how children with knowledge and experience of participation can come together with practitioners from a wide range of agencies, and share what is happening in their area. By participating in this way, they were able to identify common principles for best practice and make and present their recommendations to elected members, senior managers and trustees in the county. As a direct result of this initiative and similar work in the county, services seeking future commissioning will have to show how they have ensured that the views and opinions of children, young people and their families are included in decisions about the construction and delivery of their service.

The evidence overall demonstrates that children can and do play an active role in many aspects of service planning, delivery and review across a range of sectors. Acknowledging the role that children can play symbolizes an appreciation of children's social value (Daniel and Ivatts, 1998). However Mayall (2002) asserts that children's agency is still largely enacted at home and with friends, and that power really lies with influential professionals such as doctors, social workers, health visitors and teachers. According to Aubrey and Dahl (2006), evidence from vulnerable children suggests that 'ultimately, the education and social work agenda is controlled by professionals working to national policies that vulnerable children have little power to influence' (p.35).

In reality, children are less likely to be involved in service delivery, monitoring and evaluation, rather they participate more in generating ideas about existing and new services (Oldfield and Fowler, 2004). Research has also shown that, despite an increase in participation activity, much of this is carried out with children aged over 14 years (Kirby *et al.*, 2003; Oldfield and Fowler, 2004). There is limited evidence of involvement of children aged under 8 years (Oldfield and Fowler, 2004; Clark *et al.*, 2005). It is time to 'move beyond the rhetoric' of policy (James, 2005, p.iv) and, at a practical level, address 'professional protectionism', which can work against sharing knowledge and information with children as service users (Poulton, 1999).

HEARING CHILDREN'S VOICES: THE PRACTICE

There has never been as much guidance on involving children in service design and delivery as now. The literature is awash with principles, reports, booklets, handbooks, charters, models and standards. A number of standards developed at a national level exist across a range of sectors (*Learning to Listen*, CYPU, 2001; *National Healthy School Standard*, Health Development Agency, 1999; Charter Mark as identified by Fajerman and Treseder, 2000; *National Service Framework for Children, Young People and Maternity Services*, Department of Health and DfES, 2004; *Hear by Right*, Badham and Wade, 2005).

For example, *Hear by Right* (Badham and Wade, 2005) is a tried and tested standards framework for both statutory and voluntary sector organizations to assist them in improving their practice and policies on the involvement of children and young people. It is based on the 'Seven S' model of organizational change: shared values; strategy; structures; systems; staff; skills and knowledge; and style of leadership. Self-assessment is key to this model and it is developed across three levels specified as 'emerging', 'established' and 'advanced', with each level built on the last. With this approach, the active involvement of children and young people is embedded in service delivery and is not simply an added extra (Badham and Wade, 2005). In Scotland the Standards in Scotland's Schools Act 2000 is wide ranging and impacts on pupils' rights to have a say in their education and in the way the service is developed.

Standards have also been developed at a local level, generally only applicable to local agencies. One such example is the *Young People's Charter of Participation* (Sketchley and Walker, 2001), which was developed by children and staff from the Rotherham Participation Project in 2001 and has been piloted in many organizations. It sets out the principles, standards and action plans needed in order to promote efficient participation of children and young people. Included in the document is a checklist for organizations so that they can improve the way they encourage young people to participate in the delivery and day-to-day running of organizations. It also encourages organizations to sign up to principles, which involve developing positive attitudes towards young people, being young people-friendly, and providing suitable resources so that young people are encouraged to be involved in the organization (Rotherham Participation Project, 2001).

Though standards are an important tool in ensuring that organizations focus resources and use effective practice to involve children, Cutler (2003) asks whether having so many different standards is helpful to children. He goes on to propose that it would be better to have a single, generic standard for all organizations, with common tests resulting in a single kitemark for quality. Though it may be possible, and indeed preferable, to have a single standard, it will never be possible to provide a blueprint for effective participation by children. In fact, as Lansdown (2001) points out, this would deny children the opportunity to be actively involved in the design and development of initiatives. Operationalizing standards for children's participation in service delivery will depend on many factors, including the type of service, the context, the aim of the process and the children involved. Wright *et al.* (2006, p.6) propose a 'whole systems approach' that organizations can take to effect a change or improvement in the way in which they implement participation. They identify four aspects of service development that need to be considered.

1 A *culture* of participation needs to be established where there is a shared commitment to the involvement of children. Senior management support is important, and their backing is important for ensuring that participation initiatives are agreed and moved forward and for ensuring children's voices are acted upon (Kirby *et al.*, 2003). Oldfield and Fowler (2004), in fact, identified the commitment of senior management as being the most important action organizations can take in promoting children's participation. However, it is apparent that commitment needs to be shared and understood at all levels by staff, children and their parents/carers. In developing a culture, and in making participation by children meaningful, service organizations need to be clear about what they want to achieve and the values that underpin their work. The barriers to participation need to be identified, and steps taken to break these down. In particular it may be necessary to promote attitudinal change among adults (Oldfield and Fowler, 2004). Interestingly, though the adults in the study by Oldfield and Fowler identified this as being one of the most important actions in promoting participation, they believed that training for adults was less important than training for the children.

2 As the culture changes, it is important to develop and plan the *structures* to support it. The structures to be considered include staff, resources and the processes for decision making and planning. Partnership working, identified in Oldfield and Fowler's study (2004) as being the third most important action to achieve meaningful and effective participation, can lead to the sharing of experiences through knowledge of local and national initiatives. The purpose is to avoid duplication of effort and to explore opportunities for joint funding. Funding matters in order to provide the resources needed to implement effective and sustainable participation activities. Identifying 'champions' for children, for example, means funding specialist staff who can act as catalysts for change. Commissioning organizations can play the role of champions, by requiring those they fund to involve children in decision making about services.

3 Putting participation into *practice* requires the involvement of all children, regardless of their age, culture and ethnic origin. It means accessing the perceptions of children in hard-to-reach groups such as traveller children and the children of asylum seekers. It means hearing the voices of disabled children and those with learning difficulties. The environment for participation must be a child-friendly context in which children can express their views without fear of feeling intimidated. Different approaches to participation, involving creative and flexible methods, are needed and should be appropriate to the context and to the children involved.

4 Lastly it is important that a *review* of all the above is carried out systematically, in order to make judgements about the effectiveness of participation and the impact it has on service design and delivery. The overwhelming evidence thus far points to a lack of monitoring and evaluation in many participatory activities with children (Kirby and Bryson, 2002; Kirby *et al.*, 2003; Oldfield and Fowler, 2004; Franklin and Sloper, 2004). Regular review helps to identify the benefits of involvement for the children and for the services they use. It enables children to see the impact they have and strengthens the value adults place on children's perceptions.

THE PUBLIC HEALTH PERSPECTIVE

This chapter has discussed the importance of involving children and young people in service delivery and design. Furthermore, it has shown that services can improve when children are listened to and their views and opinions are considered and taken seriously (see, for example, Poulton, 1999; Robson, 2004). Historically, children have been viewed as 'objects to be fitted into the adult constructed work' (Davis and Jones, 1996, p.107), and this generally remains the dominant paradigm today.

Child public health practice is not simply about providing adult-designed methods for improving child health. Neither is it any longer about screening and surveillance alone. It is, instead, about improving child health across whole population groups.

At its best, child public health practice is a social model of medicine incorporating challenges that demand an understanding of the social, economic and psychosocial culture of childhood. Neither health education nor health-promotion initiatives will have the positive consequences we anticipate if the child's own perspective is missing. As Oakley *et al.* (1995) argue, contemporary health promotion with children and young people is not based on what children and young people know, believe or want to know. As a result, their voices have been silenced. We might well add to that finding the likelihood that improving child health actually requires us to find ways of gaining admission to the child's perspective.

CONCLUSION

This chapter has provided an overview of the case for, and importance of, participation by children in service design and delivery. The benefits to children and to the services they use are well documented, and the increase in participatory initiatives to hear their voices is evident across all voluntary and statutory organizations, at both a local and national level. Furthermore, it has shown that services can improve when children are listened to and their views and opinions are considered and taken seriously (Poulton, 1999; Robson, 2004). However the reality is not always as effective as it could be and many barriers exist which mitigate against children's voices being heard and listened to. Historically, children have been viewed as 'objects to be fitted into the adult constructed work' (Davis and Jones, 1996, p.107) and this generally remains the dominant paradigm today.

Participation by children in service delivery will not happen without planning. However, it is also important to recognize that participation is a dynamic process that develops over time and needs input from all levels of service provider organizations, including staff, management, children and parents, but also from within the network of service provider organizations in the public and voluntary sectors.

KEY POINTS

- Children's participation depends largely on the attitude of adults around them and the interpretation those adults place on the term 'participation'.
- Children have indicated that they want to be involved in decisions about matters affecting them; more importantly, they want to be listened to by adults.
- A range of policies in the UK underpins the growing regard for the role of children as social actors. The most important of these is the Children Act (2004).

- By failing to really hear young voices, in relation to service delivery and design, we run the risk of excluding children and young people from some services and thus compromising health improvement.
- The UK has seen a significant increase in the level of participation by children in service development and delivery across a range of statutory and voluntary organizations.
- In order for participation to be put into practice, the involvement of all children and young people is required without prejudice. This also means ensuring the environment is child friendly, and that different creative approaches to participation are taken.

REFERENCES

Alderson P (1993) *Children's Consent to Surgery.* Buckingham: Open University Press.

Aubrey C, Dahl S (2006) Children's voices: the views of vulnerable children on their service providers and the relevance of services they receive. *British Journal of Social Work* 36:21–39.

Badham B, Wade H (2005) *Hear by Right: standards for the active involvement of children and young people.* Leicester: National Youth Agency.

Borland M, Hill M, Laybourne A, Stafford A (2001) *Improving Consultation with Children and Young People in Relevant Aspects of Policy Making and Legislation in Scotland.* Glasgow: University of Glasgow.

Cavat J, Sloper P (2004) The participation of children and young people in decisions about UK service development. *Child: Care, Heath and Development.* 30:613–21.

Chawla L, Kjorholt AT (1996) *Children as Special Citizens. PLA Notes 25.* London: IIED.

Chief Secretary to the Treasury (2003) *Every Child Matters* (Cm 5860). London: Stationery Office. www.everychildmatters.gov.uk/_content/documents/EveryChildMatters.pdf (accessed 17 January 2007).

Children and Young People's Unit (CYPU) (2001) *Learning to Listen: core principles for the involvement of children and young people.* London: HMSO.

Clark A, Kjorholt AT, Moss P (eds) (2005) *Beyond Listening. Children's perspectives on early childhood services.* Bristol: The Policy Press.

Curtis K, Liabo K, Roberts H, Barker M (2004) Consulted but not heard: a qualitative study of young people's views of their local health service. *Health Expectations* 7:149–56.

Cutler D (2003) *Organisational Standards and Young People's Participation in Public Decision Making.* London: Carnegie Young People Initiative.

Daniel P, Ivatts J (1998) *Children and Social Policy.* Hampshire: Palgrave.

Davis A, Jones LJ (1996) Children in the urban environment: an issue for the new public health agenda. *Health and Place* 2:107–13.

Deakin G, Jones A, Brunwin T, Mortimor E (2004) *Improve your Connexions: the Connexions Service customer satisfaction survey: summary of wave 2 survey results for all phase 1 Connexions partnerships: research brief no. RBX10-04.* Nottingham: DfES Publications.

Department for Education and Skills (2004) *Every Child Matters: the next steps.* Nottingham: DfES Publications. www.everychildmatters.gov.uk/_ content/documents/EveryChildMattersNextSteps.pdf (accessed 17 January 2007).

Department for Education and Skills (2005) *Youth Matters.* Nottingham: DfES Publications.

Department of Health (1995) *Child Health in the Community: a guide to good practice.* London: HMSO.

Department of Health (1999) *The Quality Protects Programme. Transforming children's services.* London: HMSO

Department of Health (2000) *Research and Development for a First Class Service.* London: HMSO.

Department of Health and Department for Education and Skills (2004) *National Service Framework for Children, Young People and Maternity Services.* London: Department of Health. www.dh.gov.uk/PolicyAndGuidance/ HealthAndSocialCareTopics/ChildrenServices/ChildrenServicesInformati on/ChildrenServicesInformationArticle/fs/en?CONTENT_ID=4089111 &chk=U8Ecln (accessed 17 January 2007).

Doorbar P (1995) *Children's Views of Health Care in Portsmouth and South East Hampshire.* Portsmouth: Portsmouth and SE Hampshire Health Authority and Pat Doorbar and Associates.

Doorbar P (1996) *Well Now! The report of the second stage of the children's views project.* Portsmouth: Portsmouth and SE Hampshire Health Authority and Pat Doorbar and Associates.

Edwards M (1996) *Institutionalising Children's Participation in Development. PLA Notes 25.* London: IIED.

Fajerman L, Treseder P (2000) *Children are Service Users too. A guide to consulting children and young people.* London: Save the Children.

Franklin A, Sloper P (2004) *Participation of Disabled Children and Young People in Decision-making within Social Services Departments in England.* York: Social Policy Research Unit.

Hart RA (1992) *Children's Participation: from tokenism to citizenship.* Florence: UNICEF, ICDC.

Hart C, Chesson R (1998) Children as consumers. *British Medical Journal* 316:1600–3.

Health Development Agency (1999) *National Healthy School Programme.* London: Health development Agency.

Hill M (1997) Participatory research with children. *Child and Family Social Work* 2:171–83.

Hill M, Davis J, Prout A, Tisdall K (2004) Moving the participation agenda forward. *Children and Society* 18:77–96.

HM Government (2004) *Every Child Matters: change for children.* Nottingham: DfES Publications. www.everychildmatters.gov.uk/_content/documents/ Every%20Child%20Matinserts.pdf (accessed 17 January 2007).

Hodgkin R, Newell P (1996) *Effective Government Structures for Children.* London: Calouste Gulbenkian Foundation.

Hodgson D (1996) *Young People's Participation in Social Work Planning: a resource pack.* London: National Children's Bureau.

James A (2005) Foreword. In: Clark A, Kjorholt AT, Moss P (eds) *Beyond Listening. Children's perpsectives on early childhood services.* Bristol: The Policy Press, pp.iii–v11.

James A, Prout A (eds) (1997) *Constructing and Deconstructing Childhood: contemporary issues in the sociological study of childhood* (2e). London: Falmer Press.

James A, Jenks C, Prout A (1998) *Theorizing Childhood.* Cambridge: Polity Press.

Johnson V (1996) *Starting a dialogue on children's participation. PLA Notes 25.* London: IIED.

Johnson V, Ivan-Smith E (1998) Children and young people's participation: the starting point. In: Johnson V, Ivan Smith E, Gordon G, Pridmore P, Scott P (eds) *Children and Young People's Participation in the Development Process.* London: Intermediate Technology Publications, pp.5–8.

Kirby P, Bryson S (2002) *Measuring the Magic? Evaluating and researching young people's participation in decision-making.* London: Carnegie Young People Initiative.

Kirby P, Lanyon C, Cronin K, Sinclair R (2003) *Building a Culture of Participation. Involving children and young people in policy, service planning, delivery and evaluation.* Nottingham: DfES Publications.

Kirwan N, Marshall L, Plummer J (2005) *Not just Ticking the Box: developing a participation plan for all children and young people in Essex to make sure they can have their say and be involved in decision-making about the things that affect their lives.* Chelmsford: Essex County Council

Lansdown G (1995) *Taking Part. Children's participation in decision making.* London: IPPR.

Lansdown G (2001) *Promoting Children's Participation in Democratic Decision-making.* Florence: UNICEF

Laws S (1998) *Hear Me! Consulting with young people on mental health services.* London: The Mental Health Foundation.

Lee N (1999) The challenge of childhood: distributions of childhood's ambiguity in adult institutions. *Childhood* 6:455–74.

Lee N (2001) *Childhood and Society. Growing up in an age of uncertainty.* Buckingham: Open University Press.

Lightfoot J, Sloper P (2001) *Involving Children and Young People with a Chronic Illness or Physical Disability in Local Decisions about Health Services Development. Phase one: Report on National Survey of Health Authorities and NHS Trusts.* York: University of York.

Lightfoot J, Sloper P (2003) Having a say in health: involving young people with a chronic illness or physical disability in local health services development. *Children and Society* 17:277–90.

Mayall B (1996) *Children, Health and the Social Order.* Buckingham: Open University Press.

Mayall B (2002) *Towards a Sociology for Childhood. Thinking from children's lives.* Buckingham: Open University Press.

Moules T (2005) *Whose Quality Is It? Children and young people's participation in monitoring the quality of care in hospital: a participatory research study.* Unpublished PhD thesis. Cambridge and Chelmsford: Anglia Ruskin University

Moules CTM, Kirwan N (2005) *Children's Fund Essex Evaluation of the Non-use of Service. Year 1 Report.* Centre for Research in Health and Social Care, Cambridge and Chelmsford: Anglia Ruskin University.

Nagel J (1987) *Participation.* Englewood, NJ: Prentice-Hall.

Oakley A, Bendelow G, Barnes J, Buchanan M, Hussain OAN (1995) Health and cancer prevention: knowledge and beliefs of children and young people. *British Medical Journal* 310:1029–33.

Oldfield C, Fowler C (2004) *Mapping Children and Young People's Participation in England.* Research Report No 854. London: National Youth Agency.

Poulton BC (1999) User involvement in identifying health needs and shaping and evaluating services: is it being realized? *Journal of Advanced Nursing* 30:1289–96.

Phillips B (2000) *The End of Paternalism? Child Beneficiary participation and project effectiveness.* Masters' dissertation. The Hague: Institute of Social Studies.

RBA Research Ltd (2002) *Are Young People being Heard?* London: BT and Childline

Reach – Youth Action Network. www.youthactionnetwork.org.uk/index.php?option=com_content&task=view&id=29&Itemid=43 (accessed 17 January 2007).

Robson E (2004) *Youngsters give Views on Hearing System* www.eveningtelegraph.co.uk/output/2004/06/29/story6072918t0.shtm

Rotherham Participation Project (2001) *Young People's Charter of Participation.* London: The Children's Society.

Sinclair R (1998) Involving children in planning their care. *Child and Family Social Work* 3:37–142.

Sketchley L, Walker R (2001) *Young People's Charter of Participation.* London: The Children's Society.

Stafford A, Laybourn A, Hill M (2003) 'Having a say': children and young people talk about consultation. *Children and Society* 17:361–73.

Street C, Herts B (2005) *Putting Participation into Practice: working in services to promote the mental health and well-being of children and young people.* London: Young Minds.

Street C, Stapelkamp C, Taylor E, Malek M, Kurtz Z (2005) *Minority Voices.* London: Young Minds.

Thoburn J (1992) *Participation in Practice – Involving Families in Child Protection.* Norwich: Univesrity of East Anglia.

Treseder P (1997) *Empowering Children and Young People: promoting involvement in decision making.* London: Children's Rights Office/Save the Children.

Weithorn L, Campbell S (1982) The competency of children and adolescents to make informed treatment decisions. *Child Development* 53:1589–98.

Willow C (1997) *Hear! Hear! Promoting children and young people's democratic participation in local government.* London: LGIU.

Woolcombe D (1996) *The Process of Empowerment: lessons from the work of Peace Child International. PLA Notes No 25.* London: IIED.

Wright P, Turner C, Clay D, Mills H (2006) *The Participation of Children and Young People in Developing Social Care.* London: SCIE.

Wyness M (2000) *Contesting Childhood.* London: Falmer Press.

Acts of Parliament

This Act is published by HMSO in London, and can be accessed from the UK Parliament website (www.publications.parliament.uk).

Children Act 2004

Scottish Act of Parliament

This Act is published by the Sationery Office in Edinburgh.
Standards in Scotland's Schools Act 2000

INDEX

Note: page numbers in **bold** refer to figures, tables or boxes.